Neuroanesthesia

Editors

JEFFREY R. KIRSCH
CYNTHIA A. LIEN

ANESTHESIOLOGY CLINICS

www.anesthesiology.theclinics.com

Consulting Editor
LEE A. FLEISHER

March 2021 • Volume 39 • Number 1

ELSEVIER

1600 John F. Kennedy Boulevard • Suite 1800 • Philadelphia, Pennsylvania, 19103-2899

http://www.theclinics.com

ANESTHESIOLOGY CLINICS Volume 39, Number 1
March 2021 ISSN 1932-2275, ISBN-13: 978-0-323-79624-8

Editor: Joanna Collett
Developmental Editor: Arlene Campos

Anesthesiology Clinics (ISSN 1932-2275) is published quarterly by Elsevier Inc., 360 Park Avenue South, New York, NY 10010-1710. Months of issue are March, June, September, and December. Periodicals postage paid at New York, NY and at additional mailing offices. Subscription prices are $100.00 per year (US student/resident), $368.00 per year (US individuals), $455.00 per year (Canadian individuals), $957.00 per year (US institutions), $1000.00 per year (Canadian institutions), $100.00 per year (Canadian student/resident), $225.00 per year (foreign student/resident), $488.00 per year (foreign individuals), and $1000.00 per year (foreign institutions). To receive student and resident rate, orders must be accompanied by name of affiliated institution, date of term, and the *signature* of program/residency coordinator on institutions letterhead. Orders will be billed at individual rate until proof of status is received. Foreign air speed delivery is included in all *Clinics'* subscription prices. All prices are subject to change without notice. POSTMASTER: Send address changes to *Anesthesiology Clinics,* Elsevier Health Sciences Division, Subscription Customer Service, 3251 Riverport Lane, Maryland Heights, MO 63043. Customer Service (orders, claims, online, change of address): Elsevier Health Sciences Division, Subscription Customer Service, 3251 Riverport Lane, Maryland Heights, MO 63043. **Tel:1-800-654-2452 (U.S. and Canada); 314-447-8871 (outside U.S. and Canada). Fax: 314-447-8029. E-mail: journalscustomerservice-usa@elsevier.com (for print support); journalsonlinesupport-usa@elsevier.com (for online support).**

Reprints. For copies of 100 or more of articles in this publication, please contact the Commercial Reprints Department, Elsevier Inc., 360 Park Avenue South, New York, NY 10010-1710. Tel.: 212-633-3874; Fax: 212-633-3820; E-mail: reprints@elsevier.com.

Anesthesiology Clinics, is also published in Spanish by McGraw-Hill Inter-americana Editores S. A., P.O. Box 5-237, 06500 Mexico D. F., Mexico.

Anesthesiology Clinics, is covered in *MEDLINE/PubMed (Index Medicus), Current Contents/Clinical Medicine, Excerpta Medica, ISI/BIOMED*, and *Chemical Abstracts*.

Contributors

CONSULTING EDITOR

LEE A. FLEISHER, MD
Professor of Anesthesiology and Critical Care, Professor of Medicine, Perelman School of Medicine, University of Pennsylvania, Philadelphia, Pennsylvania

EDITORS

JEFFREY R. KIRSCH, MD, FASA
Professor, Department of Anesthesiology, Associate Dean Faculty Affairs, Medical College of Wisconsin, Milwaukee, Wisconsin

CYNTHIA A. LIEN, MD
John P. Kampine Professor and Chair, Department of Anesthesiology, Medical College of Wisconsin, Milwaukee, Wisconsin

AUTHORS

MARIA BUSTILLO, MD
Associate Professor of Clinical Anesthesiology, Department of Anesthesiology, Weill Cornell Medicine, Weill Cornell Medical College, New York, New York

MICHAEL R. CHICOINE, MD
Professor, Department of Neurosurgery, Washington University School of Medicine, St Louis, Missouri

LANE CRAWFORD, MD
Assistant Professor of Clinical Anesthesiology, Division of Multispecialty Adult Anesthesiology, Vanderbilt University Medical Center, Nashville, Tennessee

BRENDA G. FAHY, MD, MCCM
Professor, Associate Chair for Faculty Affairs and Professional Development, Program Director for Combined Adult Cardiothoracic Anesthesiology and Critical Care Medicine Fellowship, Department of Anesthesiology, University of Florida College of Medicine, Gainesville, Florida

STACY L. FAIRBANKS, MD
Associate Professor of Anesthesiology, Froedtert & the Medical College of Wisconsin, Milwaukee, Wisconsin

BRIAN GIERL, MD
University of Pittsburgh Medical Center, Pittsburgh, Pennsylvania

WILLIAM L. GROSS, MD, PhD
Assistant Professor, Department of Anesthesiology, Medical College of Wisconsin, Milwaukee, Wisconsin

GABRIEL KLEINMAN, MD
Assistant Professor, Oregon Health & Science University, Portland, Oregon

JAMES KURFESS, MD
Department of Anesthesiology, Neuroanesthesia Clinical Fellow, Yale University, New Haven, Connecticut

DEAN LAOCHAMROONVORAPONGSE, MD, MPH
Assistant Professor, Department of Anesthesiology and Perioperative Medicine, Oregon Health & Science University, Portland, Oregon

BRIAN P. LEMKUIL, MD
San Diego, California

LETHA MATHEWS, MBBS
Professor of Clinical Anesthesiology, Division of Neuroanesthesiology, Vanderbilt University Medical Center, Nashville, Tennessee

KIMBERLY M. MAUER, MD
Medical Director, Comprehensive Pain Center, Associate Professor of Anesthesiology and Perioperative Medicine, Anesthesiology and Perioperative Medicine, Oregon Health & Science University, Portland, Oregon

NICHOLAS MEIER, MD
Department of Anesthesiology, Assistant Professor, Medical College of Wisconsin, Children's Hospital of Wisconsin, Milwaukee, Wisconsin

BASMA A. MOHAMED, MBChB
Assistant Professor, Department of Anesthesiology, University of Florida College of Medicine, Gainesville, Florida

DOROTHEE MUELLER, MD
Assistant Professor of Anesthesiology, Division of Critical Care Medicine, Vanderbilt University Medical Center, Nashville, Tennessee

PRISCILLA NELSON, MD
Associate Professor of Clinical Anesthesiology, Department of Anesthesiology, Weill Cornell Medicine, Weill Cornell Medical College, New York, New York

AUSTIN PETERS, MD, MCR
Assistant Professor, Oregon Health & Science University, Portland, Oregon

KATE PETTY, MD
University of Pittsburgh Medical Center, Pittsburgh, Pennsylvania

SHILPA RAO, MD
Assistant Professor, Department of Anesthesiology, Division of Neuroanesthesia, Yale School of Medicine, Yale University, New Haven, Connecticut

RAPHAEL H. SACHO, MD, FRCS
Assistant Professor, Department of Neurosurgery, Medical College of Wisconsin, Milwaukee, Wisconsin

KELSEY SERFOZO, MD
Clinical Lecturer, Department of Anesthesiology, University Hospital, University of Michigan Medical School, Ann Arbor, Michigan

AMIT SINGH, DO
Assistant Professor, Anesthesiology, Medical College of Wisconsin, Milwaukee, Wauwatosa, Wisconsin

VIJAY TARNAL, MBBS, FRCA
Clinical Associate Professor, Department of Anesthesiology, University Hospital, University of Michigan Medical School, Ann Arbor, Michigan

MAGNUS KNUT TEIG, BMedSci (Hons), MBChB, MRCP, FRCA, EDIC, FFICM
Assistant Professor of Anesthesia and Neurosurgery, Department of Anesthesiology, University of Michigan, Ann Arbor, Michigan

MARIE A. THEARD, MD
Assistant Professor, Department of Anesthesiology and Perioperative Medicine, Oregon Health & Science University, Portland, Oregon

MIRIAM M. TREGGIARI, MD, PhD, MPH
Professor and Vice Chair of Clinical Research, Department of Anesthesiology, Yale School of Medicine, Yale University, New Haven, Connecticut

KAMILA VAGNEROVA, MD
Assistant Professor, Department of Anesthesiology and Perioperative Medicine, Oregon Health & Science University, Portland, Oregon

SUKHBIR WALHA, MD
Assistant Professor of Anesthesiology, University of Colorado School of Medicine, Aurora, Colorado

YIFAN XU, MD, PhD
Resident, Department of Anesthesiology and Perioperative Medicine, Oregon Health & Science University, Portland, Oregon

ALEXANDER T. YAHANDA, MS
Department of Neurosurgery, Washington University School of Medicine, St Louis, Missouri

Contents

Foreword: The Actions that Define Us: Our Response to Critical Events   xiii

Lee A. Fleisher

Preface: Evolving Neuroanesthesia Practice   xv

Jeffrey R. Kirsch and Cynthia A. Lien

Intracranial Vascular Procedures   1

William L. Gross and Raphael H. Sacho

Anesthesia for intracranial vascular procedures is complex because it requires a balance of several competing interests and potentially can result
in significant morbidity and mortality. Frequently, periods of ischemia,
where perfusion must be maintained, are combined with situations that
are high risk for hemorrhage. This review discusses the basic surgical
approach to several common pathologies (intracranial aneurysms, arteriovenous malformations, and moyamoya disease) along with the goals for
anesthetic management and specific high-yield recommendations.

**Perioperative and Anesthetic Considerations for Patients with Degenerative Spine
Disease**   19

Basma A. Mohamed and Brenda G. Fahy

The demand for spine surgery has dramatically increased over the last 2
decades. As the population ages and surgical and anesthetic techniques
advance, the perioperative care of spine surgery patients poses challenges to anesthesiologists. Perioperative outcomes in terms of a
decrease in complication rates and total health care expenditures have
directed perioperative care to focus on enhanced recovery after surgery
protocols, which many institutions have adopted. The role of anesthesiologists in the care of patients undergoing spine surgery is expanding
beyond intraoperative care; consequently, a multidisciplinary approach
is the best direction for optimal patient care.

Anesthesia for Carotid Endarterectomy, Angioplasty, and Stent   37

Priscilla Nelson and Maria Bustillo

Anesthetic management of carotid artery disease requiring carotid endarterectomy or carotid stenting is complex and varies widely, but relies on
excellent communication between the anesthesia and surgical team
throughout the procedure to ensure appropriate cerebral perfusion. With
a systematic approach to vascular access and hemodynamic and neurologic monitoring, anesthesia can be applied to maximize cerebral perfusion while minimizing the risk of postoperative hemorrhage or
hyperperfusion.

Anesthetic Considerations for Pediatric Craniofacial Surgery   53

Nicholas Meier

Anesthetic management of craniosynostosis remains a challenging experience. It requires input and collaboration from multiple specialties to improve patient outcomes. Understanding the surgical corrective techniques and the underlying risks of each is essential to providing the best care to this patient population. The propensity for significant blood loss necessitates fundamental knowledge of pediatric resuscitation and the development of perioperative transfusion protocols that have been shown to reduce transfusion requirements in the peri-operative period.

Anesthetic Management of Asleep and Awake Craniotomy for Supratentorial Tumor Resection   71

Yifan Xu and Kamila Vagnerova

Understanding how anesthetics impact cerebral physiology, cerebral blood flow, brain metabolism, brain relaxation, and neurologic recovery is crucial for optimizing anesthesia during supratentorial craniotomies. Intraoperative goals for supratentorial tumor resection include maintaining cerebral perfusion pressure and cerebral autoregulation, optimizing surgical access and neuromonitoring, and facilitating rapid, cooperative emergence. Evidence-based studies increasingly expand the impact of anesthetic care beyond immediate perioperative care into both preoperative optimization and minimizing postoperative consequences. New evidence is needed for neuroanesthesia's role in neurooncology, in preventing conversion from acute to chronic pain, and in decreasing risk of intraoperative ischemia and postoperative delirium.

Anesthetic Management of Patients Undergoing Open Suboccipital Surgery   93

Kelsey Serfozo and Vijay Tarnal

The posterior cranial fossa with its complex anatomy houses key pathways regulating consciousness, autonomic functions, motor and sensory pathways, and cerebellar centers regulating balance and gait. The most common posterior fossa pathologies for which neurosurgical intervention may be necessary include cerebellopontine angle tumors, aneurysms, and metastatic lesions. The posterior cranial fossa can be accessed from variations of the supine, lateral, park-bench, prone, and sitting positions. Notable complications from positioning include venous air embolism, paradoxic air embolism, tension pneumocephalus, nerve injuries, quadriplegia, and macroglossia. An interdisciplinary approach with careful planning, discussion, and clinical management contributes to improved outcomes and reduced complications.

Acute Ischemic Stroke   113

Kate Petty, Brian P. Lemkuil, and Brian Gierl

Anesthesiologists provide care to acute and subacute ischemic stroke (IS) patients and stroke survivors in interventional radiology, intensive care, and operating rooms. These encounters will become more frequent following studies that have extended the treatment window from last known well time for fibrinolytic and endovascular thrombectomy (EVT).

The number of stroke centers certified to quickly and effectively initiate treatment of IS patients and the number of patients connected to them by telehealth continue to grow. This article reviews IS pathophysiology, assessment, treatment, pathology, and complications; anesthetic management during EVT; perioperative stroke management; and how anesthesia has an impact on patients with prior stroke.

Anesthesia for Acute Spinal Cord Injury   127
Shilpa Rao and Miriam M. Treggiari

The spinal cord extends from the base of the skull to the first lumbar vertebrae from which it continues as cauda equina. Injuries to the spinal cord can lead to significant short- and long-term morbidities. Depending on the level of injury, morbidities may include acute hemodynamic changes, weakness of respiratory muscles and ventilator dependence, and loss of bowel and bladder function. Acute spinal cord injury with cord compression is a surgical emergency. Important anesthetic implications include airway stabilization and management, fluid management, and maintenance of spinal cord perfusion pressure at all times.

Spinal Cord Tumor Surgery   139
Sukhbir Walha and Stacy L. Fairbanks

A spinal cord tumor is any tumor involving the spinal cord or immediate surrounding area. Tumors typically are classified as extradural, intradural extramedullary, or intramedullary intradural. Many spinal cord tumor resections attempt to balance tumor removal with preservation of neurologic function. It is important that anesthesiologists be familiar with the common perioperative risks involved in resection of spinal cord tumors as well as how to form an anesthetic plan that takes intraoperative neuromonitoring and patient comorbidities into consideration. Other risks of prolonged spinal tumor resection include postoperative visual loss, acute on chronic pain, and delayed awakening.

Anesthetic Management of Patients Undergoing Intravascular Treatment of Cerebral Aneurysms and Arteriovenous Malformations   151
Magnus Knut Teig

Arteriovenous malformation (AVM) rupture risk is a complex calculation, and the risks of rupture are influenced by the location and anatomy of the AVM, as well as any history of recurrence. Endovascular treatment of AVMs commonly includes embolization using a liquid embolizate of ethyl vinyl alcohol copolymer. The technique has been enhanced by the invention of detachable tip microcatheters. Embolization may be curative or may be used as part of multimodal therapy for AVMs to reduce their size before open or radiosurgery approaches. These therapies and the consideration necessary to plan for and effectively anesthetize patients undergoing them are discussed.

Decompressive Surgery for Patients with Traumatic Brain Injury   163

Austin Peters and Gabriel Kleinman

> Traumatic brain injury, which is a clinical spectrum, requires a thorough evaluation and strict monitoring for clinical deterioration owing to ongoing secondary injury and raised intracranial pressure. Once the intracranial pressure has been treated with maximal medical therapy, surgical decompression is necessary and must be initiated rapidly. Anesthetic management of surgical decompression must balance reduction of the intracranial pressure, maintenance of cerebral perfusion pressures, avoidance of secondary injuries, and optimization of surgical conditions.

Pain Management in Neurosurgery: Back and Lower Extremity Pain, Trigeminal Neuralgia   179

Yifan Xu, Kimberly M. Mauer, and Amit Singh

> Interventional anesthetic techniques are an integral component of a biopsychosocial approach and multidisciplinary treatment. Injection techniques are often used to diagnose disorders, decrease the need for surgery, or increase the time to surgery. The role of neural blockade techniques using local anesthetics and steroids in the assessment and treatment of pain continues to be refined. With the current opioid crisis and an aging population with increasing medical comorbidities, there is an emphasis on the use of nonopioid, nonsurgical, and multimodal therapies to treat chronic pain. This article reviews indications, goals, and methods of common injection techniques.

Basics of Neuromonitoring and Anesthetic Considerations   195

Shilpa Rao, James Kurfess, and Miriam M. Treggiari

> It is important anesthesiologists understand the pharmacologic interactions of anesthetics and monitoring of evoked potentials or electroencephalography. Intravenous and inhaled anesthetics have varying degrees of influence on different monitoring modalities and can affect amplitude and latency of evoked potentials or voltage and frequency of electroencephalography. Sudden and abrupt changes in monitoring are concerning and should be evaluated promptly. The source of the changes is related to sudden modifications of anesthesia delivery, variations in vital parameters, or the result of surgical manipulation. Identifying sources of abnormal signals and determining the reason for the change should be addressed immediately and corrected accordingly.

Intraoperative MRI for Adult and Pediatric Neurosurgery   211

Dean Laochamroonvorapongse, Marie A. Theard, Alexander T. Yahanda, and Michael R. Chicoine

> Intraoperative MRI (iMRI) technology and its use in both adult and pediatric neurosurgery have advanced significantly over the past 2 decades, allowing neurosurgeons to account for brain shift and optimize resection of brain lesions. Combining the risks of the MR environment with those of the operating room creates a challenging, zero-tolerance environment for the anesthesiologist. This article provides an overview of the currently

available iMRI systems, the neurosurgical evidence supporting iMRI use, and the anesthetic and safety considerations for iMRI procedures.

Anesthetic Considerations for Functional Neurosurgery   **227**

Lane Crawford, Dorothee Mueller, and Letha Mathews

Functional neurosurgery is a rapidly growing field that uses surgical resection, ablation, or neuromodulation to treat an assortment of neurologic and psychiatric disorders, the most common of which are movement disorders and epilepsy. Anesthesiologists caring for patients undergoing neurofunctional procedures should be aware of the anesthetic implications of patients' underlying disease as well as procedure-specific concerns, such as the effects of anesthetics on intraoperative neuromonitoring and limited access to patients due to stereotactic frames or intraoperative imaging.

ANESTHESIOLOGY CLINICS

FORTHCOMING ISSUES

June 2021
**Enhanced Recovery after Surgery and
Perioperative Medicine**
Michael Scott, Anton Krige, and Michael
Grocott, *Editors*

September 2021
Anesthesiologists in Time of Disaster
Lee Fleisher and Jesse Raiten, *Editors*

RECENT ISSUES

December 2020
Management of Critical Events
Alex A. Hannenberg, *Editor*

September 2020
Pediatric Anesthesia
Alison Perate and Vanessa Olbrecht,
Editors

SERIES OF RELATED INTEREST

Neurosurgery Clinics

THE CLINICS ARE AVAILABLE ONLINE!
Access your subscription at:
www.theclinics.com

Foreword

The Actions that Define Us: Our Response to Critical Events

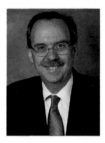

Lee A. Fleisher, MD
Consulting Editor

As anesthesiologists, we are used to hearing that our job is 99% boredom and 1% sheer terror. While many of us believe that this description is far from accurate, our ability to "rescue" a patient who is having a complication and recovery and learn after a critical event is paramount. The method by which we learn to address such events is continuing to evolve as our knowledge of human cognitive traps evolves. In this issue of *Anesthesiology Clinics*, experts in the field describe some of these general concepts and approaches. This is further enhanced by articles addressing specific events by true experts in their respective fields.

In deciding who could assemble a group of experts and provide a vision for this issue, one name came to mind. Alexander Hannenberg, MD has been a leader in our specialty for decades. I personally met Alex while he was leading the American Society of Anesthesiologists (ASA) efforts in quality and quality measurement for the AMA Physician Consortium for Performance Improvement. He has also served as a past president of the ASA and as its Chief Quality Officer. He is now Clinical Professor of Anesthesiology at Tufts University School of Medicine and is a faculty member in the Safe Surgery Program at Ariadne Labs. He has also given much of his time as a founding board member to the important Lifebox USA. He has assembled

Anesthesiology Clin 39 (2021) xiii–xiv
https://doi.org/10.1016/j.anclin.2020.12.002
1932-2275/21/© 2020 Published by Elsevier Inc.

an amazing group of authors to teach us how to learn and do the best for our patients every day.

Lee A. Fleisher, MD
Perelman School of Medicine at
University of Pennsylvania
3400 Spruce Street, Dulles 680
Philadelphia, PA 19104, USA

E-mail address:
Lee.Fleisher@uphs.upenn.edu

Preface

Evolving Neuroanesthesia Practice

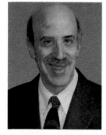 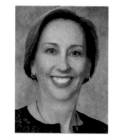

Jeffrey R. Kirsch, MD, FASA   Cynthia A. Lien, MD

Editors

The goal of writing this issue was to provide an up-to-date management approach to the patient with neurologic disease that is amenable to treatment through surgical or intravascular intervention. It is critical that the anesthesia care provider stay current on evolving surgical and interventional approaches to the management of patients with neurologic disease. Those diseases that we considered most important to address in this issue were tumors, trauma, and congenital problems in the cranium and in the spine. We were pleased to be able to recruit expert authors who practice at some of the busiest academic medical centers in the world.

For neurovascular disease, we have included articles to address anesthetic management for both open and intravascular approaches. While not covered in this issue, over the past several months the impact of a COVID-19 infection on neurologic health has been recognized and needs to be mentioned. Unfortunately, COVID-19 significantly increases the rate of stroke in infected individuals with no history of vascular disease. This is a relatively new disease, and we are still learning about it, but it appears that infected patients may have a greater need for anesthesia and intravascular intervention.

There are separate articles to address the anesthetic management of intracranial and spinal cord tumors and trauma to the spinal cord and the head. Although these articles focus primarily on diseases of adult patients, the concepts are generally transferable to pediatric patients. There is one article that focuses on a primarily pediatric topic, as it relates to the anesthetic management for children with craniosynostosis.

The current practices discussed in these articles reflect current management, and they are evolving as our understanding of the pathophysiology of neurologic disease increases. That being said, there is a desperate need for additional research to improve the anesthesia care in patients with neurologic disease. The editors and authors have decided to donate all the royalties related to the sale of this issue to the Foundation for

Anesthesiology Clin 39 (2021) xv–xvi
https://doi.org/10.1016/j.anclin.2020.12.001
1932-2275/21/© 2020 Published by Elsevier Inc.

Anesthesia Education and Research to support the studies that will further improve our care of patients with these disease entities.

DEDICATION

Jeffrey R. Kirsch, MD, FASA: I dedicate this issue to my wife, Robin, for her unwavering love and support, and to my grandchildren, Noa, Romi, Mika, and Daniel Reese, who are my shining stars.

Cynthia A. Lien, MD: For my husband, Dan, and our two daughters, Erika and Christina, for their steadfast encouragement and understanding.

Jeffrey R. Kirsch, MD, FASA
Department of Anesthesiology
Medical College of Wisconsin
8700 W Wisconsin Avenue
Anesthesiology, 3rd Floor
Administrative Suite
Milwaukee, WI 53226, USA

Cynthia A. Lien, MD
Department of Anesthesiology
Medical College of Wisconsin
8700 W Wisconsin Avenue
Anesthesiology, 3rd Floor
Administrative Suite
Milwaukee, WI 53226, USA

E-mail addresses:
jekirsch@mcw.edu (J.R. Kirsch)
clien@mcw.edu (C.A. Lien)

Intracranial Vascular Procedures

William L. Gross, MD, PhD[a],*, Raphael H. Sacho, MD[b]

KEYWORDS

- Intracranial aneurysm • Subarachnoid hemorrhage • Arteriovenous malformation
- Moyamoya

KEY POINTS

- When ischemia is suspected, mean arterial pressure should be maintained at or above baseline levels.
- Systolic blood pressure generally should be kept under 160 mm Hg both intraoperatively and postoperatively to minimize hemorrhagic risk.
- Euvolemia almost always is optimal, with strict avoidance of hypovolemia.
- Short periods of induced hypotension using adenosine can be extremely helpful to facilitate surgical control of bleeding.
- Interventions to reduce intracranial pressure that also reduce cerebral blood flow (eg, hyperventilation) should be minimized.

INTRODUCTION

Open craniotomies to treat intracranial vascular pathologies are among the most complex neurosurgical procedures, with significant potential for morbidity and mortality. Many of these procedures require a delicate balance of interventions to control bleeding, while maintaining sufficient perfusion to critical brain areas. Because this balance can be changed dramatically by anesthetic techniques, the anesthetic management during vascular procedures can contribute significantly to outcomes. This review discusses important points in the general management of all open intracranial vascular procedures, with special emphasis on 3 diseases: intracranial aneurysms, arteriovenous malformations (AVMs), and moyamoya disease.

BACKGROUND
Intracranial Aneurysms

Intracranial aneurysms, when ruptured, produce the multisystem disease aneurysmal subarachnoid hemorrhage (aSAH). In contrast to its traumatic counterpart, aSAH

---

[a] Department of Anesthesiology, Medical College of Wisconsin, 8701 West Watertown Plank Road, Milwaukee, WI 53132, USA; [b] Department of Neurosurgery, Medical College of Wisconsin, 8701 West Watertown Plank Road, Milwaukee, WI 53132, USA
* Corresponding author.
E-mail address: bgross@mcw.edu

Anesthesiology Clin 39 (2021) 1–18
https://doi.org/10.1016/j.anclin.2020.10.001   **anesthesiology.theclinics.com**
1932-2275/21/© 2020 Elsevier Inc. All rights reserved.

frequently involves significant derangement to electrolytes and cardiac function and has a high morbidity and mortality. The primary causes of death and disability from aSAH are from the initial hemorrhage, delayed cerebral ischemia (DCI), and rebleeding before the aneurysm is secured.[1] Therefore, reducing rates of rebleeding and DCI are the highest-impact interventions anesthesiologists can contribute to the care of aSAH patients. Treatment of unruptured aneurysms carries a much lower rate of morbidity but follows similar principles with regard to avoiding perioperative aneurysm rupture.

Incidence and presentation
Aneurysms are present in approximately 2% to 5% of the adult population, with 90% of them in the anterior circulation.[2] Incidence of aSAH varies significantly by country but is approximately 9 per 100,000, with overall mortality at approximately 50% to 60%.[3–5] Approximately 12% of patients die before ever reaching the hospital.[6] Cumulative early mortality in the first day, including prehospital, is approximately 25%, and a total of 40% within the first week, primarily driven by rebleeding.[6] Patients with intracranial aneurysms may present emergently after rupture or electively to treat an unruptured aneurysm. Hemorrhage presents with the classic clinical syndrome of a thunderclap, sudden severe headache, nausea, and nuchal rigidity. Unruptured aneurysms can be discovered incidentally on imaging or more rarely because of symptoms related to the mass effect of the aneurysm (eg, cranial nerve palsies or vision changes).

Timing of intervention
Given the large morbidity and mortality due to rebleeding of a ruptured aneurysm, early treatment is essential.[5,7] Performing surgery within the first few days of aSAH has been shown to improve mortality and functional outcome and reduce rates of DCI.[8,9] There is evidence that a large proportion of the early rebleeding happens within 2 hours of presentation, suggesting immediate intervention may improve outcomes.[10] Whether an open surgical clipping or endovascular treatment is appropriate depends on multiple patient and aneurysm characteristics and is beyond the scope of this review. Although endovascular treatments are continuing to evolve and improve, there still are patients who may benefit from open surgical approaches (eg, wide-necked, anterior circulation aneurysms in a young patient).

Surgical techniques/temporary clipping
The general surgical approach to aneurysm clipping requires a mechanism to reduce blood flow during critical parts of the procedure. Applying aneurysm clips to an inflated, perfused aneurysm is technically difficult and risks rupture. Additionally, in the event of rupture, blood flow to the aneurysm must be reduced to allow the surgeon to perform the arterial repair. Consideration of how to control flow to the aneurysm is a critical part of the surgical plan.

Frequently, flow reduction is achieved through proximal control, by applying temporary clips to vessels that feed or exit the aneurysm. Before extensive manipulation, temporary clips are applied to isolate the aneurysm from circulation. Depending on the location and duration of application, temporary clips may create hypoperfusion of distal cortex, causing ischemia. In observational studies, temporary clip application has not been associated with increased postoperative deficits[11]; however, given the potential, it is prudent to minimize the time they are applied and maximize cerebral protection during temporary clipping. If proximal control is difficult to achieve, several other techniques can be used. There are case reports of very large aneurysms being treated using cardiopulmonary bypass and deep hypothermic arrest[12] with acceptable results. There also have been reports of successful use of transvenous pacing wires to implement controlled hypotension through rapid ventricular pacing.[13]

Adenosine-induced asystole

Alternatively, brief episodes of hypotension can be induced reliably through bolus doses of adenosine, a commonly available medication. These can be particularly effective during acute, unexpected intraprocedural rupture and can be implemented without any prior planning. The brief circulatory arrest creates a short (approximately 30 seconds) period of minimal hemorrhage, which allows the surgeon to visualize the bleeding point and achieve hemostasis. Adenosine also can be used proactively for aneurysms where proximal control is technically difficult to obtain, for example, in paraclinoid or other skull base aneurysms.[14] Adenosine first was introduced to intracranial aneurysm surgery by Groff and colleagues in 1999[15]; several case series have shown that it is effective and safe for use in aneurysm clipping[14,16] as well as in AVM treatment.[17]

Adenosine traditionally has been used as an atrioventricular nodal blocking agent at lower doses (6 mg–12 mg) to abort supraventricular tachycardias. At higher doses, it produces a dose-dependent period of asystole and profound hypotension. In 2 dose-response studies, doses in the range of 0.24 mg/kg to 1.76 mg/kg (ideal body weight) of adenosine produced a linear increase in duration of asystole and profound hypotension.[16,17] The bolus dose of adenosine can be approximated to about 1 mg per second of asystole desired.[14] A bolus dose in the range of 0.3 mg/kg to 0.4 mg/kg, usually dosed by ideal body weight, reliably produced approximately 30 seconds to 45 seconds of profound hypotension to facilitate securing of the aneurysm.[16] Although these doses are higher than typically used for other indications, it has been shown that using this weight-based formula is safe and produces more timely results than escalating doses based on response.[18]

Adenosine can be given in any peripheral intravenous (IV) catheter but should be given as a rapid bolus dose in the largest, most proximal IV access available. In cases of adenosine anticipated to be used, pacing pads frequently are placed in cases of sustained arrythmias; however, there are no published reports of them being required. Depending on the access site, asystole should be achieved within 20 seconds. Arrythmias can develop (most commonly atrial fibrillation) but usually are transient (<1 minute) and self-terminating. Adenosine has a reliably short half-life of less than 10 seconds,[19] so drug-induced effects reverse quickly. Aside from cardiac effects, bronchospasm also has been reported,[19] so care must be taken in patients with severe reactive airway disease. Overall, adenosine is a safe and reliable drug that all anesthesiologists involved with intracranial vascular procedures should be comfortable administering.

Arteriovenous Malformations

Intracranial AVMs are congenital malformations usually diagnosed either in childhood or young adults. They can, however, present at any age. The initial presenting symptom in 45% to 70% of adults is headache, seizures, or hemorrhage.[20] Mortality from the initial hemorrhage is estimated to be approximately 10% to 30%.[21] The primary cause of morbidity in these patients is hemorrhage, which is estimated to occur in approximately 1% of patients per year.[22] In patients with AVMs that already have bled, rebleeding occurs in approximately 16% of patients in the first year and in an additional 8% in every subsequent year.[23,24]

AVMs belong to a larger family of vascular malformations, including venous and cavernous malformations. The term AVM commonly is used generically to refer to many kinds of intracranial vascular malformations. The classic parenchymal AVMs discussed, however, are more specifically designated pial AVMs, because their arterial supply is derived from pial vessels.[25] Primary symptoms include ischemia from vascular steal, seizures, and bleeding.

Therapeutic options

Treatment of AVMs can be performed by open surgical resection, endovascular embolization, or stereotactic radiation or with a combination of multiple modalities. The approach to unruptured AVM management is complex and needs to be tailored based on patient and AVM characteristics as well as institutional expertise. Attempts to study the natural history of AVMs have been met with difficulty and some controversy.[26,27] In some cases, the natural history of the disease may be more favorable than intervention.[28] For many AVMs, however, microsurgical resection with or without presurgical embolization remains an excellent therapeutic option.

The Spetzler-Martin grading scale often is used to help stratify surgical risk and can help with the selection of appropriate surgical candidates (discussed later [**Table 1**]). Younger patients with Spetzler-Martin grade 1 or grade 2 and some with grade 3 generally are good candidates for microsurgical AVM resection. Given that treatment of large AVMs can have high rates of complications,[28] patient preference also is a large factor in deciding treatment options. Although intervention on some AVMs may have a statistically large perioperative morbidity, it may be reasonable in some patients, given the increased quality of life, removing the worry of long-term hemorrhagic risk. Because of the significantly higher propensity for rebleeding in ruptured AVMs, greater consideration of surgical resection is given to these patients.

Moyamoya Disease

Named after the angiographic puff of smoke seen in this disease, the primary lesion in moyamoya disease is chronic, progressive stenosis of the distal internal carotid artery. Ischemia following this stenosis induces the large number of small-caliber collaterals that lead to the smoky appearance on angiogram. Although partial perfusion occurs through these collaterals, cerebral blood flow (CBF) still is restricted and highly dependent on blood pressure (BP). Transient ischemic attacks and strokes are common, along with hemorrhage of the fragile collateral vessels.

Treatment is performed either by direct anastomosis of an extracranial artery (usually the superior temporal artery) to the middle cerebral artery (ie, extracranial-intracranial bypass) or through indirect means by placement of a perfused vascular tissue (eg, superficial temporal artery [pial synangiosis], muscle, or omentum) on the brain surface.[29] The combination of the presence of this vascular tissue with the ischemic brain causes angiogenesis to occur and eventually create anastomoses

Table 1
Grading scale for arteriovenous malformations to predict postoperative deficits developed by Spetzler and Martin

Component		Score
Size	<3 cm	1
	3–6 cm	2
	>6 cm	3
Location	Noneloquent	0
	Eloquent	1
Venous drainage	Superficial	0
	Deep	1

Final score is total sum of risk factors, ≥4 is associated with significant deficits.

with the underlying brain. In a series of 34 symptomatic adult patients, the 5-year risk of stroke from untreated moyamoya disease was 65%. After direct revascularization, 84% of patients have symptomatic improvement and 77% after indirect.[30]

CLINICAL GRADING & EVALUATION
Subarachnoid Hemorrhage Grading

Determining the clinical severity at presentation of aSAH is helpful for overall prognostication. Historically, the Hunt and Hess scale was used to grade the degree of neurologic impairment; however, it has been criticized for being too subjective and having low inter-rater reliability.[31] Because of this, 2 other scales based on the commonly used Glasgow Coma Scale (GCS) score were developed: World Federation of Neurological Surgeons (WFNS) and Prognosis on Admission of Aneurysmal Subarachnoid Hemorrhage (PAASH) scales (**Table 2**). Both are simple transformations of the GCS into different clinical grades; however, the PAASH grades has been shown to be more aligned with categories of outcome.[32] Although the GCS score was not designed for SAH, its inter-rater reliability, simplicity, and widespread use make it useful.

Arteriovenous Malformations Grading

Grading of AVMs is done to predict likelihood of postoperative deficits with open surgical resection using the Spetzler-Martin grading scale,[33] shown in **Table 1**. It is higher risk to resect AVMs that are larger, have deep venous drainage, and are located near eloquent cortex (sensorimotor or language). The original case series showed 4% overall risk of major postoperative deficits with surgical treatment of grade 3 or less AVMs and 19% risk for grade 4 or greater. These associations have been confirmed in recent studies as well.[26]

Moyamoya Grading

The traditional grading scale for moyamoya disease, proposed by Suzuki and colleagues[34], is based solely on angiographic features; however, it has limited clinical

Table 2
Clinical grading scales for aneurysmal subarachnoid hemorrhage

Grade	Hunt and Hess	World Federation of Neurologic Surgeons	Prognosis on Admission of Aneurysmal Subarachnoid Hemorrhage
I	Mild headache	GCS 15	GCS 15
II	Severe headache with only cranial nerve palsies	GCS 13–14, no focal neurologic deficits	GCS 11–14
III	Lethargic, mild focal neurologic deficits	GCS 13–14, with focal deficits	GCS 8–10
IV	Stuporous, severe deficits	GCS 7–12	GCS 4–7
V	Comatose, posturing	GCS <7	GCS 3

WFNS and PAASH have been shown to be simpler and better correlated with outcome.

utility in isolation.[29] Recently the Berlin moyamoya grading scale was proposed,[35] which correlates more closely with risks of postoperative ischemic deficits (**Table 3**). This scale combines angiographic, magnetic resonance imaging (MRI), and perfusion features to stratify patients from mild to severe: grades I (1–2 points), II (3–4 points), and III (5–6 points). Preoperative symptoms are seen in 15% to 20% of grade I patients versus 90% of grade III patients.[35,36] In a validation study, 0/40 (0%) of grade I or grade II patients had perioperative neurologic complications, whereas complications were seen in 12/30 (40%) of grade III patients.[36] Using the Berlin grading system, an anesthesiologist can appropriately stratify patients' perioperative risk and apply extra vigilance to those patients at highest risk.

GOALS
Common Principals

Vascular neurosurgery cases require a balance of maintaining adequate perfusion while minimizing bleeding risk. Because of the need for close management of BP, arterial lines are standard in most cases. Multiple large-gauge IV lines are required both for drips and fluid resuscitation. The volume of blood that can be lost, even from small caliber intracranial blood vessels, can be surprising, given that the brain receives such a large proportion of the cardiac output (CO) and bleeding cannot be controlled easily with direct pressure.

The potential instability of these cases usually requires general endotracheal anesthesia; however, there have been a few series demonstrating awake techniques for neurologic monitoring in aneurysms[37] and AVMs.[38] Similar to many neurosurgical cases, high-dose intraoperative opiates can be helpful to minimize sympathetic stimulation; remifentanil is popular because of its short half-time. In many intracranial vascular cases, 0.5 minimum alveolar concentration volatile anesthetic, an opiate infusion, and paralysis provide a good balance of anesthesia, intracranial pressure (ICP) control, and adequate monitoring conditions. Inhalational versus IV anesthetic agents can cause minor differences in regional perfusion,[39] although no clinical differences are observed.[40]

Open Aneurysm Clipping

Although very different clinical scenarios, anesthetic management of ruptured and unruptured aneurysms follows similar general principles with regard to monitoring and BP management. The primary goals of both cases are close control of BP to prevent either an initial or recurrent aneurysmal bleed. Because they vary substantially in their risk of morbidity and mortality, however, a significantly higher level of vigilance

Table 3		
The Berlin moyamoya grading scale to predict clinical symptoms and perioperative morbidity		
Diagnostic Modality		**Points**
Digital subtraction angiography	Occlusive lesion	1
	+ Intracranial compensation	2
	+ Extracranial compensation	3
MRI	No ischemia, hemorrhage, or atrophy	0
	Ischemia, hemorrhage, or atrophy	1
Perfusion	No steal phenomenon	0
	Steal phenomenon	2

Final score is the sum of individual points, grade III (5–6) being associated with increased perioperative risk.

and strictness is indicated during the care of ruptured aneurysms. Additionally, patients with ruptured aneurysms present to the operating room with several comorbid complications not present in elective cases, including hydrocephalus, cardiac effects, and electrolyte abnormalities.

In an otherwise healthy elective aneurysm clipping, a postinduction arterial line is reasonable, if hemodynamic stability is reasonably assured through liberal use of opiates (eg, remifentanil) or antihypertensives (eg, esmolol). Ruptured aneurysms universally require preinduction arterial lines to assure hemodynamic control. Elective aneurysms rarely require more advanced access, whereas a ruptured aneurysm with multiple vasoactive drips may require a central line and occasionally could benefit from a pulmonary artery catheter to target inotropes and volume status (discussed later).

Of particular note are patients presenting for semiurgent clipping after a sentinel bleed. Sentinel bleeds are diagnosed in patients who present with a clinical syndrome suggestive of aSAH (headache, nausea, and nuchal rigidity) but are found to have an unruptured aneurysm. These phenomena have been noted in approximately 40% of aSAH cases and occur approximately 2 weeks to 4 weeks before frank rupture.[41,42] The mechanism of the headache is thought to be related to an aneurysmal leak and suggests it may be easier for the aneurysm to rupture. These cases present to the operating room similar to elective cases; however, they should be treated more aggressively given their increased potential for rupture.

Postoperatively, bleeding risks are reduced, but a smooth emergence still is indicated. BP goals can be liberalized to maximize perfusion, but large spikes from pain or sympathetic medications still should be avoided to reduce hemorrhagic risk.

DISCUSSION
Blood Pressure Management

The critical balance of perfusion and hemorrhagic risk makes BP control one of the primary concerns of vascular cases. Given that perfusion of tissues generally correlates with the time-averaged pressure, mean arterial pressure (MAP) is typically used for perfusion goals. In contrast, prevention of hemorrhage is related to reducing the magnitude of the pressure wave transmitted to potential bleeding sources, so systolic BP (SBP) goals are typical.

Although the association between MAP and CBF relies on several variables (eg, intracranial vascular tone) that are difficult to observe, general statements can be made regarding MAP goals. It generally is accepted that maintaining MAP within 20% of baseline values maintains adequate CBF in patients who are not undergoing active ischemia. Patients at risk for ischemia may need much tighter control, however. Moyamoya patients are particularly sensitive to drops in their BP and should be maintained at or above their baseline MAP. Temporary clipping during aneurysm surgery is another instance where ischemia is possible, and it frequently is recommended to increase the MAP by 10% during these periods of time, although there is a lack of clinical evidence to show a difference in outcomes. In contrast, intentionally inducing hypotension has been shown to worsen outcomes in aSAH[43] and is discouraged by the guidelines.[7] A retrospective analysis of 1099 aSAH patients looking at the association of time below MAP thresholds (as low as 60 mm Hg), however, did not show a significant correlation with postoperative neurologic outcome.[44] Because this was a retrospective study, it is difficult to make strong claims, but it suggests that within BP ranges of current clinical practice, MAP is not strongly associated with outcome. Given the complex relationship between MAP and CBF, and the current lack of evidence supporting specific MAP goals, in situations of suspected ischemia, neuro-monitoring may be helpful to exclude neurologic injury (discussed later).

In contrast to ischemic risk, hemorrhagic risk has been quantitatively studied in several disease states. Patients with intracranial vascular lesions frequently present significantly hypertensive, compensating for reduced CBF. Postoperative hemorrhage after craniotomy has been associated significantly with SBP greater than 160 mm Hg during emergence or within 12 hours postoperatively.[45] In addition, a meta-analysis of aSAH found a significantly increased rate of rebleeding with SBP greater than 160 mm Hg,[46] and, in a series of 134 aSAH patients, treating hypertension dropped rebleeding rates from 33% to 15%.[47] Overall, keeping the SBP less than 160 mm Hg appears consistently associated with a reduction in perioperative hemorrhagic risk.

Fluid Management

Historically, recommendations for various degrees of hypervolemia and hypovolemia have been made for different vascular pathologies, but a growing amount of basic science and clinical evidence suggests that maintaining euvolemia during most vascular procedures appears optimal. Although MAP is easier to measure, optimizing perfusion of the brain (ie, CBF) is the primary goal. Systemic MAP can be increased either by modulating systemic vascular resistance or CO. In states of lowered CO (eg, due to hypovolemia), increasing modulating systemic vascular resistance (eg, through a phenylephrine infusion) increases MAP without a corresponding increase in peripheral perfusion. Although the regulation of the cerebral vasculature is complex, and its response may differ slightly from systemic effects,[48] there is growing evidence that cerebral vessels respond in ways similar to vasoconstrictive agents. For example, increasing MAP using phenylephrine may not increase CBF as much as other interventions that support CO,[49,50] such as maintaining euvolemia. Because of these effects, optimizing volume status rather than relying on pressors may lead to improved CBF at a similar BP.

Fluid management in aneurysmal subarachnoid hemorrhage

Fluid management is complex, particularly in aSAH patients, because they are both very susceptible to ischemia and very likely to become hypovolemic. Hypovolemia has been associated with increased rates of DCI and poor long-term disability outcomes.[51,52] The primary causes of hypovolemia in aSAH patients are cerebral salt wasting and iatrogenic causes (eg, mannitol administration). Using invasive monitoring, severe hypovolemia has been found in 17% of aSAH patients.[53] Although hypervolemia has been a traditional component of the hypervolemia, hemodilution, and hypertension (HHH) DCI therapy, this has fallen out of favor given evidence that hypervolemia does not improve CBF or outcomes compared with euvolemia and may increase complications.[54–56] In addition, hemodilution (with or without volume expansion) has been shown experimentally to increase CBF but also results in a concomitant decrease in total oxygen delivery[57] and does not improve outcomes.[56] Although the induced hypertension component of HHH therapy has been associated with improved CBF in some trials,[56] a recent randomized controlled trial (RCT) showed no CBF change in aSAH patients whose BP was augmented with norepinephrine.[58]

Based on standard monitoring using arterial lines and central venous pressure, clinicians tend to under-resuscitate aSAH, suggesting advanced CO monitoring may be indicated in these patients.[53] A combination of fluid balance, central venous pressure, and arterial waveform analysis (using FloTrac; Edwards Lifesciences, Irvine, CA), versus invasive CO methods (eg, pulmonary artery catheters or transpulmonary dilutional measurements) have shown consistently better hemodynamic measurements and reductions in DCI using more advanced CO monitors.[59,60] A recent RCT compared using transpulmonary CO (PiCCO$_2$ [Pulse Contour Cardiac Output, v2]; PULSION, Munich, Germany) to guide fluid resuscitation versus standard management and showed significantly lower rates of DCI (13% vs 32%, respectively) and more likely good outcomes (Glasgow Outcome Scale = 5; 66% vs 44%, respectively) using CO measurements to guide fluid resuscitation. Currently, the data comparing clinical outcomes have been limited to invasive monitors, although the same logic may apply to other noninvasive measurements of CO (eg, transthoracic echocardiography). Although advanced CO monitoring currently is not standard of care, the evidence is building that it may improve outcome, particularly in aSAH patients at higher risk for DCI.

Fluid management in moyamoya disease

Moyamoya patients are extremely sensitive to reductions in CBF, so BP and fluid management traditionally have been aggressive during the perioperative period.[61] Primarily due to clinical experience, hypervolemia is classically recommended, with some centers preadmitting patients for aggressive IV hydration.[62] In contrast to aSAH, most moyamoya disease patients do no present with concurrent cardiopulmonary disfunction and, therefore, likely tolerate larger fluid challenges. Specific evidence supporting a particular goal is lacking, however.

Cardiac Effects

In the context of acute vascular diseases (eg, a ruptured aneurysm), catecholamine surge can induce a reversible stress-related cardiomyopathy (SRC). Although classically SRC is associated with aSAH, it occasionally can be seen in several other neurologic conditions, including seizure, meningitis, and ischemic stroke.[63] The precise incidence of SRC after aSAH is difficult to ascertain because most patients do not have echocardiograms performed, but it is estimated to occur in 1% to 5% of aSAH patients.[64,65] The classic form of SRC is Takotsubo cardiomyopathy, also called apical ballooning syndrome, named after the dilation and hypokinesis of apical and midventricular myocardial segments. Although this is the classic presentation, many morphologic variants exist that do not follow this pattern. Common among all of them is an acute reduction in systolic left ventricular function that completely reverses with time.

The mechanism of SRC is not completely clear but appears to be due to myocardial stunning due to calcium overload within the myocytes and a large production of oxygen free radicals, without any evidence of necrosis.[66] At the time of diagnosis, circulating levels of epinephrine are greater than 30 times normal.[66] In most cases, acute ST elevation is seen, along with the expected progression of T-wave inversion and Q waves. The clinical and electrocardiogram findings of Takotsubo cardiomyopathy are indistinguishable from a myocardial infarction,[67] although electrocardiogram findings in SRC are more transient. It is estimated that 4% to 6% of women who present with acute coronary syndrome have Takotsubo cardiomyopathy.[66] Cardiac enzymes also can be elevated but not to the same degree as a ST elevation myocardial infarction of the same magnitude. SRC and acute coronary syndrome, however, generally are distinguishable on echocardiography, given the noncoronary distribution of hypokinesis in SRC.

Patients with SRCs should be managed similarly to other patients in systolic heart failure.[68] Serial echocardiography usually is necessary to guide treatment, along with advanced monitoring (eg, pulmonary artery catheters) as indicated. Inotropic support frequently is required, along with strict management of fluids to avoid overloading the heart. Although SRC patients present with a clinical picture similar to other systolic heart failure patients, their prognosis generally is good because the cardiac deficits usually are completely reversible. In a retrospective review of 30 patients with Takotsubo cardiomyopathy who had ejection fractions between 22% and 65%, no association was found with outcome and cardiac impairment,[69] suggesting aggressive treatment should not be withheld because of concern for cardiac complications.

Intracranial Pressure Management

General management of increased ICP in intracranial vascular procedures is similar to general neuroanesthesia practice, with a few caveats. Mannitol and hyperosmotics frequently are administered; however, care must be given to the diuretic effects of mannitol and its overall effect on fluid balance. Patients presenting after rupture of a vascular lesion frequently require an external ventricular drain. Regarding ruptured aneurysms, there is a theoretic risk of causing a rerupture with aggressive drainage, but data supporting this are conflicting.[70–72] Overall, given the known risk of increased ICP, CSF drainage to below 20 mm Hg generally is recommended, with avoidance of over-drainage.

Hyperventilation to achieve hypocapnia is used widely in neuroanesthesia to lower ICP; however, its use in vascular cases must be judicious given the reduction in CBF. The aggressive use of hyperventilation in the context of brain ischemia has been associated with a greater risk of harm[73] and hyperventilation of aSAH patients to less than a $Paco_2$ of 35 mm Hg in the intensive care unit is associated with poor outcomes,[74] although this relationship was not seen intraoperatively during aneurysm clipping,[44] likely due to the small number of hyperventilated patients in this sample.

Patients with moyamoya disease are particularly sensitive to the effects of hyperventilation. Children with moyamoya disease have been observed to experience transient ischemic attacks in association with crying episodes,[75] which correlate with decreases in CBF.[76] In contrast, permissive hypercapnia in aSAH patients produces increases in CBF,[77] suggesting that raising the EtCO2 actually could be protective in times of reduced CBF (assuming ICP is otherwise controlled).

Neurologic Monitoring

Although much of the focus of anesthetic management in neurosurgical cases is on maintaining perfusion to the brain, classic models based on MAP and ICP are loose approximations and do not consider the complex dynamics of cerebral vascular tone.[78] For this reason, in cases of possible brain ischemia, more direct monitoring of regional CBF or brain function may be indicated.

Neurophysiologic monitoring has been used in many forms of neurosurgery. The most common types of monitoring applied to intracranial vascular procedures are electroencephalography (EEG) and somatosensory evoked potentials (SSEPs). SSEPs used to predict stroke after aneurysm clipping have been shown to have a 94% negative predictive value but a 25% positive predictive value.[79] Similar results have been seen using SSEPs for predicting stroke after carotid endarterectomy.[80] Theoretically, the lower positive predictive value could be because when real SSEP changes associated with ischemia were observed, intraoperative modifications prevented the eventual development of a postoperative strokes (therefore, the changes were counted as false positive). Using SSEPs, however, has not been shown to improve overall outcome.[81] If local perfusion to a region is not able to be increased with increases in MAP, for example, due to a lack of collateral blood supply, detection of ischemia may not lead to reductions in stroke. EEG and SSEPs frequently are used in other intracranial cases as well; however, robust data supporting a clinical benefit are lacking.

Neuroprotection

To minimize the effects of ischemic periods, various neuroprotective techniques have been attempted, the most popular being propofol administration and hypothermia. Both techniques are used widely but have limited evidence of their effectiveness.

Propofol
In addition to reducing the cerebral metabolic rate and decreasing ICP, animal studies have suggested propofol may have direct neuroprotective properties. There is mixed evidence from a large number of studies using cell cultures and animal models of cerebral ischemia supporting the ability of propofol to reduce infarct size after ischemic insults to the brain.[82] Clinically, propofol boluses of approximately 1 mg/kg to 2 mg/kg frequently are used prior to ischemic events (eg, applying temporary clips) to induce burst suppression on EEG, although doses in this range frequently cause significant hypotension that must be mitigated with vasopressors. If EEG-based neuromonitoring is used, fractionated doses of propofol can be titrated until burst suppression is observed on EEG. Although burst suppression theoretically may minimize neural damage, to date, no studies have shown differences in clinical outcomes.[7]

Intraoperative hypothermia
Hypothermia has been attempted in many clinical contexts as a neuroprotectant, given the significant reduction in cerebral metabolism than can be achieved. So far, the only clinical condition that has shown a clear benefit has been post–cardiac arrest.[83] Hypothermia has been tested in several neurologic pathologies but consistently has failed to show improvement in outcomes. Intraoperative hypothermia (33°C) was tested in an RCT of 1001 patients undergoing aneurysm clipping, and no difference in outcomes were observed.[84] An RCT with 500 severe traumatic brain injury patients also failed to show neurologic improvement with postinjury hypothermia.[85] Overall, hypothermia has a strong theoretic motivation and has been implemented safely in intracranial vascular patients, but no improvement of outcome ever has been demonstrated so there is little evidence to support its use.[7]

Medications

Antiepileptic drugs
Seizures after craniotomies are common and in the postoperative period may contribute to perioperative complications.[7] The incidence varies substantially by pathology, but overall 22% of intracranial vascular patients experience seizures postoperatively, 7% within the first week.[86] Anterior circulation aneurysms and AVMs carry a higher risk, possibly as high as 40% to 50%, within the first 5 postoperative years.[86,87] Several studies have looked at prophylactic use of antiepileptic drugs (AEDs); however, they do not appear to be consistently effective at preventing postoperative seizures.[88] In addition, the use of prophylactic AEDs in aSAH patients has been shown to be associated with increased complications and worsened outcomes.[89] In spite of a lack of strong evidence, the reasonable concern of significant perioperative morbidity from a seizure leads to their continued use in some centers. This ambivalence is represented in the aSAH guidelines, where the American guidelines state prophylactic AEDs may be considered[7] whereas the European guidelines state there is no evidence supporting their use.[5]

Steroids

Similar to other neurologic conditions, the glucocorticoid hydrocortisone has been tried in aSAH to reduce the neural inflammatory response but greatly increases the rates of complications and has not been shown to improve outcome.[90,91] In contrast, 0.3 mg/ d to 0.4 mg/d of the mineralocorticoid fludrocortisone has been shown to reduce the amount of natriuresis in aSAH and help maintain fluid balance.[92,93] Although there is limited evidence supporting its use, these studies suggest fludrocortisone may be helpful in maintaining euvolemia in pathologies that are prone to salt wasting.

Antifibrinolytics (tranexamic acid/aminocaproic acid)

Because of the success of using antifibrinolytics in trauma and obstetric hemorrhage, there has been interest applying them to intracranial hemorrhage. Several studies have been done on aSAH patients, in an attempt to prevent aneurysmal rebleeding. Antifibrinolytic therapy significantly decreases early rebleeding but also increases ischemic events, leading to overall similar mortality.[94] Two small trials have been published that administered tranexamic acid[95] and aminocaproic acid[96] only during the period of time immediately after presentation and demonstrated a significant reduction in rebleeding, although overall outcomes were not improved. In a large RCT of 2325 intracerebral hemorrhage patients randomized to receive tranexamic acid, mortality also was reduced in the first week, but 90-day mortality was unchanged. Taken together, antifibrinolytics may be indicated at times of increased hemorrhagic risk (eg, before securing a ruptured aneurysm), but overall do not seem to improve outcome.

SUMMARY

Intracranial vascular pathologies are complex and keeping these patients safe through surgical interventions not always is straightforward. The primary concerns of the anesthesiologist for these patients focus on optimizing perfusion during times of ischemia while simultaneously minimizing the risk of hemorrhage. There are not many simple answers to management questions in these patients, which requires thoughtful application of the principles presented here.

CLINICAL CARE POINTS

- Maintain SBP less than 160 mm Hg in all patients with a concern for hemorrhage.
- Optimize fluid status toward euvolemia in all patients.
- In patients with demonstrated ischemia (eg, moyamoya disease), maintain preoperative MAP and liberally maintain fluid status.
- Significant hyperventilation (end-tidal CO_2 <30) rarely is indicated, except in emergent situations.
- Adenosine is a safe and useful emergency medication that all anesthesiologists should be familiar with.
- Neuromonitoring and neuroprotection with propofol and hypothermia are used widely but may have limited effectiveness in preventing postoperative deficits.

DISCLOSURE

The authors have no conflicts of interest to disclose.

REFERENCES

1. Kassell NF, Torner JC, Jane JA, et al. The International Cooperative Study on the timing of aneurysm surgery: part 2: surgical results. J Neurosurg 1990;73(1): 37–47.
2. Rinkel GJE, Djibuti M, Algra A, et al. Prevalence and risk of rupture of intracranial aneurysms. Stroke 1998;29(1):251–6.
3. Broderick JP, Brott TG, Duldner JE, et al. Initial and recurrent bleeding are the major causes of death following subarachnoid hemorrhage. Stroke 1994;25(7): 1342–7.
4. Locksley HB. Natural history of subarachnoid hemorrhage, intracranial aneurysms and arteriovenous malformations. J Neurosurg 1966;25(3):321–4.
5. Steiner T, Juvela S, Unterberg A, et al. European Stroke Organization guidelines for the management of intracranial aneurysms and subarachnoid haemorrhage. Cerebrovasc Dis 2013;35(2):93–112.
6. Huang J, van Gelder JM. The probability of sudden death from rupture of intracranial aneurysms: a meta-analysis. Neurosurgery 2002;51(5):1101–5 [discussion: 1105–7].
7. Connolly ES, Rabinstein AA, Carhuapoma JR, et al. Guidelines for the management of aneurysmal subarachnoid hemorrhage: a guideline for healthcare professionals from the American Heart Association/american Stroke Association. Stroke 2012;43(6):1711–37.
8. Öhman J, Heiskanen O. Timing of operation for ruptured supratentorial aneurysms: a prospective randomized study. J Neurosurg 1989;70(1):55–60.
9. Solomon RA, Onesti ST, Klebanoff L. Relationship between the timing of aneurysm surgery and the development of delayed cerebral ischemia. J Neurosurg 1991;75(1):56–61.
10. Ohkuma H, Tsurutani H, Suzuki S. Incidence and significance of early aneurysmal rebleeding before neurosurgical or neurological management. Stroke 2001;32(5): 1176–80.
11. Jabre A, Lindsay S. Temporary vascular occlusion during aneurysm surgery. Surg Neurol 1987;27(1):47–62.
12. Levati A, Tommasino C, Moretti MP, et al. Giant intracranial aneurysms treated with deep hypothermia and circulatory arrest. J Neurosurg Anesthesiol 2007; 19(1):25–30.
13. Whiteley JR, Payne R, Rodriguez-Diaz C, et al. Rapid ventricular pacing: a novel technique to decrease cardiac output for giant basilar aneurysm surgery. J Clin Anesth 2012;24(8):656–8.
14. Powers CJ, Wright DR, McDonagh DL, et al. Transient adenosine-induced asystole during the surgical treatment of anterior circulation cerebral aneurysms: technical note. Oper Neurosurg (Hagerstown) 2010;67(2):ons461–70.
15. Groff MW, Adams DC, Kahn RA, et al. Adenosine-induced transient asystole for management of a basilar artery aneurysm: case report. J Neurosurg 1999;91(4): 687–90.
16. Bebawy JF, Gupta DK, Bendok BR, et al. Adenosine-induced flow arrest to facilitate intracranial aneurysm clip ligation. Anesth Analg 2010;110(5):1406–11.
17. Hashimoto T, Young WL, Aagaard BD, et al. Adenosine-induced ventricular asystole to induce transient profound systemic hypotension in patients undergoing endovascular therapy: dose–response characteristics. Anesthesiology 2000; 93(4):998–1001.

18. Lee SH, Kwun BD, Kim JU, et al. Adenosine-induced transient asystole during intracranial aneurysm surgery: indications, dosing, efficacy, and risks. Acta Neurochir 2015;157(11):1879–86.
19. Faulds D, Chrisp P, Buckley MM-T. Adenosine: an evaluation of its use in cardiac diagnostic procedures, and in the treatment of paroxysmal supraventricular tachycardia. Drugs 1991;41(4):596–624.
20. Söderman M, Andersson T, Karlsson B, et al. Management of patients with brain arteriovenous malformations. Eur J Radiol 2003;46(3):195–205.
21. Aoun SG, Bendok BR, Batjer HH. Acute management of ruptured arteriovenous malformations and dural arteriovenous fistulas. Neurosurg Clin N Am 2012; 23(1):87–103.
22. Stapf C, Mast H, Sciacca RR, et al. Predictors of hemorrhage in patients with untreated brain arteriovenous malformation. Neurology 2006;66(9):1350–5.
23. Gross BA, Du R. Rate of re-bleeding of arteriovenous malformations in the first year after rupture. J Clin Neurosci 2012;19(8):1087–8.
24. Beecher JS, Lyon K, Ban VS, et al. Delayed treatment of ruptured brain AVMs: is it ok to wait? J Neurosurg 2018;128(4):999–1005.
25. Geibprasert S, Pongpech S, Jiarakongmun P, et al. Radiologic assessment of brain arteriovenous malformations: what clinicians need to know. Radiographics 2010;30(2):483–501.
26. Wong J, Slomovic A, Ibrahim G, et al. Microsurgery for ARUBA trial (a randomized trial of unruptured brain arteriovenous malformation)-eligible unruptured brain arteriovenous malformations. Stroke 2016;48(1):136–44.
27. Amin-Hanjani S. ARUBA results are not applicable to all patients with arteriovenous malformation. Stroke 2014;45(5):1539–40.
28. Mohr JP, Parides MK, Stapf C, et al. Medical management with or without interventional therapy for unruptured brain arteriovenous malformations (ARUBA): a multicentre, non-blinded, randomised trial. Lancet 2013;383(9917):614–21.
29. Acker G, Fekonja L, Vajkoczy P. Surgical management of Moyamoya disease. Stroke 2018;49(2):476–82.
30. Park S-E, Kim J-S, Park EK, et al. Direct versus indirect revascularization in the treatment of moyamoya disease. J Neurosurg 2017;129(2):480–9.
31. Degen LAR, Mees SMD, Algra A, et al. Interobserver variability of grading scales for aneurysmal subarachnoid hemorrhage. Stroke 2011;42(6):1546–9.
32. van Heuven AW, Mees SMD, Algra A, et al. Validation of a prognostic subarachnoid hemorrhage grading scale derived directly from the glasgow coma scale. Stroke 2008;39(4):1347–8.
33. Spetzler RF, Martin NA. A proposed grading system for arteriovenous malformations. J Neurosurg 1986;65(4):476–83.
34. Suzuki J, Takaku A. Cerebrovascular "moyamoya" disease. Disease showing abnormal net-like vessels in base of brain. Arch Neurol 1969;20(3):288–99.
35. Czabanka M, Peña-Tapia P, Schubert GA, et al. Proposal for a new grading of Moyamoya disease in adult patients. Cerebrovasc Dis 2011;32(1):41–50.
36. Kashiwazaki D, Akioka N, Kuwayama N, et al. Berlin grading system can stratify the onset and predict perioperative complications in adult moyamoya disease. Neurosurgery 2017;81(6):986–91.
37. Abdulrauf SI, Vuong P, Patel R, et al. "Awake" clipping of cerebral aneurysms: report of initial series. J Neurosurg 2017;127(2):311–8.
38. Gamble AJ, Schaffer SG, Nardi DJ, et al. Awake craniotomy in arteriovenous malformation surgery: the usefulness of cortical and subcortical mapping of language function in selected patients. World Neurosurg 2015;84(5):1394–401.

39. Villa F, Iacca C, Molinari AF, et al. Inhalation versus endovenous sedation in subarachnoid hemorrhage patients. Crit Care Med 2012;40(10):2797–804.
40. Lee JW, Woo JH, Baik HJ, et al. The effect of anesthetic agents on cerebral vasospasms after subarachnoid hemorrhage: a retrospective study. Medicine 2018;97(31):e11666.
41. Leblanc R. The minor leak preceding subarachnoid hemorrhage. J Neurosurg 1987;66(1):35–9.
42. Juvela S. Minor leak before rupture of an intracranial aneurysm and subarachnoid hemorrhage of unknown etiology. Neurosurgery 1992;30(1):7–11.
43. Hitchcock ER, Tsementzis SA, Dow AA. Short- and long-term prognosis of patients with a subarachnoid haemorrhage in relation to intra-operative period of hypotension. Acta Neurochir 1984;70(3–4):235–42.
44. Akkermans A, van Waes JA, Peelen LM, et al. Blood pressure and end-tidal carbon dioxide ranges during aneurysm occlusion and neurologic outcome after an aneurysmal subarachnoid hemorrhage. Anesthesiology 2019;130(1):92–105.
45. Basali A, Mascha EJ, Kalfas I, et al. Relation between perioperative hypertension and intracranial hemorrhage after craniotomy. Anesthesiology 2000;93(1):48–54.
46. Tang C, Zhang T-S, Zhou L-F. Risk factors for rebleeding of aneurysmal subarachnoid hemorrhage: a meta-analysis. PLoS One 2014;9(6):e99536.
47. Wijdicks EFM, Vermeulen M, Murray GD, et al. The effects of treating hypertension following aneurysmal subarachnoid hemorrhage. Clin Neurol Neurosurg 1990;92(2):111–7.
48. van Lieshout JJ, Secher NH. Point:counterpoint: sympathetic activity does/does not influence cerebral blood flow. Point: sympathetic activity does influence cerebral blood flow. J Appl Physiol (1985) 2008;105(4):1364–6.
49. Nissen P, Brassard P, Jørgensen TB, et al. Phenylephrine but not ephedrine reduces frontal lobe oxygenation following anesthesia-induced hypotension. Neurocrit Care 2010;12(1):17–23.
50. Koch KU, Mikkelsen IK, Aanerud J, et al. Ephedrine versus phenylephrine effect on cerebral blood flow and oxygen consumption in anesthetized brain tumor patients: a randomized clinical trial. Anesthesiology 2020;133(2):304–17.
51. Yoneda H, Nakamura T, Shirao S, et al. Multicenter prospective cohort study on volume management after subarachnoid hemorrhage. Stroke 2018;44(8):2155–61.
52. Watanabe A, Tagami T, Yokobori S, et al. Global end-diastolic volume is associated with the occurrence of delayed cerebral ischemia and pulmonary edema after subarachnoid hemorrhage. Shock 2012;38(5):480–5.
53. Hoff R, Rinkel G, Verweij B, et al. Blood volume measurement to guide fluid therapy after aneurysmal subarachnoid hemorrhage. Stroke 2009;40(7):2575–7.
54. Lennihan L, Mayer SA, Fink ME, et al. Effect of hypervolemic therapy on cerebral blood flow after subarachnoid hemorrhage : a randomized controlled trial. Stroke 2000;31(2):383–91.
55. Togashi K, Joffe AM, Sekhar L, et al. Randomized pilot trial of intensive management of blood pressure or volume expansion in subarachnoid hemorrhage (IMPROVES). Neurosurgery 2015;76(2):125–35.
56. Dankbaar JW, Slooter AJ, Rinkel GJ, et al. Effect of different components of triple-H therapy on cerebral perfusion in patients with aneurysmal subarachnoid haemorrhage: a systematic review. Crit Care 2010;14(1):R23.
57. Ekelund A, Reinstrup P, Ryding E, et al. Effects of Iso- and hypervolemic hemodilution on regional cerebral blood flow and oxygen delivery for patients with

vasospasm after aneurysmal subarachnoid hemorrhage. Acta Neurochir 2002; 144(7):703–13.

58. Gathier CS, Dankbaar JW, van der Jagt M, et al. Effects of induced hypertension on cerebral perfusion in delayed cerebral ischemia after aneurysmal subarachnoid hemorrhage. Stroke 2018;46(11):3277–81.

59. Mutoh T, Ishikawa T, Nishino K, et al. Evaluation of the FloTrac uncalibrated continuous cardiac output system for perioperative hemodynamic monitoring after subarachnoid hemorrhage. J Neurosurg Anesthesiol 2009;21(3):218–25.

60. Mutoh T, Kazumata K, Terasaka S, et al. Early intensive versus minimally invasive approach to postoperative hemodynamic management after subarachnoid hemorrhage. Stroke 2014;45(5):1280–4.

61. Kansha M, Irita K, Takahashi S, et al. Anesthetic management of children with Moyamoya disease. Clin Neurol Neurosurg 1997;99:S110–3.

62. Parray T, Martin TW, Siddiqui S. Moyamoya disease. J Neurosurg Anesthesiol 2011;23(2):100–9.

63. Morris NA, Chatterjee A, Adejumo OL, et al. The risk of takotsubo cardiomyopathy in acute neurological disease. Neurocrit Care 2019;30(1):171–6.

64. Abd TT, Hayek S, Cheng J, et al. Incidence and clinical characteristics of takotsubo cardiomyopathy post-aneurysmal subarachnoid hemorrhage. Int J Cardiol 2014;176(3):1362–4.

65. Lee VH, Connolly HM, Fulgham JR, et al. Tako-tsubo cardiomyopathy in aneurysmal subarachnoid hemorrhage: an underappreciated ventricular dysfunction. J Neurosurg 2006;105(2):264–70.

66. Richard C. Stress-related cardiomyopathies. Ann Intensive Care 2011;1(1):39.

67. Prasad A, Lerman A, Rihal CS. Apical ballooning syndrome (Tako-Tsubo or stress cardiomyopathy): a mimic of acute myocardial infarction. Am Heart J 2008; 155(3):408–17.

68. Bybee KA, Prasad A. Stress-related cardiomyopathy syndromes. Circulation 2008;118(4):397–409.

69. Inamasu J, Ganaha T, Nakae S, et al. Therapeutic outcomes for patients with aneurysmal subarachnoid hemorrhage complicated by Takotsubo cardiomyopathy. Acta Neurochir 2016;158(5):885–93.

70. Paré L, Delfino R, Leblanc R. The relationship of ventricular drainage to aneurysmal rebleeding. J Neurosurg 1992;76(3):422–7.

71. McIver JI, Friedman JA, Wijdicks EFM, et al. Preoperative ventriculostomy and rebleeding after aneurysmal subarachnoid hemorrhage. J Neurosurg 2002;97(5): 1042–4.

72. Hellingman CA, van den Bergh WM, Beijer IS, et al. Risk of rebleeding after treatment of acute hydrocephalus in patients with aneurysmal subarachnoid hemorrhage. Stroke 2007;38(1):96–9.

73. Curley G, Kavanagh BP, Laffey JG. Hypocapnia and the injured brain: more harm than benefit. Crit Care Med 2010;38(5):1348–59.

74. Williamson CA, Sheehan KM, Tipirneni R, et al. The association between spontaneous hyperventilation, delayed cerebral ischemia, and poor neurological outcome in patients with subarachnoid hemorrhage. Neurocrit Care 2015;23(3): 330–8.

75. Bakdash T, Cohen AR, Hempel JM, et al. Moyamoya, dystonia during hyperventilation, and antiphospholipid antibodies. Pediatr Neurol 2002;26(2):157–60.

76. Takeuchi S, Tanaka R, Ishii R, et al. Cerebral hemodynamics in patients with Moyamoya disease. A study of regional cerebral blood flow by the 133Xe inhalation method. Surg Neurol 1985;23(5):468–74.

77. Westermaier T, Stetter C, Kunze E, et al. Controlled hypercapnia enhances cerebral blood flow and brain tissue oxygenation after aneurysmal subarachnoid hemorrhage: results of a phase 1 study. Neurocrit Care 2016;25(2):205–14.

78. Panerai RB. The critical closing pressure of the cerebral circulation. Med Eng Phys 2003;25(8):621–32.

79. Wicks RT, Pradilla G, Raza SM, et al. Impact of changes in intraoperative somatosensory evoked potentials on stroke rates after clipping of intracranial aneurysms. Neurosurgery 2012;70(5):1114–24.

80. Nwachuku EL, Balzer JR, Yabes JG, et al. Diagnostic value of somatosensory evoked potential changes during carotid endarterectomy: a systematic review and meta-analysis. JAMA Neurol 2015;72(1):73–80.

81. Greve T, Stoecklein VM, Dorn F, et al. Introduction of intraoperative neuromonitoring does not necessarily improve overall long-term outcome in elective aneurysm clipping. J Neurosurg 2019;132(4):1–9.

82. Adembri C, Venturi L, Pellegrini-Giampietro DE. Neuroprotective effects of propofol in acute cerebral injury. CNS Drug Rev 2007;13(3):333–51.

83. Arrich J, Holzer M, Havel C, et al. Hypothermia for neuroprotection in adults after cardiopulmonary resuscitation. Cochrane Database Syst Rev 2016;(2). https://doi.org/10.1002/14651858.cd004128.pub4.

84. Todd MM, Hindman BJ, Clarke WR, et al, Investigators IH for AST (IHAST). Mild intraoperative hypothermia during surgery for intracranial aneurysm. N Engl J Med 2005;352(2):135–45.

85. Cooper DJ, Nichol AD, Bailey M, et al. Effect of early sustained prophylactic hypothermia on neurologic outcomes among patients with severe traumatic brain injury. JAMA 2018;320(21):2211.

86. Foy PM, Copeland GP, Shaw MDM. The incidence of postoperative seizures. Acta Neurochir 1981;55(3–4):253–64.

87. Shaw MDM, Foy PM. Epilepsy after craniotomy and the place of prophylactic anticonvulsant drugs: discussion paper. J R Soc Med 1990;84(4):221–3.

88. Jos MAK, Onno PMT, Alphons GHK, et al. Effectiveness of antiepileptic prophylaxis used with supratentorial craniotomies: a meta-analysis. Seizure 1996;5(4):291–8.

89. Rosengart AJ, Huo D, Tolentino J, et al. Outcome in patients with subarachnoid hemorrhage treated with antiepileptic drugs. J Neurosurg 2007;107(2):253–60.

90. Katayama Y, Haraoka J, Hirabayashi H, et al. A randomized controlled trial of hydrocortisone against hyponatremia in patients with aneurysmal subarachnoid hemorrhage. Stroke 2007;38(8):2373–5.

91. Hashi K, Takakura K, Sano K, et al. Intravenous hydrocortisone in large doses in the treatment of delayed ischemic neurological deficits following subarachnoid hemorrhage–results of a multi-center controlled double-blind clinical study. No To Shinkei 1988;40(4):373–82 [in Japanese].

92. Mori T, Katayama Y, Kawamata T, et al. Improved efficiency of hypervolemic therapy with inhibition of natriuresis by fludrocortisone in patients with aneurysmal subarachnoid hemorrhage. J Neurosurg 1999;91(6):947–52.

93. Hasan D, Lindsay KW, Wijdicks EF, et al. Effect of fludrocortisone acetate in patients with subarachnoid hemorrhage. Stroke 1989;20(9):1156–61.

94. Roos YBWEM, Rinkel GJ, Vermeulen M, et al. Antifibrinolytic therapy for aneurysmal subarachnoid haemorrhage. Cochrane Database Syst Rev 2003;(2). https://doi.org/10.1002/14651858.cd001245.

95. Hillman J, Fridriksson S, Nilsson O, et al. Immediate administration of tranexamic acid and reduced incidence of early rebleeding after aneurysmal subarachnoid hemorrhage: a prospective randomized study. J Neurosurg 2002;97(4):771–8.
96. Leipzig TJ, Redelman K, Horner TG. Reducing the risk of rebleeding before early aneurysm surgery: a possible role for antifibrinolytic therapy. J Neurosurg 1997; 86(2):220–5.

Perioperative and Anesthetic Considerations for Patients with Degenerative Spine Disease

Basma A. Mohamed, MBChB, Brenda G. Fahy, MD, MCCM*

KEYWORDS

- Enhanced recovery after surgery • Anesthesia management for spine surgery
- Degenerative spine disease • Adult spine deformity
- Postoperative complications for spine surgery • Low back pain

KEY POINTS

- Perioperative management of patients undergoing spine surgery focuses on enhanced recovery after surgery through optimization of all phases of care.
- Preoperative evaluation of patients undergoing spine surgery includes a multisystem approach with an emphasis on the impact of the spine disorder on cardiopulmonary function, pain, and psychosocial aspects.
- Airway management planning is critical for patients with cervical spine disease.
- Perioperative hemodynamic goals and planning should be dedicated to optimizing volume status and using goal-directed fluid therapy and blood transfusion management.
- Perioperative care includes early identification of risk factors for postoperative complications and appropriate measures to reduce risk and prevent further complications.

INTRODUCTION

Degenerative spine disease, a common and debilitating disease, causes pain and disability, and it increases health care costs. In North America, low back pain prevalence from degenerative spine disease is ~4.5%,[1] and the number of spine surgeries performed has been dramatically increasing over the last 2 decades. This increase in prevalence is caused by an aging population and advances in surgical techniques, including minimally invasive procedures. The advancement in surgical and anesthetic techniques allows patients with multiple comorbidities and complicated spine disorders to be surgical candidates and further increases demand.[2]

Department of Anesthesiology, University of Florida College of Medicine, 1600 Southwest Archer Road, PO Box 100254, Gainesville, FL 32610, USA
* Corresponding author.
E-mail address: bfahy@anest.ufl.edu

Anesthesiology Clin 39 (2021) 19–35
https://doi.org/10.1016/j.anclin.2020.11.005
1932-2275/21/© 2020 Elsevier Inc. All rights reserved.

anesthesiology.theclinics.com

The prevalence of surgically treated degenerative cervical spine disease with myelopathy is ~1.6 per 100,000[3]; however, the actual prevalence is likely higher because of difficulty with diagnosis, and it is expected to increase as the population ages. Degenerative cervical changes with aging include disc herniation, ligament hypertrophy, ligament ossification, and osteophyte formation.[4] These changes cause neurologic symptoms and deficits, requiring surgery to be urgent. As a result, providers have less time to optimize patient comorbidities.

The chronic nature of degenerative spine disease and the need for conservative treatment before proceeding with surgery result in patients with chronic pain, opioid dependence, and sometimes poor functional status. In addition, the prevalence of degenerative spine disease in members of the geriatric population, who often have complex morbidity profiles, poses several challenges for anesthesiologists. Complex patients require a comprehensive perioperative management plan to address the effects of aging, the associated and possibly poorly treated comorbidities, the complexity of spine surgery, and the potential for perioperative surgical and medical complications to provide safe perioperative care. The introduction of enhanced recovery after surgery (ERAS) clinical pathways for spine surgery has been attractive to surgeons and perioperative management teams in different institutions. Early studies have shown that ERAS protocols enable faster recovery, increase patient satisfaction, decrease hospital length of stay, and reduce overall health care expenditure.[5,6] This article describes the perioperative anesthetic considerations for patients undergoing surgery for degenerative spine disease and adult spine deformity.

PREOPERATIVE EVALUATION AND MANAGEMENT OF SPINE SURGERY PATIENTS

Preoperative evaluation of patients undergoing spine surgery should focus on spinal disorder, surgical planning, and implications of the associated comorbidities. In addition to a standard preoperative anesthesia evaluation, which includes a detailed history and physical examination, evaluation and optimization of comorbidities, appropriate tests, and imaging, the anesthesiologist should focus on the impact of the spine disorder on the overall health status of the patient. This focus entails a clear understanding of the underlying spine disease, duration of symptoms, and impact on multiple organ systems to optimize possible comorbidities. This preoperative evaluation should focus on airway, cardiopulmonary, and preoperative pain/psychological evaluations.

Airway Evaluation

Airway examinations deserve special attention for patients undergoing spine surgery, especially for patients with cervical degenerative spine disease, to plan appropriate airway management. In addition to standard airway evaluation, further evaluation should be dedicated to cervical spine disorder. **Box 1** details preoperative airway evaluation of nontraumatic cervical spine disease.

Cardiopulmonary Evaluation

A preoperative cardiac evaluation, risk stratification, and medication management based on the 2014 and 2016 American College of Cardiology and American Heart Association guidelines for cardiac evaluation should be performed before noncardiac surgery.[7,8] In addition, preoperative cardiac evaluation for patients undergoing spine surgery should focus on functional capacity, antiplatelet and anticoagulation management, and possible cor pulmonale and right ventricular dysfunction resulting from thoracolumbar spine deformity (**Box 2**). Preoperative pulmonary evaluation should focus

---

Box 1
Preoperative considerations for airway evaluation for cervical spine disease

- Impaired extension of the craniocervical junction
  - Reduced mouth opening and difficulty with mandibular protrusion (prognathism)

- The presence or absence of Lhermitte sign
  - Produced by flexion and extension of the neck causing an electrical sensation that runs down the back into the upper extremities from posterior column involvement
  - Suggests spinal cord compression caused by cervical spine disorder
  - Alerts the anesthesiologist to maintain neutral head position during intubation

- Evaluation for myelopathy or spinal canal stenosis

- Evaluation of coexisting diseases that can affect airway management
  - Rheumatoid arthritis and Down syndrome with atlantoaxial instability (AAI)
  - Evaluation of cervical radiographic images to assess for AAI in the rheumatoid arthritis population

Data from Fleisher LA, Fleischmann KE, Auerbach AD, et al. 2014 ACC/AHA guideline on perioperative cardiovascular evaluation and management of patients undergoing noncardiac surgery: a report of the American College of Cardiology/American Heart Association Task Force on practice guidelines. J Am Coll Cardiol. 2014;64:e77–137; with permission.

Box 2
Preoperative cardiac considerations specific to spine surgery patients

Instructions on preoperative antiplatelet therapy
1. Safe to continue aspirin for patients with coronary artery disease or stroke
2. Discontinue clopidogrel or prasugrel per the American College of Cardiology/American Heart Association recommendations

Instructions for preoperative anticoagulation therapy
1. Discontinue direct oral anticoagulants 72 hours before surgery
2. Discontinue warfarin 5 to 7 days before surgery
3. Bridge using parenteral anticoagulation if high risk for thromboembolism

Evaluate for cor pulmonale and right ventricular dysfunction
1. High-risk patients have thoracolumbar adult spine deformity
2. Preliminary evaluation of pulmonary hypertension (transthoracic echocardiography)
3. Further evaluation by pulmonary hypertension specialized center

Evaluate functional capacity
1. Underestimated by patients because of spine disorder and debilitating pain
2. Duke Activity Status Index for metabolic equivalents

Data from Levine GN, Bates ER, Bittl JA, et al. 2016 ACC/AHA Guideline Focused Update on Duration of Dual Antiplatelet Therapy in Patients With Coronary Artery Disease: A Report of the American College of Cardiology/American Heart Association Task Force on Clinical Practice Guidelines: An Update of the 2011 ACCF/AHA/SCAI Guideline for Percutaneous Coronary Intervention, 2011 ACCF/AHA Guideline for Coronary Artery Bypass Graft Surgery, 2012 ACC/AHA/ACP/AATS/PCNA/SCAI/STS Guideline for the Diagnosis and Management of Patients With Stable Ischemic Heart Disease, 2013 ACCF/AHA Guideline for the Management of ST-Elevation Myocardial Infarction, 2014 AHA/ACC Guideline for the Management of Patients With Non-ST-Elevation Acute Coronary Syndromes, and 2014 ACC/AHA Guideline on Perioperative Cardiovascular Evaluation and Management of Patients Undergoing Noncardiac Surgery. Circulation. 2016;134:e123–55; with permission.

on optimization of coexisting pulmonary disease, identification of patient-related risk factors for postoperative pulmonary complications, and evaluation of patients with adult spine deformity, which might result in restrictive lung disease and associated complications (**Box 3**). At present, no recommendations for routine preoperative pulmonary function tests or chest imaging exist, necessitating that providers obtain appropriate tests based on the suspicion of any underlying lung disease.

Preoperative Pain and Psychological Evaluation

Patients presenting for spine surgery often experience pain and psychological symptoms related to clinical impairment and poor quality of life after conservative management fails to alleviate pain. Patients with chronic, disabling pain may experience anxiety, depression, catastrophizing, and kinesophobia, which can be predictors of poor patient outcomes.[9–12] Patients scheduled for spine surgery benefit from a preoperative evaluation focusing on preoperative psychological factors with possible interventions (**Box 4**).

At present, ERAS protocols in spine surgery focus on the implementation of physical prehabilitation, pain and neuroscience education, cognitive behavior therapy, and cognitive prehabilitation for brain health.[13–15] Additional preoperative considerations for patients undergoing spine surgery should focus on the evaluation of the geriatric population, neurologic and musculoskeletal evaluation, in addition to nutrition and diabetes management (**Box 5**).[16]

INTRAOPERATIVE MANAGEMENT OF SPINE SURGERY PATIENTS
Anesthetic Technique

Anesthetic management for spine surgery focuses on multiple aspects, including the choice of the anesthetic technique (general vs regional anesthesia), with medications

---

Box 3
Preoperative pulmonary evaluation for spine surgery patients

Optimization of coexisting pulmonary disease
1. Perform detailed history and pulmonary examination
2. Evaluate functional capacity to rule out lung disease
3. Evaluate pulmonary symptoms of coexisting connective tissue disease
4. Perform pulmonary diagnostic imaging, if indicated
5. Perform pulmonary function tests, if indicated
6. Treat exacerbation of coexisting lung disease
7. Consult with the pulmonologist if optimization required

Patient risk factors for postoperative pulmonary complications
1. Old age
2. Chronic obstructive pulmonary disease
3. Congestive heart failure
4. Obstructive sleep apnea
5. American Society of Anesthesiologists physical status greater than II
6. Smoking
7. Upper respiratory infection

Evaluation of pulmonary disease in adult patients with spine deformity (kyphosis or kyphoscoliosis)
1. Restrictive lung disease on pulmonary function test
2. Transthoracic echocardiography for evaluation of pulmonary hypertension and cor pulmonale
3. Referral to pulmonology for further evaluation and management

---

Box 4
Preoperative pain and psychological evaluation for spine surgery patients

Anxiety and depression and degree of symptom control

Degree of catastrophizing and kinesophobia
• This finding affects patient rehabilitation potential after surgery

Evaluation for risk of postoperative cognitive dysfunction or delirium

Current pain management plan
• Multimodal pain medications
• Prior pain intervention
• Is the pain controlled?

Social support system
• Discharge planning
• Rehabilitation potential in the postoperative setting

---

based on intraoperative neuromonitoring (IONM) requirements. General anesthesia is the most common technique for spine surgery. Regional anesthesia is used for select patients undergoing lumbar spine surgery. Risk factors for intraoperative blood loss include spine deformity or spine tumor surgeries and surgery involving 6 or more levels of fusion, thus requiring large-bore intravenous access and/or placement of central venous access for fluid resuscitation and potential use of vasopressors.

For general anesthesia, IONM influences the choice of volatile anesthetic versus total intravenous anesthesia (**Box 6**). Common agents used for total intravenous anesthesia are propofol, ketamine, remifentanil, and sufentanil. Other adjuncts include dexmedetomidine and lidocaine infusions. Volatile anesthetics should be avoided when transcranial motor evoked potential is required because of their significant effect on the amplitude of evoked potentials.[17] Neuromuscular blocking agents are usually required during the early stage of surgery (incision and exposure). Their continuation may not be feasible when motor evoked potentials and electromyography are used for IONM.

Box 5
General preoperative considerations specific to spine surgery patients

Preoperative geriatric evaluation
1. Assessment of functional capacity and frailty
2. Mini-Cog cognitive assessment
3. Address polypharmacy
4. Assessment of multiple comorbidities

Neurologic evaluation
1. Preexisting neurologic deficits to guide intraoperative neuromonitoring and postoperative expectation
2. Neurologic deficits caused by cervical spine disease to guide airway management

Musculoskeletal evaluation
1. Joint stiffness and range of motion for appropriate positioning
2. Patients with connective tissue disease need multisystem evaluation (rule out kidney disease)
3. Perioperative management of immunosuppressive medications

Nutrition and diabetes
1. Diabetes control: evaluation of hemoglobin A1c
2. Malnutrition: prealbumin, albumin, and lymphocyte count
3. Osteoporosis: appropriate treatment

Box 6
Anesthetic considerations for optimization of intraoperative neuromonitoring

Somatosensory evoked potential (SSEP)
1. Inhalational anesthetic technique is acceptable.
2. Neuromuscular blockade (NMB) does not affect SSEP.
3. It is usually used for adult spine deformity or degenerative spine disease surgery (eg, thoracolumbar and cervical surgeries).
4. It is not commonly used for isolated lumbar spine surgery.

Motor evoked potential
1. It is best if volatile anesthesia is avoided.
2. Total intravenous anesthesia is the anesthetic technique of choice.
3. Optimize blood pressure for myelopathy and thoracic deformity surgery to optimize evoked potential.
4. NMB should be avoided. It can be used for airway and positioning then reversed.

Electromyography
1. It is used in lumbar spine surgery (transforaminal lumbar interbody fusion, extreme lateral interbody fusion).
2. Avoid NMB.

General considerations
1. Blood pressure goals are within 10% to 20% of baseline. May augment if evoked potential is symmetrically abnormal.
2. Avoid boluses of anesthetics. Address hypertension using vasodilators not anesthetics.
3. Balance total intravenous anesthesia using low-dose propofol, opioid infusion, and ketamine as an adjunct at a subanesthetic dose.
4. Avoid acidosis and hypothermia.

Regional anesthesia for selective patients undergoing lumbar spine surgery requires the patient, surgeon, and anesthesiologist to agree on the anesthetic technique. The patient must tolerate prone positioning without respiratory or airway compromise. In a systematic review and meta-analysis of spinal anesthesia compared with general anesthesia for lumbar spine surgery, Zorrilla-Vaca and collegaues[18] analyzed 15 trials involving 961 patients and showed that spinal anesthesia was superior to general anesthesia in preventing postoperative nausea and vomiting and decreasing length of hospital stay and blood loss.

Airway Management

Patients undergoing elective cervical spine surgery for degenerative spine disease should undergo careful airway evaluation (see **Box 1**). Many patients undergoing elective spine surgery have a stable spine alignment, but in-line stabilization and minimizing extreme range of cervical motion is recommended. In contrast, patients with rheumatoid arthritis presenting with atlantoaxial instability may pose a challenge for anesthesiologists, and a careful airway management plan, including a backup plan, should be established before induction of anesthesia. Many patients scheduled for lumbar or thoracolumbar spine surgery have similar cervical spine disorders. **Fig. 1** suggests an algorithmic approach for airway management in patients with cervical spine disease that can be adapted for specific patients.

Positioning

The most common position for spine surgery is prone. Goals of prone positioning include facilitating surgical exposure while preventing position-related complications (eg, postoperative visual loss, increased blood loss, peripheral nerve injury). Prone

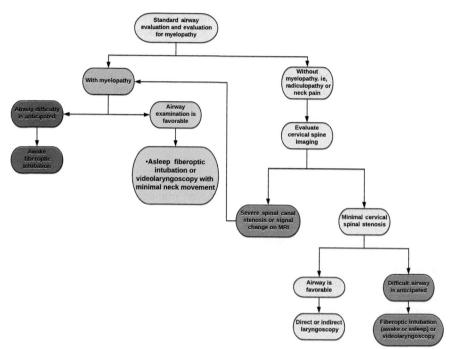

Fig. 1. A suggested algorithm for airway management for patients with cervical spine disease with decisions for individual patients based on professional medical judgment.

positioning is usually accomplished using a specialized surgical table (eg, Jackson spinal table); a prone frame (eg, Wilson frame); or padding, including gel pads, a chest roll, and prone headrest. This position avoids abdominal compression and inferior vena cava compression, which may increase blood loss and compromise ventilation, mainly in obese patients. It also avoids excessive thoracic compression and increased intrathoracic pressure, which may increase airway pressures and decrease cardiac output (CO). Additional goals of prone positioning include ensuring adequate support for the head and face to avoid ocular compression and providing adequate extremity positioning, including padding and maintaining neutral arm and leg positions to avoid peripheral nerve injury. Prone positioning also maintains adequate pressure-point padding, mainly for prolonged procedures,[19] and avoids hyperextension and hyperflexion in the head position, which may compromise venous drainage, or extreme rotation of the cervical spine. Either a gel foam pad or a Mayfield head holder can be used for the posterior surgical approach. Ensure 2 fingerbreadths in the space between the angle of the mandible and suprasternal notch.

Supine positioning is used for an anterior approach for cervical (anterior cervical decompression and fusion) and lumbar spine (anterior interbody lumbar fusion) surgery. In addition to simple supine positioning, surgeons use traction of the head to distract the cervical spine to allow placement of the bone graft, decompression, and fusion.

Demand for minimally invasive procedures led to the introduction of the extreme lateral interbody fusion procedure, which requires lateral positioning. Positioning goals include confirming the 90° position of the patient using radiographs. The table and the patient should be flexed to increase the distance between the iliac crest and the rib cage.[20] Lateral decubitus can also be used for an anterior approach of the upper thoracic spine and retroperitoneal approach of the thoracolumbar junction. Special considerations for lateral decubitus include positioning the dependent arm to prevent brachial plexus injury or vascular compression. An axillary roll is recommended. In addition, the nondependent arm should usually be positioned outstretched in front of the patient and supported on a pillow or padded armrest. Head positioning requires a neutral cervical spine and padded headrest to prevent obstruction to the endotracheal tube and/or cerebral venous drainage.

Monitoring

Intraoperative monitoring during spine surgery focuses on hemodynamic monitoring and goal-directed fluid therapy, blood transfusion management, and IONM. Anesthetic considerations are required for optimization of IONM (see **Box 6**).

Hemodynamic monitoring and goal-directed fluid therapy

The choice of invasive hemodynamic monitoring with an arterial line is determined by the procedure and patient comorbidities. Procedures where an arterial line is useful include a prolonged procedure (ie, >4 hours) or when the anesthesiologist anticipates increased blood loss/large fluid shifts; a spine disorder associated with neurologic deficits (eg, myelopathy); and anticipated spinal cord compromise requiring close blood pressure monitoring to maintain spinal perfusion pressure (eg, thoracolumbar spine deformity surgery, cervical spine deformity, or severe spinal canal stenosis). Patient-related factors include coexisting severe cardiac disease, severe pulmonary comorbidity or the need for lung isolation, and severe renal disease. The threshold for arterial line placement should be low given anticipated hemodynamic instability caused by prone positioning or excessive blood loss and the expected frequent laboratory testing to guide fluid/blood transfusion management.

Minimally invasive CO monitors using arterial waveform pulse contour analysis (pulse pressure variation [PPV] or stroke volume variation [SVV]) or transesophageal Doppler are widely used for spine surgery. Indications include guiding fluid therapy and choice of vasopressors, inotropes, or volume resuscitation to optimize hemodynamic instability and monitoring CO for patients with severe cardiac comorbidities. Minimally invasive CO monitors introduced the concept of goal-directed fluid therapy as part of ERAS protocols. Small trials and observational studies have shown that goal-directed fluid therapy is associated with a shorter length of stay, earlier resumption of bowel activity, and improved postoperative respiratory performance.[21]

Despite the expected changes that occur with SVV and PPV in the prone position, following the trend of these parameters can predict fluid responsiveness in that position. PPV and SVV can also guide fluid therapy and volume responsiveness so that patients adequately receive volume resuscitation while avoiding unnecessary volume overload, which may cause bowel edema, pulmonary congestion, and airway and facial edema. Intraoperative goal-directed fluid therapy guided by PPV or SVV may minimize the need for continued postoperative fluid resuscitation or postoperative vasopressors and prevent unnecessary use of vasopressors in the postoperative period.[22]

Regarding choice of fluids, there are no consensus guidelines or evidence to support the use of colloids versus crystalloids. However, Ramchandran and colleagues[23] found in a propensity score–matched analysis that administration of crystalloid to colloid in a ratio more than 3:1 was independently associated with delayed extubation in patients who underwent multilevel thoracic or lumbar spine fusion. A lower ratio of colloid administration was also considered a risk factor for postoperative visual loss.[24,25]

Monitoring for venous air embolism is an additional consideration. Case reports of cardiac arrest in the prone position for spine surgery have shown that venous air embolism is the most common cause.

Perioperative blood transfusion management

Complex spine surgery often requires transfusion of blood products for increased blood loss and dilutional coagulopathy. This finding is common in procedures that include multilevel spine fusion, adult spine deformity surgery (eg, scoliosis correction), and revision surgeries. Studies have shown an association between transfusion and increased morbidity, mortality, length of hospital stay, and health care expenditure.[26,27] The anesthesiologist should discuss different modalities to minimize blood loss and blood transfusion requirements with the surgical team.

Preoperative measures include following antiplatelet and anticoagulant recommendations (see **Box 2**). Preoperative anemia evaluation and management should follow the current recommendations for perioperative blood management by the American Society of Anesthesiologists (ASA)[28] and Network for Advancement of Transfusion Alternatives.[29]

Intraoperative measures include the use of antifibrinolytic agents: tranexamic acid (TXA) and aminocaproic acid. In a systematic review of 18 randomized and 18 non-randomized controlled trials including 2572 patients comparing TXA versus placebo, TXA was effective in reducing intraoperative and postoperative blood loss and transfusion rate.[30] The patient population included adult spine deformity, cervical decompression and fusion, and adolescent idiopathic scoliosis surgeries. Another systematic review and meta-analysis evaluating topical TXA use during spine surgery found that TXA was effective in decreasing total blood loss and drainage volume without increasing the risks of deep vein thrombosis (DVT), pulmonary embolism, or hematoma formation.[31] TXA dosing involves 15 mg/kg on incision and repeating every 3 hours.[32] Recent meta-analyses have found that antifibrinolytics decrease intraoperative, postoperative, and total blood loss during spine surgery.[33–35] The evidence for aminocaproic acid is less convincing. A meta-analysis of 293 patients from 4 randomized controlled trials (RCTs) showed that aminocaproic acid reduced the rate of blood transfusion but not the total blood loss or blood transfusion amount.[34]

Another intraoperative consideration is cell salvage. Studies evaluating the use of cell salvage during adult spine deformity surgery have shown decreased total blood transfusion. The costs of setting up a cell salvage unit is equivalent to 2 units of blood transfusion; thus, cell salvage should be dedicated to patients with expected blood loss of 500 to 600 mL.[2,32]

There is some controversy regarding the impact of preoperative autologous blood donation on the reduction of allogenic transfusion, with most studies showing a mild reduction in the rate of transfusion. Per the ASA recommendations on blood management, if autologous blood donation is recommended by the perioperative team, the patient should be offered this option only if there is enough time for erythropoietic reconstitution.[28]

Furthermore, patient positioning is important intraoperatively. Inadequate prone positioning whether via a frame or table can cause increases in intra-abdominal pressure, intrathoracic pressure, and venous pressure to the inferior vena cava and epidural veins, leading to increased surgical bleeding in spine surgery. Evidence suggests superior outcomes for the Jackson spinal table because of its ability to reduce intra-abdominal pressure, thus reducing intraoperative blood loss.[36,37]

Perioperative Pain Management

Recently, there has been growing interest in multimodal analgesia in spine surgery patients, mostly as part of an ERAS protocol to minimize opioid use. That method avoids potential long-term opioid-related complications such as ileus, respiratory depression, and chronic opioid dependence. As a result, multiple pharmacologic agents have been introduced as part of a multimodal analgesia pathway for spine surgery.

Multimodal analgesia

Several studies have shown that nonsteroidal antiinflammatory drugs (NSAIDs) could effectively reduce postoperative pain and opioid consumption in spine surgeries. A meta-analysis of 408 patients from 8 studies showed a reduction of the visual analog scale (VAS) score at 24 hours.[38] Bone nonunion and bleeding are among the primary concerns of using NSAIDs in spine surgery. In a systematic review including 12,895 orthopedic and spine surgery patients, the data were conflicting on the nonunion risk of NSAIDs.[39] Overall, although the current evidence suggests that NSAIDs are an effective analgesic after spine surgery, NSAIDs should be used with caution mainly for spine fusion surgery; high doses and prolonged use should be avoided.[2] Acetaminophen's effectiveness on pain score and opioid consumption in the first 24 hours postoperatively is controversial. Two small RCTs showed a statistically significant reduction in VAS scores, but they found no reduction in opioid consumption in the first 24 postoperative hours.[40,41] The use of preoperative oral gabapentin is receiving attention as part of a multimodal pain management regimen. In 2 meta-analyses of RCTs involving patients undergoing spine surgery, gabapentin was effective in reducing pain scores and postoperative opioid consumption. Per the meta-analysis, there was no difference between the groups in side effects (dizziness, somnolence, or sedation).[42,43]

Ketamine and methadone

Ketamine has been reported to reduce postoperative opioid consumption. In a meta-analysis of 14 RCTs consisting of 649 patients, Pendi and colleagues[44] found that perioperative ketamine as an adjunct pain medication reduced postoperative opioid requirements up to 24 hours after spine surgery. The ASA consensus guidelines recommend intravenous ketamine for invasive painful procedures including spine surgery (eg, scoliosis). Moderate evidence supports using subanesthetic intravenous doses up to 0.35 mg/kg followed by an infusion of up to 1 mg/kg as adjuncts for perioperative pain management.[45]

Methadone is an alternative opioid with a long half-life. When used as a single intraoperative dose, it provides stable blood concentration, avoiding fluctuations associated with repeated injections of other long-acting opioids (eg, morphine, hydromorphone). Methadone has multiple advantages for patients undergoing spine surgery. In small doses (5–10 mg), it acts like a shorter-acting opioid, lasting 3 to 4 hours. When 20 mg or more is given, it has a longer effect similar to its elimination half-life (35 hours). Methadone activates NMDA (N-methyl-D-aspartate) receptors and inhibits reuptake of serotonin and norepinephrine, which can contribute to improved postoperative mood. Trials evaluating methadone doses of 0.2 mg/kg on postoperative pain control and postoperative opioid consumption have revealed a reduction in opioid requirements by greater than 50%, lower pain score, and higher overall satisfaction compared with other opioids (eg, sufentanil or hydromorphone).[46–48] Dunn and colleagues[49] found that intraoperative methadone was associated with an increased risk of postoperative respiratory depression and recommended observation in an appropriate postoperative setting.

Systemic lidocaine

An RCT studying the effects of systemic lidocaine versus placebo for lumbar discec-tomy, a minimally invasive procedure,[50] showed reductions in postoperative pain scores and fentanyl patient-controlled anesthesia (PCA) dosing up to 48 hours post-operatively. Another RCT of 116 complex spine surgery patients[51] found reductions in pain scores and morphine PCA doses with systemic lidocaine compared with the placebo but no difference in postoperative 30-day complication rates. Notably, sys-temic lidocaine was the only intraoperative analgesic medication in this trial. Another trial, by Dewinter and colleagues,[52] showed that lidocaine failed to add postoperative analgesic benefits when combined with opioid-based anesthetic technique. The use of systemic lidocaine as a perioperative analgesia adjunct for spine surgery requires further investigation.

Local anesthesia

Although not commonly used in practice, the effect of epidural analgesia compared with intravenous PCA following spine surgery was evaluated in a meta-analysis of 17 RCTs including 938 patients. The analysis showed that epidural analgesia reduced postoperative pain scores and opioid consumption. A disadvantage was the epidural impact on motor functions affecting neurologic examinations.[53] Lipo-somal bupivacaine for subcutaneous infiltration after spinal decompression did not reduce pain scores or postoperative opioid consumption compared with bupi-vacaine hydrochloride.[54] However, a meta-analysis of 11 studies including 438 pa-tients using intramuscular local anesthetic infiltration during closure for lumbar spine surgery showed reduced postoperative analgesic requirements and a longer time to first analgesic requests.[55] The erector spinae block for patients undergoing spine surgery has been reported only in case reports involving lumbar spine fusion and scoliosis surgery. In these case reports, the investigators used opioid-free anesthesia.[56–58]

POSTOPERATIVE MANAGEMENT OF SPINE SURGERY PATIENTS

ERAS represents a perioperative, multidisciplinary, evidence-based care approach to decrease postoperative complications, length of hospital stay, and readmission rate and improve functional recovery. In a systematic review, Dietz and col-leagues[59] analyzed 19 studies reporting that ERAS improved pain scores and decreased postoperative opioid consumption without influencing complications or readmission rates. However, it decreased direct, indirect, and total costs. ERAS protocol implementation in postoperative care focuses on early mobilization and physical therapy, adequate postoperative multimodal pain management to minimize opioid side effects, early nutrition and bowel regimen to prevent ileus, and preemptive strategies in high-risk patients (eg, ambulation and DVT prophy-laxis to prevent DVT and pulmonary embolism, avoidance of a urinary catheter to decrease the incidence of urinary tract infections, prophylactic antibiotics to pre-vent surgical site infection).[60–62]

Multimodal analgesia started preoperatively continues intraoperatively using keta-mine and local anesthesia infiltration as opioid adjuncts. The postoperative focus in-cludes acetaminophen, NSAIDs in certain populations, and gabapentinoids, in addition to oral/intravenous opioids. The anesthesiologist as a perioperative consul-tant should evaluate each patient for the potential risk of postoperative complications (**Box 7**). Early identification of risk factors guides the team to discuss prevention methods.

Box 7
Postoperative complications after spine surgery

Venous thromboembolism
1. There are no consensus guidelines recommending the routine use of chemical prophylaxis.
2. The benefits of chemical thromboprophylaxis outweigh the risk of bleeding.

Postoperative pulmonary complications (PPCs)
1. The PPC rate after lumbar spine was reported as 5.7%.
2. PPC include lung collapse, atelectasis, and pneumonia.
3. Risk factors are chronic obstructive pulmonary disease, smoking, and diabetes.

Postoperative ileus
1. The incidence ranges from 2.6% to 8.4%.
2. Risk factors include male gender, anterior surgical approach, more than 9 levels of fusion, electrolyte disorders, and pathologic weight loss.
3. Impact: it increases length of stay and health care costs.

Delirium
1. The incidence ranges from 3.3% to 77%.
2. Risk factors include age greater than 65 years, female gender, polypharmacy, abnormal laboratory tests (low albumin level, low hemoglobin level, and low hematocrit), surgery duration, intraoperative blood loss, postoperative fever, functional impairment, and sleep disorders.

Postoperative visual loss
1. The incidence is 1.9 per 10,000 in a report by Nandyala and colleagues.[63]
2. Prevention:
   - Optimization of patient's hemodynamic status
   - Adequate volume resuscitation
   - Maintaining high normal blood pressure for hypertensive patients
   - Invasive monitoring of blood pressure in high-risk patients
   - Use of vasopressors as indicated on a case-by-case basis
   - Avoid extreme neck flexion or extension

Data from Nandyala SV, Marquez-Lara A, Fineberg SJ, et al. Incidence and risk factors for perioperative visual loss after spinal fusion. Spine. 2014;14:1866-72.

SUMMARY

As the population ages and surgical and anesthetic techniques advance, the demand for surgery for degenerative spine disease will continue to increase and the complexity of patient comorbidities will continue to pose challenges to anesthesiologists and perioperative teams. The perioperative outcomes in the form of decreases in the complication rate, 30-day readmission rate, and total health care expenditure have guided the perioperative care plan to focus on ERAS. Many institutions have adopted different pathways of the ERAS protocol, which involves preoperative risk stratification and optimization, intraoperative measures to enhance patient recovery, and postoperative measures to prevent further complications and optimize potential patient rehabilitation after hospital discharge. The anesthesiologist's role in the perioperative care of patients undergoing spine surgery is expanding beyond the intraoperative phase of care; currently, a multidisciplinary approach involving medicine consultants, nursing, and physical therapy in addition to the surgical and anesthesiology team is the optimal plan for patient care.

DISCLOSURE

The authors have no sources of funding or conflicts of interest to declare.

CLINICS CARE POINTS

- The chronic nature of degenerative spine disease and the need for conservative treatment before proceeding with surgery result in patients with chronic pain, opioid dependence, and sometimes poor functional status.
- Airway examinations deserve special attention for patients undergoing spine surgery, especially for patients with cervical degenerative spine disease, to plan appropriate airway management.
- Patients with chronic, disabling pain may experience anxiety, depression, catastrophizing, and kinesophobia, which can be predictors of poor patient outcomes.
- For general anesthesia, intraoperative neuromonitoring (IONM) influences the choice of volatile anesthetic versus total intravenous anesthesia.
- Regional anesthesia for selective patients undergoing lumbar spine surgery requires the patient, surgeon, and anesthesiologist to agree on the anesthetic technique.
- The most common position for spine surgery is prone. Goals of prone positioning include facilitating surgical exposure while preventing positioning-related complications (e.g., postoperative visual loss, increased blood loss, peripheral nerve injury).
- Intraoperative monitoring during spine surgery focuses on hemodynamic monitoring and goal-directed fluid therapy, blood transfusion management, and IONM.
- Studies have shown an association between transfusion and increased morbidity, mortality, length of hospital stay, and healthcare expenditure.
- Recently, there has been growing interest in multimodal analgesia in spine surgery patients, mostly as part of an ERAS protocol to minimize opioid use.
- ERAS represents a perioperative, multidisciplinary, evidence-based care approach to decrease postoperative complications, length of hospital stay, and readmission rate and improve functional recovery.
- The anesthesiologist's role in the perioperative care of patients undergoing spine surgery is expanding beyond the intraoperative phase of care; currently, a multidisciplinary approach involving medicine consultants, nursing, and physical therapy in addition to the surgical and anesthesiology team is the optimal plan for patient care.

REFERENCES

1. Ravindra VM, Senglaub SS, Rattani A, et al. Degenerative lumbar spine disease: estimating global incidence and worldwide volume. Global Spine J 2018;8: 784–94.
2. Alboog A, Bae S, Chui J. Anesthetic management of complex spine surgery in adult patients: a review based on outcome evidence. Curr Opin Anaesthesiol 2019;32:600–8.
3. Davies BM, Mowforth OD, Smith EK, et al. Degenerative cervical myelopathy. BMJ 2018;360:k186.
4. Kovalova I, Kerkovsky M, Kadanka Z, et al. Prevalence and imaging characteristics of nonmyelopathic and myelopathic spondylotic cervical cord compression. Spine 2016;41:1908–16.
5. Dagal A, Bellabarba C, Bransford R, et al. Enhanced perioperative care for major spine surgery. Spine 2019;44:959–66.

6. Ali ZS, Flanders TM, Ozturk AK, et al. Enhanced recovery after elective spinal and peripheral nerve surgery: pilot study from a single institution. J Neurosurg Spine 2019;1–9. https://doi.org/10.3171/2018.9.SPINE18681.

7. Fleisher LA, Fleischmann KE, Auerbach AD, et al. 2014 ACC/AHA guideline on perioperative cardiovascular evaluation and management of patients undergoing noncardiac surgery: a report of the American College of Cardiology/American Heart Association Task Force on practice guidelines. J Am Coll Cardiol 2014; 64:e77–137.

8. Levine GN, Bates ER, Bittl JA, et al. 2016 ACC/AHA guideline focused update on duration of dual antiplatelet therapy in patients with coronary artery disease: a report of the American College of Cardiology/American Heart Association Task Force on clinical practice guidelines: an update of the 2011 ACCF/AHA/SCAI guideline for percutaneous coronary intervention, 2011 ACCF/AHA guideline for coronary artery bypass graft surgery, 2012 ACC/AHA/ACP/AATS/PCNA/SCAI/ STS guideline for the diagnosis and management of patients with stable ischemic heart disease, 2013 ACCF/AHA guideline for the management of ST-elevation myocardial infarction, 2014 AHA/ACC guideline for the management of patients with non-ST-Elevation Acute Coronary Syndromes, and 2014 ACC/AHA guideline on perioperative cardiovascular evaluation and management of patients under-going noncardiac surgery. Circulation 2016;134:e123–55.

9. Burgess LC, Arundel J, Wainwright TW. The effect of preoperative education on psychological, clinical and economic outcomes in elective spinal surgery: a sys-tematic review. Healthcare (Basel) 2019;7:48.

10. Ellis DJ, Mallozzi SS, Mathews JE, et al. The relationship between preoperative expectations and the short-term postoperative satisfaction and functional outcome in lumbar spine surgery: a systematic review. Global Spine J 2015;5: 436–52.

11. Menendez ME, Neuhaus V, Bot AGJ, et al. Psychiatric disorders and major spine surgery: epidemiology and perioperative outcomes. Spine 2014;39:E111–22.

12. Celestin J, Edwards RR, Jamison RN. Pretreatment psychosocial variables as predictors of outcomes following lumbar surgery and spinal cord stimulation: a systematic review and literature synthesis. Pain Med 2009;10:639–53.

13. Culley DJ, Crosby G. Prehabilitation for prevention of postoperative cognitive dysfunction? Anesthesiology 2015;123:7–9.

14. Angus M, Jackson K, Smurthwaite G, et al. The implementation of enhanced re-covery after surgery (ERAS) in complex spinal surgery. J Spine Surg 2019;5: 116–23.

15. Gometz A, Maislen D, Youtz C, et al. The effectiveness of prehabilitation (prehab) in both functional and economic outcomes following spinal surgery: a systematic review. Cureus 2018;10:e2675.

16. Frei BW, Woodward KT, Zhang MY, et al. Considerations for clock drawing scoring systems in perioperative anesthesia settings. Anesth Analg 2019;128: e61–4.

17. Macdonald DB, Skinner S, Shils J, et al, American Society of Neurophysiological Monitoring. Intraoperative motor evoked potential monitoring - a position state-ment by the American Society of Neurophysiological Monitoring. Clin Neurophy-siol 2013;124:2291–316.

18. Zorrilla-Vaca A, Healy RJ, Mirski MA. A comparison of regional versus general anesthesia for lumbar spine surgery: a meta-analysis of randomized studies. J Neurosurg Anesthesiol 2017;29:415–25.

19. Cottrell J, Patel P. Neurosurgical diseases and trauma of the spine and spinal cord anesthetic considerations. In: Cottrell J, Patel P, editors. Cottrell and Patel's neuroanesthesia. 2nd edition. Philadelphia: Elsevier; 2016. p. 389–90.
20. Ozgur BM, Aryan HE, Pimenta L, et al. Extreme Lateral Interbody Fusion (XLIF): a novel surgical technique for anterior lumbar interbody fusion. Spine 2006;6: 435–43.
21. Bacchin MR, Ceria CM, Giannone S, et al. Goal-directed fluid therapy based on stroke volume variation in patients undergoing major spine surgery in the prone position: a cohort study. Spine 2016;41:E1131–7.
22. Min JJ, Lee J-H, Hong KY, et al. Utility of stroke volume variation measured using non-invasive bioreactance as a predictor of fluid responsiveness in the prone position. J Clin Monit Comput 2017;31:397–405.
23. Ramchandran S, Day LM, Line B, et al. The impact of different intraoperative fluid administration strategies on postoperative extubation following multilevel thoracic and lumbar spine surgery: a propensity score matched analysis. Neurosurgery 2019;85:31–40.
24. Nickels TJ, Manlapaz MR, Farag E. Perioperative visual loss after spine surgery. World J Orthop 2014;5:100–6.
25. Lee LA. Perioperative visual loss and anesthetic management. Curr Opin Anaesthesiol 2013;26:375–81.
26. Basques BA, Anandasivam NS, Webb ML, et al. Risk factors for blood transfusion with primary posterior lumbar fusion. Spine 2015;40:1792–7.
27. Aoude A, Nooh A, Fortin M, et al. Incidence, predictors, and postoperative complications of blood transfusion in thoracic and lumbar fusion surgery: an analysis of 13,695 patients from the American College of Surgeons National Surgical Quality Improvement Program database. Global Spine J 2016;6:756–64.
28. American Society of Anesthesiologists Task Force on Perioperative Blood Management. Practice guidelines for perioperative blood management: an updated report by the American Society of Anesthesiologists Task Force on Perioperative Blood Management*. Anesthesiology 2015;122:241–75.
29. Goodnough LT, Maniatis A, Earnshaw P, et al. Detection, evaluation, and management of preoperative anaemia in the elective orthopaedic surgical patient: NATA guidelines. Br J Anaesth 2011;106:13–22.
30. Hui S, Xu D, Ren Z, et al. Can tranexamic acid conserve blood and save operative time in spinal surgeries? A meta-analysis. Spine 2018;18:1325–37.
31. Luo W, Sun R-X, Jiang H, et al. The efficacy and safety of topical administration of tranexamic acid in spine surgery: a meta-analysis. J Orthop Surg Res 2018; 13:96.
32. Pennington Z, Ehresman J, Westbroek EM, et al. Interventions to minimize blood loss and transfusion risk in spine surgery: a narrative review. Clin Neurol Neurosurg 2020;196:106004.
33. Yuan Q-M, Zhao Z-H, Xu B-S. Efficacy and safety of tranexamic acid in reducing blood loss in scoliosis surgery: a systematic review and meta-analysis. Eur Spine J 2017;26:131–9.
34. Yuan L, Zeng Y, Chen Z-Q, et al. Efficacy and safety of antifibrinolytic agents in spinal surgery: a network meta-analysis. Chin Med J 2019;132:577–88.
35. Li G, Sun T-W, Luo G, et al. Efficacy of antifibrinolytic agents on surgical bleeding and transfusion requirements in spine surgery: a meta-analysis. Eur Spine J 2017;26:140–54.
36. Malhotra A, Gupta V, Abraham M, et al. Quantifying the amount of bleeding and associated changes in intra-abdominal pressure and mean airway pressure in

patients undergoing lumbar fixation surgeries: a comparison of three positioning systems. Asian Spine J 2016;10:199–204.

37. Kim E, Kim H-C, Lim Y-J, et al. Comparison of intra-abdominal pressure among 3 prone positional apparatuses after changing from the supine to the prone position and applying positive end-expiratory pressure in healthy euvolemic patients: a prospective observational study. J Neurosurg Anesthesiol 2017;29:14–20.

38. Zhang Z, Xu H, Zhang Y, et al. Nonsteroidal anti-inflammatory drugs for postoperative pain control after lumbar spine surgery: a meta-analysis of randomized controlled trials. J Clin Anesth 2017;43:84–9.

39. Borgeat A, Ofner C, Saporito A, et al. The effect of nonsteroidal anti-inflammatory drugs on bone healing in humans: a qualitative, systematic review. J Clin Anesth 2018;49:92–100.

40. Shimia M, Parish M, Abedini N. The effect of intravenous paracetamol on postoperative pain after lumbar discectomy. Asian Spine J 2014;8:400–4.

41. Cakan T, Inan N, Culhaoglu S, et al. Intravenous paracetamol improves the quality of postoperative analgesia but does not decrease narcotic requirements. J Neurosurg Anesthesiol 2008;20:169–73.

42. Han C, Kuang M-J, Ma J-X, et al. The efficacy of preoperative gabapentin in spinal surgery: a meta-analysis of randomized controlled trials. Pain Physician 2017; 20:649–61.

43. Peng C, Li C, Qu J, et al. Gabapentin can decrease acute pain and morphine consumption in spinal surgery patients: a meta-analysis of randomized controlled trials. Medicine 2017;96:e6463.

44. Pendi A, Field R, Farhan S-D, et al. Perioperative ketamine for analgesia in spine surgery: a meta-analysis of randomized controlled trials. Spine 2018;43: E299–307.

45. Schwenk ES, Viscusi ER, Buvanendran A, et al. Consensus guidelines on the use of intravenous ketamine infusions for acute pain management from the American Society of Regional Anesthesia and Pain Medicine, the American Academy of Pain Medicine, and the American Society of Anesthesiologists. Reg Anesth Pain Med 2018;43:456–66.

46. Gottschalk A, Durieux ME, Nemergut EC. Intraoperative methadone improves postoperative pain control in patients undergoing complex spine surgery. Anesth Analg 2011;112:218–23.

47. Murphy GS, Szokol JW, Avram MJ, et al. Clinical effectiveness and safety of intraoperative methadone in patients undergoing posterior spinal fusion surgery: a randomized, double-blinded, controlled trial. Anesthesiology 2017;126:822–33.

48. Murphy GS, Szokol JW. Intraoperative methadone in surgical patients: a review of clinical investigations. Anesthesiology 2019;131:678–92.

49. Dunn LK, Yerra S, Fang S, et al. Safety profile of intraoperative methadone for analgesia after major spine surgery: an observational study of 1,478 patients. J Opioid Manag 2018;14:83–7.

50. Kim K-T, Cho D-C, Sung J-K, et al. Intraoperative systemic infusion of lidocaine reduces postoperative pain after lumbar surgery: a double-blinded, randomized, placebo-controlled clinical trial. Spine 2014;14:1559–66.

51. Farag E, Ghobrial M, Sessler DI, et al. Effect of perioperative intravenous lidocaine administration on pain, opioid consumption, and quality of life after complex spine surgery. Anesthesiology 2013;119:932–40.

52. Dewinter G, Moens P, Fieuws S, et al. Systemic lidocaine fails to improve postoperative morphine consumption, postoperative recovery and quality of life in

patients undergoing posterior spinal arthrodesis. A double-blind, randomized, placebo-controlled trial. Br J Anaesth 2017;118:576–85.

53. Meng Y, Jiang H, Zhang C, et al. A comparison of the postoperative analgesic efficacy between epidural and intravenous analgesia in major spine surgery: a meta-analysis. J Pain Res 2017;10:405–15.

54. Grieff AN, Ghobrial GM, Jallo J. Use of liposomal bupivacaine in the postoperative management of posterior spinal decompression. J Neurosurg Spine 2016;25: 88–93.

55. Perera AP, Chari A, Kostusiak M, et al. Intramuscular local anesthetic infiltration at closure for postoperative analgesia in lumbar spine surgery: a systematic review and meta-analysis. Spine 2017;42:1088–95.

56. Chin KJ, Dinsmore MJ, Lewis S, et al. Opioid-sparing multimodal analgesia with bilateral bi-level erector spinae plane blocks in scoliosis surgery: a case report of two patients. Eur Spine J 2019. https://doi.org/10.1007/s00586-019-06133-8.

57. Chin KJ, Lewis S. Opioid-free analgesia for posterior spinal fusion surgery using erector spinae plane (ESP) blocks in a multimodal anesthetic regimen. Spine 2019;44:E379–83.

58. Brandão J, Graça R, Sá M, et al. Lumbar erector spinae plane block: successful control of acute pain after lumbar spine surgery – a clinical report. Rev Esp Anestesiol Reanim 2019;66:167–71.

59. Dietz N, Sharma M, Adams S, et al. Enhanced recovery after surgery (ERAS) for spine surgery: a systematic review. World Neurosurg 2019;130:415–26.

60. Soffin EM, Vaishnav AS, Wetmore DS, et al. Design and implementation of an enhanced recovery after surgery (ERAS) program for minimally invasive lumbar decompression spine surgery: initial experience. Spine 2019;44:E561–70.

61. Smith J, Probst S, Calandra C, et al. Enhanced recovery after surgery (ERAS) program for lumbar spine fusion. Perioper Med (Lond) 2019;8:4.

62. Ali ZS, Ma TS, Ozturk AK, et al. Pre-optimization of spinal surgery patients: development of a neurosurgical enhanced recovery after surgery (ERAS) protocol. Clin Neurol Neurosurg 2018;164:142–53.

63. Nandyala SV, Marquez-Lara A, Fineberg SJ, et al. Incidence and risk factors for perioperative visual loss after spinal fusion. Spine 2014;14:1866–72.

Anesthesia for Carotid Endarterectomy, Angioplasty, and Stent

Priscilla Nelson, MD, Maria Bustillo, MD*

KEYWORDS

- Carotid artery disease • Carotid endarterectomy • Carotid artery stenosis • Stroke
- Cerebrovascular accident

KEY POINTS

- Carotid artery disease is common and appropriate intervention is important in the prevention of primary and secondary strokes.
- Based on degree of carotid stenosis and symptomatic or asymptomatic nature of the lesion, treatment can be medical or through surgical intervention.
- There is continued debate regarding optimal management of carotid artery disease, particularly in asymptomatic patients.
- Intervention is generally warranted in asymptomatic patients with significant stenosis who are at high risk for a subsequent neurologic event because of the lesion.
- The decision to intervene in symptomatic disease is better defined and accepted. Surgical intervention can be accomplished with an open carotid endarterectomy or an endovascular carotid angioplasty with stenting.

INTRODUCTION

Carotid artery disease accounts for 10% to 20% of all strokes. Carotid atherosclerosis typically occurs at the bifurcation of the internal and external carotid artery (**Fig. 1**), causing ischemic symptoms, which can be due to hemodynamically significant stenosis or emboli. Emboli from carotid artery disease usually lodge in the middle cerebral artery; however, depending on the anatomy of the circle of Willis, they can also settle in the anterior and posterior branches of the cerebral artery.[1] Appropriate intervention is important in the prevention of primary and secondary strokes.

Based on the degree of carotid stenosis and the symptomatic or asymptomatic nature of the lesion, treatment can be medical or through surgical intervention. There is continued debate regarding the optimal management of carotid artery disease, particularly in asymptomatic patients. Intervention is generally warranted

Department of Anesthesiology, Weill Cornell Medicine, Weill Cornell Medical College, 525 East 68th Street, Box 124, New York, NY 10065, USA
* Corresponding author.
E-mail address: bustilo@med.cornell.edu

Anesthesiology Clin 39 (2021) 37–51
https://doi.org/10.1016/j.anclin.2020.11.006
1932-2275/21/© 2020 Elsevier Inc. All rights reserved.

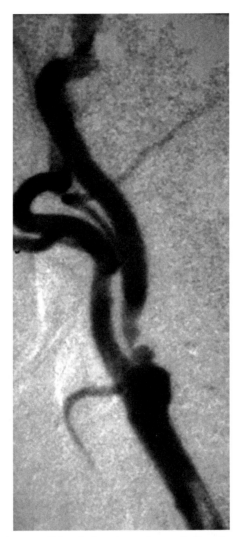

Fig. 1. Angiogram before carotid endarterectomy demonstrating stenosis in the internal carotid artery.

in asymptomatic patients with significant stenosis who are at high risk for a subsequent neurologic event because of the lesion. The decision whether or not to intervene in symptomatic disease is better defined and accepted. Surgical intervention for carotid artery atherosclerosis can be accomplished with an open carotid endarterectomy (CEA) or an endovascular carotid angioplasty with carotid stenting (CAS).

Open CEA involves making an incision in the anterolateral neck to fully expose the carotid artery to obtain proximal and distal control. The artery is then either simply clamped or a bypass tubing is placed proximal and distal to the area of disease before opening the vessel and removing the plaque causing the stenotic lesion. CAS requires obtaining vascular arterial access, most commonly through the femoral artery in the groin. A wire is then passed from the femoral artery through the aorta and into the carotid artery of interest, where balloons, emboli protection devices, and stents are inserted over the wire to address the area of stenosis. Both procedural techniques have advantages and disadvantages, the specifics of which are both well-described and evolving. The timing of intervention is important for symptomatic disease management, with early intervention (within 2 weeks, but generally after 48 hours, of a transient ischemic attack or stroke) having greater efficacy.[2] Research is ongoing as to which patients should undergo CAS and which should have a CEA. Currently, the decision is highly dependent on surgeon and institutional referral patterns. Although the initial early trials on carotid stents were stopped because of high periprocedural stroke rates, stenting technology has evolved with emboli protection devices, newer stents, and improved techniques, resulting in improved patient outcomes.

SYMPTOMATIC CAROTID DISEASE MANAGEMENT
Evidence for Carotid Endarterectomy Efficacy

CEA is still considered to be the gold standard treatment for symptomatic carotid stenosis. Landmark studies done in the 1990s demonstrated that CEA for symptomatic carotid stenosis decreased the risk of subsequent stroke when compared with medical management alone. The NASCET trial found that, in patients with greater than 70% stenosis, the 2-year risk of ipsilateral stroke was 26% in the group that was managed medically and 9% in the group that underwent CAE in addition to medical therapy. The study also demonstrated a decreased risk overall of stroke or death in patients who underwent surgical intervention.[3] The advantages of CEA also persisted in the long term,[4] a finding that was subsequently confirmed by the European Carotid Study Trial.[5] Follow-up examination of the NASCET data found no benefit of CAE when the carotid stenosis was less than 50%.[6] Pooled analyses lent further support to this conclusion.[7]

Evidence for Carotid Stenting Efficacy

CAS for symptomatic carotid stenosis is associated with a higher risk of stroke and death when compared with CEA.[8] However, CAS is generally considered a second-line choice for high-grade symptomatic carotid stenosis and is often reserved for specific indications, including patients who have a lesion that is not amenable to CEA, patients with radiation-induced stenosis, patients with stenosis occurring in the setting of previous CEA, and patients with significant comorbidities that increase the risks of general anesthesia. These recommendations are based on meta-analyses of randomized trials.[9] CAS is associated with a lower risk of periprocedural myocardial infarction, cranial nerve palsy, and surgical site hematoma.[9] The debate continues, however, regarding the use of CAS in symptomatic patients and is an area of continued research.

ASYMPTOMATIC CAROTID DISEASE MANAGEMENT

The management of asymptomatic carotid stenosis is controversial, typically involving medical management and CEA or CAS. Guidelines have been established by the American Heart Association and the American Stroke Association for the primary prevention of stroke in this patient population.[10] The recommendations include daily aspirin and a statin along with lifestyle changes in patients with low-grade stenosis and consideration of surgical intervention in asymptomatic patients with a higher grade stenosis. The use of CAS is less clearly defined.

Evidence for Medical Management Efficacy

With an enhanced understanding of the pathophysiology of the disease and available medications as well as the development of new pharmacologic agents, the medical management of carotid artery disease has advanced over the past several decades. Management typically involves the use of statins and antiplatelet agents, along with treatment of hypertension, smoking cessation, weight reduction, and tight glucose control in patients with diabetes.[11] Some experts believe that medical management may be as efficacious as surgical intervention in asymptomatic patients.[11,12] This belief is certainly a topic of debate and is the premise for the Carotid Revascularization Endarterectomy Trial (CREST)-2 trial, which randomizes patients to medical management or medical management with intervention in asymptomatic carotid stenosis. This trial is projected to end in December of 2020 and will likely provide additional level 1 evidence on this topic.[12,13]

Evidence for Carotid Endarterectomy Efficacy

CEA for asymptomatic carotid stenosis is not as advantageous as it is for symptomatic disease; however, it remains the standard intervention against which others are judged. The benefit of surgical intervention is greatest in patients who have a high degree of carotid stenosis. The ASCT trial[14] randomized patients with carotid stenosis of more than 60% to receive either an CEA and medical management or just medical management.[15,16] Study results suggest that surgical intervention for asymptomatic carotid stenosis should be done in patients who have a prolonged life expectancy and in centers with proven high volume and low morbidity CEA surgery is done, because minimizing perioperative complications is the key to gaining benefit from a marginally beneficial procedure.

Evidence for Carotid Stenting Efficacy

Multiple studies have been performed to compare CAS with CEA in both asymptomatic and symptomatic patients. Several specific, high-profile studies have demonstrated the noninferiority of CAS. These studies include the CREST[17] and the ACT-1 trial.[18] A recent meta-analysis examined randomized controlled trials and involved a subgroup analysis examining only asymptomatic patients.[19] An additional study looked specifically at asymptomatic patients.[20] Both studies demonstrated a trend toward an increased risk of periprocedural stroke with CAS. Further, a recent Cochrane Review also found evidence of a small increased risk of periprocedural stroke or death with CAS, but suggested a need for additional studies in the asymptomatic population because the data varied widely in the studies included in their review.[8]

Absolute and Relative Contraindications to Revascularization

Although the debate continues as to the advantages of CEA and CAS in general populations, there are patients for whom the risk of CEA is too high. In these cases, stenting may be the better option. The absolute contraindication to both CAS and CEA is total or near total occlusion of the carotid artery.[21,22] Patients who are at high risk for CEA-associated morbidity include those with contralateral carotid occlusion, severe coronary artery disease, concurrent tracheostomy, prior radical neck dissection, neck radiation, contralateral vocal cord paralysis, and a lesion that is not accessible owing a location that is either too high or too low in the carotid artery.[22] Patients at high risk for CAS include patients with a visible thrombus at the level of the lesion, active infection, inability to obtain vascular access, severely calcified plaque, severely calcified aortic arch, near occlusion of the carotid artery, inability to deploy a cerebral protection device, and a tortuous carotid artery.

PREOPERATIVE EVALUATION FOR CAROTID STENTING AND CAROTID ENDARTERECTOMY

Atherosclerosis in the carotid arteries is indicative of atherosclerosis throughout the body.[23] Although the timing of surgery is important to prevent stroke, it is important to still consider medical optimization in the patient, to the extent possible. Preoperative optimization should include blood pressure control, blood glucose control, an assessment to ensure euvolemia (particularly in patients with heart failure), determination of baseline electrolytes, and an electrocardiogram.[23] An echocardiogram is usually part of the initial stroke workup and can help to guide subsequent anesthetic therapy. Typically, a stress test is not warranted. A complete understanding of the patient's renal function, and whether or not there is dysfunction, is necessary because the contrast typically administered during stenting can be nephrotoxic. Aspirin, beta-blockers, and statins should be continued on the day of surgery.

ANESTHETIC CONSIDERATIONS
Intraoperative Management for Carotid Endarterectomy

Carotid endarterectomy procedural overview
CEA is an open surgical procedure (**Fig. 2**).[24] The procedure is initiated with an incision along the anterior or medial aspect of the sternocleidomastoid muscle. The dissection is carried through the subcutaneous tissues and platysma, with the sternocleidomastoid

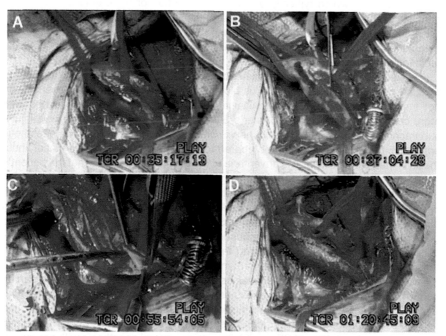

Fig. 2. Overview of CEA surgical procedure. (*A*) The carotid artery is circumferentially isolated above and below the carotid bifurcation. (*B*) The carotid artery is clamped (if no shunt is used). (*C*) The artery is incised and the plaque removed. (*D*) The arteriotomy is closed longitudinally.

being retracted and the carotid sheath entered. Most commonly, the carotid artery is then exposed and circumferentially cleared above and below the level of the plaque. The vessel is clamped, and a longitudinal incision is made, exposing the plaque, which is then removed. The vessel is subsequently closed primarily or a vascular patch is placed, which increases the vessel diameter. Shunts are occasionally used to allow continued distal flow during carotid cross-clamping. Some surgeons use an eversion technique where the vessel is completely divided and everted for plaque removal, followed by circumferential repair of the vessel.[25]

Intraoperative Care for Carotid Endarterectomy

CEA can be performed either with general anesthesia or with minimal sedation and local/regional anesthesia, although most commonly general anesthesia is used.[26,27] Available data suggest minimal differences in outcomes based on anesthetic choice or whether a patient is awake or receiving general anesthesia.[28] A recent meta-analysis demonstrated no outcome advantage when comparing CEA performed under general or local/regional anesthesia, in terms of perioperative stroke, myocardial infraction, or 30-day mortality.[29] A meta-analysis that combined both retrospective studies and randomized control trials demonstrated a small advantage when comparing local/regional anesthesia to general anesthesia in terms of postoperative stroke, transient ischemic attack, myocardial infraction, and mortality.[30] An additional recent retrospective review reported a higher incidence of pneumonia and a greater need for blood transfusion in the general anesthesia group when propensity matched with patients who had local anesthesia.[31] Studies have shown that, when using local/regional anesthesia, patients have better hemodynamic stability and do not encounter the hypotension, which typically occurs with induction or hypertension with emergence.[32] Further, there may be a lower incidence of postoperative cognitive delirium during the hospital stay for patients who had CEA without general anesthesia. Ideally as an anesthesiologist, one should be skilled in both methods, because the chosen technique depends largely on the patient, the surgeon, and intuition practice.

If a regional anesthetic is the chosen approach, superficial cervical plexus block is typically used.[33] Deep cervical plexus blocks typically are avoided because they do not improve the quality of the analgesia during surgery and are associated with more complications, including Horner's Syndrome, recurrent laryngeal nerve injury, subarachnoid block, and phrenic nerve block. As with any regional anesthetic approach, the surgeon should be prepared to supplement analgesia with local anesthesia in their surgical field. The advantage of the awake procedure is that the patient's neurologic status can be more easily monitored. The disadvantages of caring for an awake patient are due in large measure to the complications associated with deep cervical plexus blocks, which is not warranted for this procedure.[34] Patients having awake procedures must be cooperative. Should the patient request a conversion to general anesthesia or should a complication, such as respiratory arrest, cerebrovascular accident, or stroke, occur during the procedure, conversion to general anesthesia would be required with emergent intubation.

Should general anesthesia be chosen as the anesthetic for the procedure, it can be performed with total intravenous anesthesia or a balanced technique if short-acting anesthetics are used to allow for prompt emergence from anesthesia for a thorough neurologic evaluation.[23] Studies do not demonstrate an advantage of one technique over another in the setting of CEA.[35,36] When using general anesthesia with neurologic monitoring like an electroencephalogram (EEG), one must ensure a steady state of anesthesia throughout the procedure at a dose that does not suppress the EEG. Care must be taken to not use the anesthetic agents to treat hemodynamic instability.

For example, increasing the anesthetic agent to treat a high blood pressure (taking advantage of the vasodilatory effect of the agents) will suppress an EEG signal and not allow appropriate monitoring for ongoing ischemia.

During general anesthesia, the patient's airway should be secured with an endotracheal tube. Ventilation should aim for normocapnia, because hypocapnia may lead to cerebral vasoconstriction and hypercapnia may lead to a steal phenomenon because blood vessels to the normal brain dilate and shunt blood away from the area at risk for ischemia. During emergence, the presence of an endotracheal tube may be associated with hypertension and coughing, which can lead to the formation of a neck hematoma and potentially a hemorrhagic stroke. Upon emergence from general anesthesia, the anesthesia provider should use an anesthetic that minimizes coughing, such as remifentanil or for a deep extubation with, for example, dexmedetomidine.

Intraoperative Management for Carotid Stents

Carotid stenting procedure overview

There are 4 main steps to CAS, including (1) percutaneous arterial access, (2) angiography, (3) placement of an embolic protection device, and (4) stent placement and dilation.[23,24] Percutaneous access is most commonly achieved via the common femoral artery or radial artery. Angiography is performed to ascertain anatomy within the aorta, aortic arch, and carotid and cerebral arteries (**Fig. 3**). After the initial angiographic imaging, the patient is anticoagulated. Typically, heparin is administered and titrated to an activated clotting time of 250 to 300seconds.[37] After anticoagulation, the guidewire and sheath are placed. Then, an embolic protection device is placed and the stent is positioned and deployed (**Fig. 4**). Angioplasty is performed to ensure that the stent is adherent to the wall of the carotid artery. The artery is then assessed for postdeployment perfusion (**Fig. 5**).

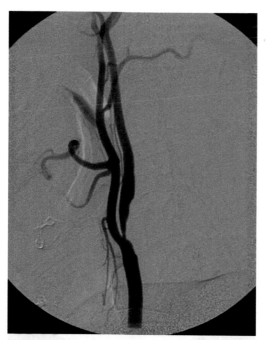

Fig. 3. Angiograph before a CAS procedure demonstrating stenosis of the internal carotid just distal to the bifurcation.

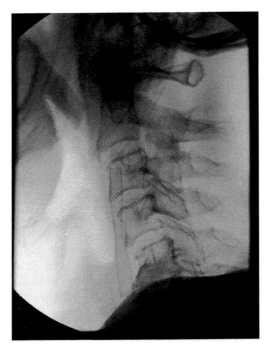

Fig. 4. The stent is placed over a wire and confirmed to be in the appropriate position.

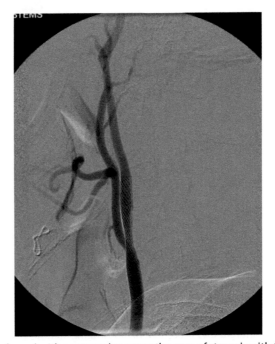

Fig. 5. Flow is confirmed with contrast dye across the area of stenosis with the stent in place.

Intraoperative anesthetic care for carotid stenting

CAS is usually performed with the patient awake and under sedation.[26,27] Patients should be made comfortable to the extent possible without depressing respiration. Minimal sedation is preferable to moderate and deep sedation because the patient needs to be able to communicate and follow commands. Ischemia from emboli or hypoperfusion is readily detectable in a patient who is awake. Because it is common for patients to experience pain during stent deployment and angioplasty, the anesthesiologist needs to be ready to manage this sudden change in the patient's level of comfort.

Intraoperative hemodynamic monitoring and management

Standard American Society of Anesthesiologists monitors along with an intra-arterial catheter are required for CAS or CEA.[23] Usually there is no need for central access and 1 to 2 peripheral intravenous lines should suffice. The arterial line is often placed before the cervical plexus block or induction of general anesthesia for beat-to-beat blood pressure monitoring and control, because large swings in blood pressure can occur with carotid manipulation. The anesthesia provider should know what the patient's normal variation in blood pressure is with sleep and wakefulness and speak with the surgeon before the carotid artery is clamped during endarterectomy to determine blood pressure goals while the carotid is clamped. Typically, elevation of the blood pressure from the patient's baseline (approximately 20%), during clamping of the carotid artery, may be indicated to ensure recruitment of collateral circulation through the circle of Willis.[37]

Because carotid surgery and stenting can lead to wide swings in blood pressure, one should have short-acting vasoactive agents readily available to increase and decrease the patient's blood pressure.[37] As mentioned elsewhere in this article, the use of volatile anesthetic agents to treat hypertension is not recommended. Typically, phenylephrine and nicardipine infusions can be prepared before beginning the anesthetic in the event that sustained infusions are required in addition to intermittent dosing.

When patients are receiving general anesthesia for surgical treatment of carotid artery disease, it is important to be in constant communication with the neuromonitoring team and the surgeon to ensure that the blood pressure goals that had been decided on allow for adequate cerebral perfusion as determined by neuromonitoring.

For CAS, the blood pressure goal at the start of the procedure is normotension. When catheters and guidewires are being placed, vasospasm can occur.[38] This event is usually treated with short-acting intra-arterial vasodilators. During intra-arterial treatment of vasospasm, the systemic blood pressure can fall and may require treatment with short-acting vasopressors. During manipulation of the carotid artery, it is common to observe bradycardia from baroreceptor activation.[37] This event is usually self-limited and can be treated with a muscarinic antagonist such as atropine. After stent placement, the systolic blood pressure should be maintained between 100 mm Hg and 150 mm Hg.

Once the plaque is removed or stented, blood pressure should be returned to the normotensive state so as to not cause a hemorrhagic cerebral infarction. If the patient is awake, hypertension during clot removal may be associated with headache and facial flushing.[39]

Fluid management

Fluid resuscitation is also important to consider in caring for a patient undergoing a carotid procedure. Generally, given the short duration of the surgery, most patients do not require more than a liter of intravenous fluid. Placement of a Foley catheter should be considered, because intravenous contrast that is administered during the procedure by the surgeon or interventionalist can have diuretic effects. A full bladder at the conclusion of the procedure can lead to hypertension, which can cause adverse patient outcomes, as described elsewhere in this article.[23]

Cerebral perfusion monitoring

Cerebral perfusion monitoring is used in many centers to assess ischemic or embolic events during CEA and CAS. Detection of cerebral ischemia and emboli can be done in a variety of techniques that fall into 3 categories that monitor (1) cerebral blood flow, (2) cerebral activity, and (3) cerebral oxygen saturation.

The adequacy of cerebral blood flow is monitored using either transcranial Doppler, measurement of carotid stump pressure, or EEG. Transcranial Doppler measures blood flow velocity in the middle cerebral artery.[37] It is a surrogate measure of cerebral blood flow because the flow velocity is determined by size of the artery, which can be vasodilated or vasoconstricted depending on a variety of factors, which include the $Paco_2$, the anesthetic agent, and vasopressor use. It gives real-time feedback about embolization, because emboli have a very distinct acoustic signal.[37] The burden of emboli has been associated with postoperative stroke. The carotid stump pressure is measured distal to the carotid clamp. It is an estimate of the pressure from backflow via the circle of Willis and other collaterals.[23] This monitoring is not continuous, and typically provides a single point value reading. Controversy exists regarding the usefulness of this measure, with a recent analysis demonstrating that the stump pressure as a single criterion was not reliable in predicting mortality, stroke, or transient ischemic attacks.[40] In addition to the stump pressure being impacted by the patient's depth of anesthesia, a detractor to its routine use is that there are no standard acceptable values. High pressures are generally thought to be acceptable, whereas lower pressures may be associated with adverse deficits. The definition of a low pressure differs between institutions.

Cerebral activity monitoring

Cerebral activity monitoring includes measurement and evaluation of EEG and evoked potentials.

Electroencephalogram The EEG measures spontaneous cortical activity from the pyramidal cells of the cortex.[37,41] An unprocessed EEG is the most commonly used monitor to assess the adequacy of cerebral perfusion when general anesthesia is used. Alternatively, processed EEG, brain function monitors (such as the bispectral index or SedLine brain function monitoring [Masimo, Irvine, CA]) may have some usefulness,[37] but are limited by their processed and regional nature. Monitoring of the EEG is begun before the induction of general anesthesia and continued throughout the surgery. All anesthetics suppress EEG activity when administered in high enough doses and many will cause burst suppression. It is important to avoid very profound levels of anesthesia and burst suppression intraoperatively so that the EEG waveforms can be interpreted.[41] This monitoring gives further support to not using the anesthetic agent to treat swings in blood pressure, because increasing anesthetic depth will lead to suppression of the EEG, which falsely mimics ischemia and renders the monitoring useless. Monitoring can be particularly useful in CEA when the carotid is clamped, because unilateral flattening of the EEG signals may indicate ischemia that warrants either inducing hypertension or placing a shunt, either of which can increase the cerebral blood flow.

Evoked potentials Somatosensory evoked potentials and motor evoked potentials serve as monitors of the cortex and subcortical areas.[42] A change in the median nerve somatosensory evoked potentials during CEA is a sensitive marker of ischemia in the middle cerebral artery.[43] Tibial nerve somatosensory evoked potentials and motor evoked potentials identify ischemia to the anterior communicating artery and subcortical territories.[43] Because of the regional nature of their evaluation, a lack of change in evoked potentials does not guarantee that the patient will emerge from anesthesia free from neurologic deficits. Thus, evoked potentials are usually used in combination with transcarotid Doppler or EEG monitoring to improve the detection of cerebral ischemia and need for shunting; they are uncommonly used in isolation.

Cerebral oxygen saturation monitoring Cerebral oxygen saturation monitoring includes assessing jugular venous oxygenation (JvO_2) and cerebral oximetry. The JvO_2 measures oxygen saturation within the jugular vein. By placing a catheter into the ipsilateral jugular vein, oxygen saturation can be monitored.[23,44] Normal saturation is between 55% and 75%, and a decrease in the baseline value can indicate ongoing ischemia if all other variables remain constant.[44] The JvO_2 is directly proportional to cerebral oxygen supply and inversely proportional to cerebral oxygen consumption. Lower JvO_2 values can indicate ischemia and higher values indicate hyperemia. The limitations of the use of the JvO_2 include that it is a global monitor of cerebral perfusion, there can be mixing of extracerebral blood, and placement of a catheter into the jugular bulb may result in jugular vein thrombosis.

  Cerebral oximetry uses near infrared spectroscopy to measure oxygen saturation of the cortex because hemoglobin is the predominant chromophore that can absorb light in the near infrared range.[45] It helps with the balance of oxygen supply and demand within the local microcirculation, acting as a continuous monitor. Usually, 2 adhesive pads are applied to the forehead and baseline oxygen saturation values are obtained for the right and the left hemispheres. These values are followed and trended intraoperatively. Unfortunately, there are no established criteria with this monitor to guide shunt placement or other therapy to prevent postoperative neurologic deficits. Baseline values vary widely, and the values can be falsely affected by regional hemodynamics and extracerebral blood. Near infrared spectroscopy has low sensitivity and specificity and as such should not be used as the only determinant of ischemia in carotid surgery.[37]

Procedure conclusion and emergence
Blood pressure can be labile after carotid manipulation and must be an area of focus as the case is concluding. The systolic blood pressure should be maintained between 100 and 150 mm Hg, using short-acting vasoactive agents, as needed. An elevated blood pressure can lead to the development of a hematoma in the neck or cerebral hyperperfusion perfusion syndrome, which can lead to intracranial hemorrhage.[46] This syndrome typically presents as a severe ipsilateral headache, hypertension, seizures, or focal neurologic deficits. The incidence of cerebral hyperperfusion syndrome is between 0% and 3% after CEA and the patients at higher risk are those that had a greater extent of ipsilateral stenosis.[39] Neck hematoma after CEA can be due to inadequate hemostasis, coughing, or elevated blood pressure in the postoperative period and can lead to airway compromise. If a neck hematoma results in airway obstruction, reestablishing a secure airway can be challenging because the hematoma can distort the view of the upper airway structures during laryngoscopy. Depending on the clinical situation, surgical opening of the neck and hematoma decompression may be required before endotracheal intubation. Hematoma formation after CAS more

commonly occurs at the access site. As patients are emerging from their anesthetic, it is important to keep in mind that a slow emergence may be secondary to stroke or residual anesthetic.

Pain control

Generally, CEA and CAS are not associated with significant postoperative pain. For CEA, the surgeon typically can infiltrate local anesthetic in the surgical site. Opioids should be used judiciously because respiratory drive can be depressed postoperatively because of carotid chemoreceptor injury.[23] Typically, if the chemoreceptor is injured during the procedure, the chemoreceptor in the contralateral carotid is intact. This is one of the reasons that bilateral CEAs should not be done during the same anesthetic and that chemoreceptor function be allowed to recover after 1 CEA before the next is scheduled.

Postoperative Complications from Carotid Endarterectomy and Carotid Stenting

There are several postoperative complications that can develop from or after CEA and CAS, many of which have been discussed in the introductory section comparing techniques. These complications include stroke, myocardial infarction, hyperperfusion syndrome, renal dysfunction, carotid thrombosis, carotid restenosis, stent fracture, dissection, and access site problems.[37] It is also possible that nerve injury can occur in the surgical field, including injury to the recurrent laryngeal nerve, facial nerve, hypoglossal nerve, and the sympathetic nerves.[23]

SUMMARY

Anesthetic management of carotid artery disease requiring CEA or CAS is complex and varies widely, but relies on excellent communication between the anesthesia and surgical team throughout the procedure to ensure appropriate cerebral perfusion. With a systematic approach to vascular access and hemodynamic and neurologic monitoring, anesthesia can be applied to maximize cerebral perfusion while minimizing the risk of postoperative hemorrhage or hyperperfusion.

ACKNOWLEDGMENTS

Special thanks to Philip E. Stieg, MD, PhD, and Athos Patsalides, MD, for intraoperative procedure imaging.

REFERENCES

1. JC G. Clinical practice. Carotid stenosis. N Engl J Med 2013;369(12):1143–50.
2. Rothwell PM EM, Gutnikov SA, Warlow CP, et al. Endarterectomy for symptomatic carotid stenosis in relation to clinical subgroups and timing of surgery. Lancet 2004;363:915–24.
3. Barnett HJM, Taylor DW, Haynes RB, et al. Beneficial effect of carotid endarterectomy in symptomatic patients with high-grade carotid stenosis. N Engl J Med 1991;325:445–53.
4. Paciaroni M, Eliasziw M, Sharpe BL, et al. Long-term clinical and angiographic outcomes in symptomatic patients with 70% to 99% carotid artery stenosis. Stroke 2000;31:2037–42.
5. Cunningham EJ, Bond R, Mehta Z, et al. Long-term durability of carotid endarterectomy for symptomatic stenosis and risk factors for late postoperative stroke. Stroke 2002;33:2658–63.

6. Barnett HJ, Taylor DW, Eliasziw M, et al. Benefit of carotid endarterectomy in patients with symptomatic moderate or severe stenosis. North American Symptomatic Carotid Endarterectomy Trial Collaborators. N Engl J Med 1998;339:1415–25.
7. Rerkasem K, Rothwell PM. Carotid endarterectomy for symptomatic carotid stenosis. Cochrane Database Syst Rev 2011;(4):CD001081.
8. Muller MD, Lyrer P, Brown MM, et al. Carotid artery stenting versus endarterectomy for treatment of carotid artery stenosis. Cochrane Database Syst Rev 2020;(2):CD000515.
9. Bonati LH, Lyrer P, Ederle J, et al. Percutaneous transluminal balloon angioplasty and stenting for carotid artery stenosis. Cochrane Database Syst Rev 2012;(9):CD000515.
10. Meschia JF, Bushnell C, Boden-Albala B, et al. Guidelines for the primary prevention of stroke: a statement for healthcare professionals from the American Heart Association/American Stroke Association. Stroke 2014;45:3754–832.
11. Abbott AL. Medical (nonsurgical) intervention alone is now best for prevention of stroke associated with asymptomatic severe carotid stenosis: results of a systematic review and analysis. Stroke 2009;40:e573–83.
12. Silverman S. Management of asymptomatic carotid artery stenosis. Curr Treat Options Cardiovasc Med 2019;21:80.
13. Howard VJ, Meschia JF, Lal BK, et al. Carotid revascularization and medical management for asymptomatic carotid stenosis: protocol of the CREST-2 clinical trials. Int J Stroke 2017;12:770–8.
14. Executive Committee for the Asymptomatic Carotid Atherosclerosis Study. Endarterectomy for asymptomatic carotid artery stenosis. JAMA 1995;273:1421–8.
15. Halliday A, Mansfield A, Marro J, et al. Prevention of disabling and fatal strokes by successful carotid endarterectomy in patients without recent neurological symptoms: randomised controlled trial. Lancet 2004;363:1491–502.
16. Halliday A, Harrison M, Hayter E, et al. 10-year stroke prevention after successful carotid endarterectomy for asymptomatic stenosis (ACST-1): a multicentre randomised trial. Lancet 2010;376:1074–84.
17. Brott TG, Howard G, Roubin GS, et al. Long-term results of stenting versus endarterectomy for carotid-artery stenosis. N Engl J Med 2016;374:1021–31.
18. Rosenfield K, Matsumura JS, Chaturvedi S, et al. Randomized trial of stent versus surgery for asymptomatic carotid stenosis. N Engl J Med 2016;374:1011–20.
19. Sardar P, Chatterjee S, Aronow HD, et al. Carotid artery stenting versus endarterectomy for stroke prevention: a meta-analysis of clinical trials. J Am Coll Cardiol 2017;69:2266–75.
20. Moresoli P, Habib B, Reynier P, et al. Carotid stenting versus endarterectomy for asymptomatic carotid artery stenosis: a systematic review and meta-analysis. Stroke 2017;48:2150–7.
21. Brott TG, Halperin JL, Abbara S, et al. 2011 ASA/ACCF/AHA/AANN/AANS/ACR/ASNR/CNS/SAIP/SCAI/SIR/SNIS/SVM/SVS guideline on the management of patients with extracranial carotid and vertebral artery disease. Stroke 2011;42:e464–540.
22. Marcucci G, Accrocca F, Antonelli R, et al. High-risk patients for carotid endarterectomy: turned down cases are rare. J Cardiovasc Surg 2012;53:333–43.
23. Shalabi A, Chang J. Anesthesia for vascular surgery. Miller's Anesthesiology 2020;1825–67.e6.
24. Silva M, Choi L, Cheng C. Peripheral artery occlusive disease. Sabiston Textbook Surg 2012;1725–84.

25. Curtis JA, Johansen K. Techniques in carotid artery surgery. Neurosurg Focus 2008;24:E18.
26. Leichtle SW, Mouawad NJ, Welch K, et al. Outcomes of carotid endarterectomy under general and regional anesthesia from the American College of Surgeons' National Surgical Quality Improvement Program. J Vasc Surg 2012;56:81–8.e3.
27. Hye RJ, Voeks JH, Malas MB, et al. Anesthetic type and risk of myocardial infarction after carotid endarterectomy in the Carotid Revascularization Endarterectomy versus Stenting Trial (CREST). J Vasc Surg 2016;64:3–8.e1.
28. Vaniyapong T, Chongruksut W, Rerkasem K. Local versus general anaesthesia for carotid endarterectomy. Cochrane Database Syst Rev 2013;(4):CD000126.
29. Unic-Stojanovic D, Babic S, Neskovic V. General versus regional anesthesia for carotid endarterectomy. J Cardiothorac Vasc Anesth 2013;27:1379–83.
30. Hajibandeh S, Hajibandeh S, Antoniou SA, et al. Meta-analysis and trial sequential analysis of local vs. general anaesthesia for carotid endarterectomy. Anaesthesia 2018;73:1280–9.
31. Malik OS, Brovman EY, Urman RD. The use of regional or local anesthesia for carotid endarterectomies may reduce blood loss and pulmonary complications. J Cardiothorac Vasc Anesth 2019;33:935–42.
32. Rerkasem K, Rothwell PM. Routine or selective carotid artery shunting for carotid endarterectomy (and different methods of monitoring in selective shunting). Cochrane Database Syst Rev 2009;(6):CD000190.
33. Howell SJ. Carotid endarterectomy. Br J Anaesth 2007;99:119–31.
34. Pandit JJ, Satya-Krishna R, Gration P. Superficial or deep cervical plexus block for carotid endarterectomy: a systematic review of complications. Br J Anaesth 2007;99:159–69.
35. Yastrebov K. Intraoperative management: carotid endarterectomies. Anesthesiol Clin North Am 2004;22:265–87, vi-vii.
36. Jellish WS, Sheikh T, Baker WH, et al. Hemodynamic stability, myocardial ischemia, and perioperative outcome after carotid surgery with remifentanil/propofol or isoflurane/fentanyl anesthesia. J Neurosurg Anesthesiol 2003;15:176–84.
37. Erickson KM, Cole DJ. Carotid artery disease: stenting vs endarterectomy. Br J Anaesth 2010;105(Suppl 1):i34–49.
38. Schirmer CM, Hoit DA, Malek AM. Iatrogenic vasospasm in carotid artery stent angioplasty with distal protection devices. Neurosurg Focus 2008;24:E12.
39. Lieb M, Shah U, Hines GL. Cerebral hyperperfusion syndrome after carotid intervention: a review. Cardiol Rev 2012;20:84–9.
40. Kordzadeh A, Abbassi OA, Prionidis I, et al. The role of carotid stump pressure in carotid endarterectomy: a systematic review and meta-analysis. Ann Vasc Dis 2020;13:28–37.
41. Rampil IJ. EEG monitoring. In: Koht A, Sloan TB, Toleikis JR, editors. Monitoring the nervous system for anesthesiologists and other health care professionals. Cham (Switzerland): Springer International Publishing; 2017. p. 169–91.
42. Becker A, Amlong C, Rusy DA. Somatosensory-evoked potentials. In: Koht A, Sloan TB, Toleikis JR, editors. Monitoring the nervous system for anesthesiologists and other health care professionals. Cham (Switzerland): Springer International Publishing; 2017. p. 3–18.
43. Anastasian ZH, Ornstein E, Heyer EJ. Carotid surgery. In: Koht A, Sloan TB, Toleikis JR, editors. Monitoring the nervous system for anesthesiologists and other health care professionals. Cham (Switzerland): Springer International Publishing; 2017. p. 459–72.

44. Sharma D, Lele A. Monitoring of jugular venous oxygen saturation. In: Koht A, Sloan TB, Toleikis JR, editors. Monitoring the nervous system for anesthesiologists and other health care professionals. Cham (Switzerland): Springer International Publishing; 2017. p. 229–42.
45. Edmonds HL, Isley MR, Balzer JR. A guide to central nervous system near-infrared spectroscopic monitoring. In: Koht A, Sloan TB, Toleikis JR, editors. Monitoring the nervous system for anesthesiologists and other health care professionals. Cham (Switzerland): Springer International Publishing; 2017. p. 205–17.
46. Ascher E, Markevich N, Schutzer RW, et al. Cerebral hyperperfusion syndrome after carotid endarterectomy: predictive factors and hemodynamic changes. J Vasc Surg 2003;37:769–77.

Anesthetic Considerations for Pediatric Craniofacial Surgery

Nicholas Meier, MD

KEYWORDS

• Craniosynostosis • Pediatrics • Transfusion • Craniofacial surgery

KEY POINTS

- Anesthetic management for craniofacial surgery in infants remains a challenge.
- Understanding the different surgical approaches to complex cranial vault repair and the associated complications is an essential part of providing safe and effective anesthetic care.
- Despite advances in perioperative management, acute hemorrhage remains the primary concern during surgery.
- In-depth resuscitative knowledge is a must when caring for this patient population.

INTRODUCTION

Craniosynostosis is defined by the premature closure of one or more cranial sutures resulting in deformity of the calvarium. Depending on the affected suture(s), the resulting anatomic deformity may lead to significant morbidity, including social anxiety, increase in intracranial pressure (ICP), neurologic deficits such as hearing loss, or intellectual disability. Because of the significant morbidity associated with this disease, many infants will require surgical correction. Those with complex synostosis, defined as more than 1 affected suture, may require multiple operations for complete correction of the deformity during the first few years of life. Clinical phenotype is the primary mode of initial diagnosis. Phenotypic descriptions are used to describe the resulting anatomic defects produced by the underlying stenotic suture(s) (**Fig. 1**). A follow-up computed tomography (CT) scan with 3-dimensional reconstruction is completed to better define the involved sutures and assist with surgical planning (**Fig. 2**).

Department of Anesthesiology, Medical College of Wisconsin, Children's Hospital of Wisconsin, 9200 West Wisconsin Avenue, Milwaukee, WI 53226, USA
E-mail address: nmeier@mcw.edu

Anesthesiology Clin 39 (2021) 53–70
https://doi.org/10.1016/j.anclin.2020.10.002
1932-2275/21/© 2021 Elsevier Inc. All rights reserved.

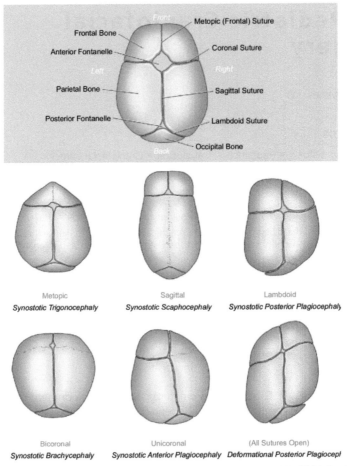

Fig. 1. Types of craniosynostosis. (*From* Buchanan EP, Xue Y, Xue AS, Olshinka A, Lam S. Multidisciplinary care of craniosynostosis. J Multidisc Healthc. 2017;10:263-270; with permission.)

BACKGROUND

In 1851, Virchow produced the first detailed documentation of craniosynostosis and noted the perpendicular nature of bone growth arrest in relation to the affected suture.[1] Craniosynostosis is broken down into 2 groups: syndromic and nonsyndromic. The incidence is 1 in 2000 to 2500 live births, with sagittal synostosis as the most common among nonsyndromic patients.[2] However, Cornelissen and colleagues[3] reported an increasing prevalence of craniosynostosis in the Netherlands without a clear explanation. Syndromic synostosis accounts for 40% of cases, while nonsyndromic synostosis accounts for around 60% of all cases.[4] **Table 1** demonstrates some of the more common associated syndromes, of which there are now over 200 associated with craniosynostosis. The syndromic synostoses are most associated with a mutation in the FGFR gene, and about 50% of mutations are de novo; most others are accounted for by autosomal dominant inheritance.[5] Multiple surgical techniques currently exist

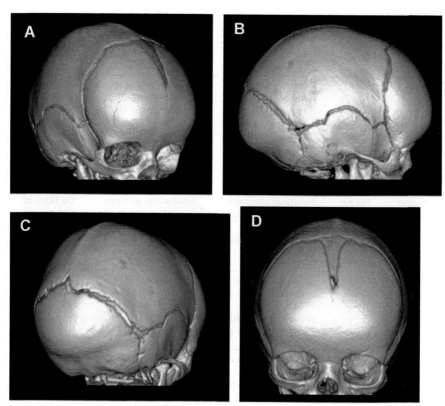

Fig. 2. Preoperative 3-dimensional reconstruction of a 6-month-old with isolated sagittal synostosis. Note the scaphocephaly with (*A*) mild frontal bossing, (*B*) prominent sagittal ridging, (*C*) occipital bun, and (*D*) bi-parietal narrowing.

depending on the type and severity of synostosis. In general, the goal is to complete surgery during the first year of life. In the 1960s, Paul Tessier presented his work with craniofacial dysmorphism, and he is now considered the father of craniofacial surgery.

SURGICAL INTERVENTION

There are 4 major surgical techniques described for repair of craniosynostosis. They include open strip craniectomy with modified Pi procedure, endoscopic strip craniectomy with post-operative helmet therapy, spring-mediated cranioplasty, and complex cranial vault remodeling procedures (fronto-orbital advancement, total calvarial remodeling, and posterior cranial vault remodeling). Given the extensive nature of these procedures and the temporally associated complications, anesthesiologists must have an in-depth knowledge of when during a given procedure critical events, such as hemorrhage, are most likely to occur.

Open Strip Craniectomy and the Modified Pi Procedure

Open strip craniectomy was first described by Dr. Lannelongue in 1890.[6] The procedure described 2 strip craniectomies running parallel just lateral to the sagittal suture. Initial surgical intervention with the simple, single-suture open craniectomy resulted

Table 1
Syndromes associated with craniosynostosis

Syndrome	Gene Mutation	Clinical Features	Neurologic Findings	Inheritance
Apert	FGFR2	Bicoronal synostosis Hand and feet syndactyly Midface hypoplasia Developmental delay Hearing loss Class III Malocclusion Exophthalmos	Variable cognitive disability, hearing loss, central nervous system (CNS) malformations	De novo or autosomal dominant
Crouzon syndrome	FGFR2 FGFR3	Bicoronal synostosis Lambdoid synostosis Shallow orbits Maxillary hypoplasia Prominent jaw Exophthalmos	Headaches, seizures, conductive hearing loss	De Novo or Autosomal Dominant
Pfieffer syndrome	FGFR1 FGFR2	Coronal ± sagittal synostosis Hypertelorism Broad thumb/hallux Partial syndactyly of fingers/toes	Hydrocephalus; Arnold-chiari malformation	Autosomal dominant
Muenke	FGFR 3	Unicoronal/bicoronal synostosis; midface hypoplasia	Macrocephaly; sensorineural hearing loss, developmental delay; intellectual disability	Autosomal dominant
Saethre-Chotzen	TWIST1 FGFR2	Coronal, lambdoid, and/or metopic synostosis, mild syndactyly, congenital heart defects	Intracranial hypertension; parietal foramina	Autosomal dominant

Data from Sawh-Martinez R, Steinbacher DM. Syndromic Craniosynostosis. Clin Past Surg. 2019;46(2):141-155; and Jezela-Stanek A, Krajewska-Walasek M. Genetic causes of syndromic cranioynostoses. Eur J Paediatr Neurol. 2013;17(3):221-224.

in delay of the deformity until later in life with poor cosmetic outcomes. The rapid skull growth seen in children was thought to contribute to this process.[7] Because of the recurrence and poor outcomes in the early stages, additional, more aggressive removal of bone into other regions of the skull were developed. In 1978, Jane and colleagues[8] described the modified Pi procedure, which extended the osteotomies posteriorly in the shape of the Greek letter Pi.

Endoscopic and Minimally Invasive Strip Craniectomy with Molded Orthotic Therapy

The endoscopic approach to strip craniectomy is a relatively new procedure first described by Jimenez and Barone in the late 1990s.[9] The goal was a less invasive procedure for simple, single-suture synostosis to reduce intraoperative complications such as hemorrhage and subsequent exposure to transfusion. The procedure, however, is accompanied by a significant and lengthy postoperative molded helmet therapy that may last 6 months or more and requires frequent readjustments as the calvarium continues to grow. For metopic synostosis repair, positioning is supine, with varying techniques for eye protection (ophthalmic lubricant or corneal protectors or both). The approach is a small 2 to 3 cm incision with dissection in the subgaleal plane posteriorly to the sagittal suture and anteriorly to the nasofrontal suture. The subperiosteal approach is typically avoided because of the increased risk of blood loss. The craniectomy ensues with dissection of the dura from the underside of the calvarium using an endoscope. At this time significant bleeding can occur from bridging veins and may necessitate patient position changes by the anesthesiologist to reduce venous bleeding and allow for surgical control.[10] The approach to sagittal synostosis is similar; however, 2 incisions (1 anteriorly and 1 posteriorly) are needed. Both approaches require extensive postoperative molded orthotic therapy to ensure proper bone and brain growth and to achieve good cosmetic results. Compared with traditional techniques, the endoscopic approach is usually complete prior to 6 months of age. Jimenez and Barone also described the minimally invasive endoscopic technique for multiple-suture, nonsyndromic patients with good overall results and safety.[11] See **Fig. 3**.

Spring-Mediated Cranioplasty

A relatively new technique by Lauritzen and colleagues in 1998 described the placement of a spring device during a less extensive procedure than complex cranial vault remodeling. The springs applied either compressing or distracting pressure to the surrounding osteotomies to promote cranial shaping and growth.[12] These springs were left in place to promote proper shaping of the skull and removed during a future procedure. On a follow-up study by the group, spring dislodgment was found to be 5%. The study concluded that results were comparable to other procedures at the time, which justified one of the main drawbacks to this surgery, an additional visit to the operating room for spring removal.[13] In 1 study, spring-mediated cranioplasty was compared with the modified-Pi procedure and showed significantly lower rates of blood loss, perioperative transfusion requirements, intensive care unit (ICU) time, operative time, recovery time, and length of hospital stay. Morphologic outcomes were similar.[14] The procedure remains as a safe and viable option for treatment of craniosynostosis. Although the risk of hemorrhage is less than seen with previously described approaches to craniosynostosis repair, the anesthesiologist should still be prepared for acute hemorrhage and venous air embolism.

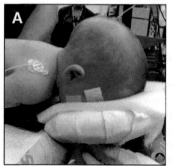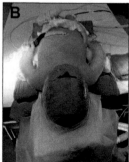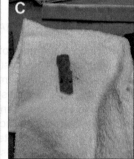

Fig. 3. (*A*) Preoperative prone positioning with horseshoe head holder for minimally invasive strip craniectomy. (*B*) Frontal and occipital incision marked with purple marking pen. (*C*) Sagittal suture craniectomy.

Complex Cranial Vault Remodeling

This group of procedures includes total calvarial remodeling, fronto-orbital advancement, and posterior cranial vault reconstruction. All 3 procedures carry a significant risk for massive hemorrhage. Therefore, a perioperative transfusion management strategy is suggested. Surgical intervention for blood loss prevention include scalp clips, bone wax, and local anesthetic infiltration with epinephrine. Osteotomies pose the highest risk of acute hemorrhage and venous air embolism during these procedures.

Fronto-Orbital Advancement

This procedure involves a zigzag, bicoronal incision (allows concealment of the scar after the hair regrows), removal of the frontal bone and orbital bandeau with subsequent reshaping and contouring of the removed bones to achieve the desired anatomy. The sculpted bone fragments are then replaced and held in place with absorbable plates or wires. Specific anesthetic considerations include triggering of the oculocardiac reflex (with subsequent bradycardia of varying degrees) when the surgeon is working near the orbit. The oculocardiac reflex is usually self-limiting when the offending stimulus is removed. Antimuscarinic treatment with atropine or glycopyrrolate is infrequently needed.

Total Calvarial Remodeling

Because of the extensive nature of this procedure, the risk for massive hemorrhage is high. Positioning for these patients can include the supine position with significant neck flexion (this is the case at this author's institution) or the prone sphinx position. Both extreme positions come with risks such as cerebral venous outflow obstruction, venous air embolism, facial edema, increased risk of bleeding, and changes in endotracheal tube position that could result in inadvertent extubation (Sphinx) or mainstem intubation (with severe neck flexion). Some institutions have opted for a staged procedure to reduce the many associated complications with this extensive procedure.

Posterior Cranial Vault Reconstruction

Posterior cranial vault remodeling is completed in the prone position with similar incisions and overall intraoperative risks as the other complex reconstructive procedures. This procedure is typically reserved for late presentation sagittal synostosis, syndromic synostosis, or children with residual deformities from prior surgery. Careful attention to positioning and management of hemorrhage is necessary.

PREOPERATIVE CONSIDERATIONS

Depending on the time of presentation and referral, most infants require surgical consultation with neurosurgical and plastic reconstructive services, as many of the described procedures are completed jointly with both surgical services contributing their expertise. These patients also require additional medical workup to optimize comorbid conditions prior to presentation to the operating room. Laboratory testing should include a complete blood count and type and screen at a minimum. If the anticipated blood loss will be significant, such as with open procedures, a type and cross match should be performed. The utility of obtaining a baseline coagulation profile may depend on whether syndromic synostosis is present or if a family history of bleeding disorders is present, and this varies by institution.

SPECIAL ANESTHETIC CONCERNS
Positioning

Minimally invasive techniques can take 2 to 4 hours; however, the more complex surgical procedures may take more than 5 hours to complete. Because of the prolonged nature of many of these procedures, strict attention to positioning and eye protection must be considered. Pressure points must be addressed whether the patient is supine or prone. Some syndromic patients may present with severe proptosis, and a strategy must be devised to keep the cornea moist if the surgeon prefers the eyes not be covered. At this author's institution, it is standard practice for the surgeon to place corneal protectors after ophthalmic ointment is used for any patient in the supine position. Some surgeons may request the eye not be covered at all, and frequent repeat application of an ophthalmic ointment is necessary. This helps to prevent desiccation and direct injury to the cornea. If the patient is prone, a horseshoe head holder is typically used, and the anesthesiologist must make sure the eyes are free from pressure. Frequent checking of the eyes is recommended during long cases in the prone position, as the surgical manipulation can cause significant head movement within the horseshoe head holder.

Venous Air Embolism

Venous air embolism (VAE) can happen anytime the operative field is above the level of the heart and a negative pressure gradient is created with an open venous system (ie, exposed dural sinus or cranial bone edge). VAE is on the differential diagnostic list for hemodynamic collapse and cardiac arrest in a patient undergoing craniofacial surgery.[15] One study of 32 patients showed the incidence, as detected by precordial Doppler ultrasound, to be 83%; however, most were of little hemodynamic significance.[16] Minimally invasive strip craniectomy has a lower incidence of VAE than open procedures based on 1 cohort of infants and neonates.[17] A low incidence of VAE during endoscopic strip craniectomy was again confirmed in a 2011 retrospective review over 5 years at a single institution. There was no change in clinical outcomes from the 2 patients who experienced VAE.[18]

Hypothermia

Hypothermia is defined by a core body temperature less than 35°C. Many factors influence the core body temperature of an infant during anesthesia including inhaled anesthetic effect, cold operating rooms, surgical irrigation with cold fluids, large volume resuscitation with room temperature crystalloids or colloids, and relatively large head to body surface area. Bleeding and increased transfusion risk are increased even with mild hypothermia (36°C).[19] A recent prospective cohort of pediatric patients revealed an incidence of 46.6% despite both active and passive warming techniques being deployed.[20] Active warming techniques include a warm operating room, radiant heat lamps, forced air convection warming devices, warm water mattresses, electronic warming blankets, and fluid warmers. Preoperative preparation to prevent intraoperative hypothermia is paramount in this population given the significant risk of hemorrhage and long duration of exposure.

Elevated Intracranial Pressure

Intracranial hypertension is one of the indications for proceeding with corrective surgery. Some children may present with intracranial hypertension to the operating room and standard precautions to limit spikes in ICP should be taken. In infants, elevated

ICP may be difficult to assess without an ophthalmologic examination or evidence seen on preoperative CT scan. Intracranial hypertension can be present in single suture craniosynostosis; however, it is more common among children with syndromic craniosynostosis, 14% and 47%, respectively.[21] In older children, signs and symptoms of elevated ICP may be nonspecific. Some may complain of headaches or other vague neurologic symptoms. A more recent retrospective study supports a higher incidence (44%) of elevated ICP in patients with isolated sagittal synostosis than previously reported.[22] In most patients presenting for corrective surgery, an inhalational induction is appropriate while keeping in mind the modifiable parameters for controlling ICP.

Hemorrhage

Acute massive hemorrhage is a risk during all surgical techniques to correct craniosynostosis because of the presence of underlying dural venous sinuses. However, the large scalp incisions, craniotomies, and multiple exposed surfaces found in complex procedures can lead to continuous and sustained blood loss over time. Blood loss of 20% to 500% of calculated circulating volume has been described.[23–26] The anesthesiologist must be prepared with a strategy to minimize loss and replace blood volume when necessary.

ANESTHETIC MANAGEMENT
Monitors

Detailed physiologic monitoring is critical during surgery for craniosynostosis. The early detection and treatment of intraoperative events such as massive hemorrhage are essential. Along with the standard American Society of Anesthesiologists (ASA) monitors, several additional monitoring systems may be considered, but ultimately the watchful and involved anesthesiologist remains the lynch pin for the care of these children.

Arterial catheters and pressure monitoring
For minimally invasive procedures where overall blood loss is less, an arterial catheter is not always necessary. However, there is still risk for serious acute hemorrhage from inadvertent puncture of dural sinuses and depending on the patient's comorbidities, an arterial catheter may be warranted. For complex cranial vault procedures where overall blood loss may constitute more than a full blood volume, an arterial catheter is standard. Assessment of volume status through electronic analysis of arterial waveforms is established in the adult critical care and operating room settings. The body of supportive evidence for arterial waveform analysis in infants and children is lacking.[27,28]

Central venous catheters and pressure monitoring
Routine placement of central venous catheters varies by institution. It is not common practice to place central venous catheters at the author's institution unless peripheral venous access is difficult to obtain, or the patient's underlying comorbidities place the patient at a potentially higher likelihood of requiring inotropic or vasopressor support. Depending on the size, central venous catheters may not be a replacement for large-bore peripheral venous access during massive hemorrhage. Central venous pressure monitoring remains a poor method for evaluating fluid responsiveness in adults.[29,30] In 2013, Stricker and colleagues[31] demonstrated that routine CVP monitoring during complex craniofacial surgery in children did not result in a decreased incidence or duration of hypotension, but that deviations of CVP below baseline were common

and most often not associated with hypotension. Based on the available data, the utility of central venous pressure monitoring is low, and central venous catheter placement should be reserved for patients with difficult peripheral access or patients with the anticipated need for pharmacologic cardiovascular support.

Precordial Doppler
Precordial Doppler, as discussed earlier, is efficacious and reliable at detecting VAE during craniofacial surgery. Its use is dependent on the institution and the availability of the device, and iy is not used regularly by anesthesiologists who care for these patients.[32]

Near infrared spectroscopy
The use of near infrared spectroscopy (NIRS) outside of adult cardiac surgery is an expanding field. The body of literature is increasing in the pediatric congenital cardiac surgery population and in pediatric intensive care units. Hoffman and colleagues[33] described the utility of 2-site (cerebral So2 and somatic So2) NIRS in the early diagnosis and reduction of the shock state in the pediatric intensive care unit. Peripheral oxygen saturation via NIRS was described as an indicator for hypoperfusion in the adult cardiac patient undergoing cardiopulmonary bypass.[34] There is only 1 study evaluating the use of NIRS during craniofacial surgery. This study found NIRS to be a useful, noninvasive monitoring technique for determining cerebral tissue oxygenation and hemodynamic parameters.[35] The risk of massive hemorrhage varies depending on the proposed surgical intervention for craniosynostosis. Somatic and cerebral oximetry may be of value in early detection and intervention of hemorrhagic shock in this patient population. Availability, unfamiliarity, and cost may be limiting factors for the use of NIRS during complex craniofacial surgery.

Intraoperative Considerations

Induction
Induction for most infants proceeds as an inhalational induction with sevoflurane and oxygen with or without nitrous oxide. If nitrous oxide is used during induction of anesthesia, it is recommended to remove it prior to incision because of the ongoing risk of venous air embolism. Syndromic synostosis may be associated with midface hypoplasia (such as Crouzon syndrome or Apert syndrome), and an underlying difficulty with mask ventilation or with airway instrumentation should be anticipated. Patients with Apert syndrome may present with tracheostomy caused by severe upper airway obstruction, which may be used for an inhalational induction.

Venous and arterial access
For less invasive procedures such as the minimally invasive approach, 2 peripheral intravenous catheters are placed, and, depending on comorbid conditions, an arterial line may be considered but is not standard practice at this author's institution. An alternative to invasive arterial pressure monitoring as a method for evaluating global systemic perfusion may include placing a regional (somatic) near infrared spectroscopy (NIRs) patch. Placement of a central venous line may be indicated if the patient is considered at high risk for VAE or there is anticipated need for pharmacologic cardiac support.

Airway
Standard instrumentation of the airway is appropriate for most nonsyndromic craniosynostosis cases. Infants with syndromic synostosis may have underlying difficult airways because of midface hypoplasia. Preparation for suspected difficult airway

should include additional direct laryngoscopy blades, availability of a video laryngoscope, or the presence of flexible fiberoptic bronchoscope. Some patients with syndromic craniosynostosis will present with tracheostomy already in place. Securement of the endotracheal tube is especially important given the multitude of positioning options for any given surgical procedure and the fact that the head of the bed may be turned 90° to 180° away from the anesthesiologist. At this author's institution, a standard oral endotracheal tube is used for most procedures and is secured with a submandibular stitch at the midline, as well as tape and small transparent dressings. RAE tubes are not necessary and may hinder suctioning during the procedure. Loss of airway in the patient with a difficult airway and with the bed rotated has the potential for catastrophe.

Maintenance
Maintenance of anesthesia includes a volatile agent such as sevoflurane, usually paired with bolus or continuous opioid infusion. Remifentanil and sufentanil are the most common options used for opioid infusion. Fentanyl is also an option, but because of its longer context sensitive half-time, may reduce the chance of postsurgical extubation. A dexmedetomidine infusion may be added as an adjunct to other anesthetics.

Extubation
Extubation readiness should always be evaluated at the conclusion of any craniofacial surgery. Positioning, duration of the procedure, large volume resuscitation, presence of a difficult airway, ongoing coagulopathy, acid-base status, the presence of preoperative upper airway obstruction, and temperature are all factors that may influence the anesthesiologist's decision to extubate. Extreme positioning may lead to facial and airway edema that requires postoperative intubation until swelling decreases. If airway edema is suspected, the anesthesiologist should consider doing a leak test prior to proceeding with extubation.

TRANSFUSION MANAGEMENT

Assessment of blood loss and subsequent overall volume status is difficult in complex cranial vault procedures for several reasons. These factors include the use of copious irrigation fluid, saturation of surgical drapes, communication from surgeons, and limitations of the available monitoring equipment. Careful attention to the whole picture, including urine output, arterial/venous blood gas analysis, ongoing surgical blood loss, volume of irrigation used, coagulation profiles, and invasive and noninvasive monitoring devices will help guide the diligent anesthesiologist in the assessment and management of the hypovolemic state frequently seen during these complex procedures. A recent observational study from the Pediatric Craniofacial Collaborative Group found that age of no more than 24 months, ASA status of at least 4. At least III, preoperative anemia, longer surgical times, avoidance of intraoperative antifibrinolytics and cell salvage, and lack of transfusion protocols were factors associated with increased allogenic blood product transfusion.[36] Thrombo-elastography is now a more readily available tool for the anesthesiologist. A study by Hass, and colleagues[37] found that using thrombo-elastography with preset thresholds reduced intra-operative transfusion requirements, which also lead to a calculated mean total cost reduction of 17.1%.

Massive Transfusion
Hypoperfusion from unrecognized hemorrhage may have end-organ consequences; however the aggressive treatment of hypovolemia with crystalloids and various blood

products may also lead to undesired effects such as dilutional anemia, dilutional coagulopathy, transfusion reactions, hypothermia, acidosis, hyperkalemia, and hypocalcemia from citrated blood products.

Dilutional coagulopathy

Dilutional coagulopathy is likely related to both consumption and dilution of clotting factors simultaneously. Fibrinolysis, thrombin generation, and clot firmness are some of the factors affected by dilution.[38] In adults, a loss of approximately 1.14 to 1.42 blood volumes can produce significant coagulopathy (which is dominated by a reduction in fibrinogen) when volume is replaced with crystalloids and PRBCs alone.[39,40] Stricker and colleagues[26] found similar postoperative coagulopathy in a craniofacial surgical population when blood loss was more than one blood volume, and those losses were replaced with crystalloid and PRBCs. A reduction in platelets, however, appears to be a late finding in dilutional coagulopathy.[26] Using donor-matched FFP prophylactically as reconstituted blood has been shown to reduce postoperative surgical drain output and improve postoperative coagulation profiles.[41]

Hyperkalemia

Hyperkalemic cardiac arrest after rapid administration of stored PRBCs has been described.[42,43] In a 2014 literature review, Lee and colleagues[44] found that the rate of transfusion, the site of infusion, and cardiac output were drivers of hyperkalemic arrest, and that measures to reduce the overall risk include anticipating and replacing blood volume before hemodynamic compromise is noted, using larger bore peripheral catheters (>23-gauge) rather than central catheters, using fresh PRBCs, and frequent monitoring of electrolytes. Irradiation also leads to an increase in potassium leakage from red blood cells (RBCs),[45] especially after 7 days.[46,47] In the most recent update from the Wake Up Safe group, when massive hemorrhage is anticipated, the recommendations include administering RBCs that have been washed, reducing the time from irradiation to administration of PRBCs, and PRBCs that are less than 7 day old.[48]

Transfusion Mitigation

Given the nature of large volume blood loss during craniosynostosis surgery, the need for transfusion is always present. Allogenic transfusion carries the risk of infection and alloimmunization. This risk increases with each new donor exposure. Many studies have looked at methods to minimize blood loss during craniofacial surgery, including the use of antifibrinolytics, cell salvage, hemodilution, erythropoietin, fibrinogen concentrates, and reinfusion of shed blood.

Transfusion protocols

The benefit of institutional perioperative transfusion protocols with multidisciplinary input has been well described.[49–54] The benefits of transfusion protocols include a reduction in blood donor exposures, transfusion waste, and transfusion volume. The transfusion protocols described differ by institution, and not all institutions will have access to each described intervention; however, creating a multidisciplinary team to address even some of the issues will likely create benefit moving forward. With the institution of perioperative protocols, some institutions have self-reported limited transfusion-free outcomes.[32] A more recent study reported a transfusion-free rate of 66% at the time of discharge with the implementation of a quality improvement protocol that included preoperative EPO, intraoperative aminocaproic acid, cell saver, and delineation of intraoperative and postoperative resuscitation and transfusion guidelines.[55]

Antifibrinolytic agents

The use of antifibrinolytic agents has been shown to reduce blood loss and transfusion requirements in major pediatric surgery with acceptable adverse effect profiles.[56] Tranexamic acid (TXA), epsilon aminocaproic acid (EACA), and aprotinin have all been studied in the pediatric craniofacial surgery population.[56-58] Tranexamic acid (TXA) has been shown to significantly reduce perioperative blood transfusion in a recent meta-analysis.[59] ε-Aminocaproic acid is another antifibrinolytic agent with the same mechanism of action as TXA. One prospective observational study showed aminocaproic acid reduced blood donor exposures, calculated surgical blood loss, and postoperative surgical drain output.[58] A recent publication showed no difference in postoperative seizure or thromboembolic events in patients who did or did not receive the antifibrinolytic agents TXA or EACA.[60] Antifibrinolytic agents should be considered in craniofacial surgery and appear to have a low incidence of side effects in this population. The low cost and relative ease of administration also make antifibrinolytics desirable for managing hemorrhage in these patients. Caution should be used in patient's deemed at a higher risk for thromboembolic events and may require a multidisciplinary discussion to assess risks and benefits.

Cell salvage techniques

Cell salvage techniques in patients undergoing complex craniofacial surgery have been studied,[61-65] and in a single -center review, there was no difference noted in allogenic blood transfusion rates with or without cell saver in patients undergoing fronto-orbital advancement; howeverm the authors did note that in the cell saver group 25% of patients did not require allogenic transfusion.[66] Other considerations in implementing a cell saver strategy is the potential need for additional personnel to operate the device, which would likely add to the already elevated cost of the machine itself.

Preoperative erythropoietin

Erythropoietin (EPO) induces proliferation and maturation of red blood cells. The use of erythropoietin is established in reducing blood transfusions in infants undergoing craniosynostosis surgery when used in combination with other techniques and therapies.[53,67-70] In 2007, the US Food and Drug Administration issued a black box warning for EPO because of growing evidence of stroke, thrombotic access complications, increased cardiovascular events, and end-stage renal disease (ESRD). In 2016, a multinational cohort study of patients with ESRD receiving erythropoiesis-stimulating agents (ESA) found reportable adverse events ranging from 3.8% to 13.3% (with stroke risk 0.6% to 1.5%) depending on the ESA dose and mean hemoglobin concentration.[71] The need for preoperative clinic visits and the relatively high cost of preoperative EPO therapy may be limiting factors for implementation, and therefore should be addressed on an institutional basis. The use of EPO remains limited.

Other Blood Component Replacement

Whole blood

Whole blood is an alternative therapy in place of reconstituted blood components. Its use may be limited by availability. Fibrin levels and fibrin polymerization were maintained up to 33 days in cold storage based on thrombo-elastography studies; however, the authors did note that although clot formed, it was slow to form and relatively weak in the absence of additional coagulation factors and platelets.[72] Leukocyte reduction filters placed during collection will result in the removal of 99.9% of platelets and leukocytes, which significantly reduces the contribution of whole blood to platelet count and activity. Whole blood has the benefit of potentially reduced the number of blood donor exposures.

Fibrinogen replacement

Fibrinogen can be found in FFP, cryoprecipitate, or as a concentrate. The relative amount of fibrinogen in FFP is low, and the required volume of administration to correct hypofibrinogenemia and its potential detrimental effects needs to be considered in the infant population. Fibrinogen concentrate administered to infants undergoing craniofacial surgery was found to improve fibrinogen polymerization and clot strength based on thrombo-elastography.[73] However, a recent double-blind study evaluating the efficacy of prophylactic high-dose fibrinogen concentrate therapy in complex cranial vault surgery found no reduction in transfusion of blood products or estimated blood loss.[74]

Recombinant activated factor VIIa

Recombinant activated factor VIIa as a rescue for life-threatening hemorrhage during craniofacial surgery has been described by Stricker and colleagues[75] without noted adverse events. Its use is also described in a critically ill infant population, with results showing a decreased need for FFP transfusion and no significant additional risk.[76] A recent review determined the rate of thrombotic events to be low (0.17%) and stable overtime in patients receiving recombinant activated factor VIIa for 1 of the 4 licensed indications. The thrombotic events were associated with older age, cardiovascular disease, and simultaneous use of activated prothrombin complex concentrates.[77]

POSTOPERATIVE MANAGEMENT

Patients who undergo minimally invasive strip craniectomies or spring mediated repairs may be admitted to the postanesthesia care unit and then discharged to the floor depending on the individual's comorbidities. Complex craniofacial surgery patients are admitted to the ICU postoperatively. Recovery time varies between patients, but the typical intensive care unit stay is 1 to 2 days. Patients may need additional transfusion in the postoperative period because of ongoing blood loss. Hyponatremia has been described as well as cerebrospinal fluid leaks and infection.

SUMMARY

Craniofacial surgery in infants and children is a well-studied field. The introduction of less-invasive surgical techniques has led to a reduction in morbidity. A deep understanding of surgical techniques, management of acute massive hemorrhage, and transfusion strategies is crucial in taking care of this pediatric surgical population. Development and implementation of detailed perioperative multidisciplinary transfusion management strategies will reduce blood volume loss, transfusion requirements, number of blood donor exposures, and in some cases result in a transfusion-free perioperative course.

CLINICAL CARE POINTS

- Anesthesiologists must be able to manage acute massive hemorrhage and have a working knowledge of the associated physiologic derangements that accompany it.
- A multidisciplinary perioperative transfusion protocol is recommended to reduce transfusion rates and number of blood donor exposures.

DISCLOSURE

None.

REFERENCES

1. Virchow R. Uever den Cretinismus, namenlich in Franken, und uer pathologische Schadelformen. Verh Phys Med Ges Wurzburg 1851;2:230.
2. Kalantar-Hormozi H, Abbaszadeh-Kasbi A, Sharifi G, et al. Incidence of familial craniosynostosis among patients with nonsyndromic craniosynostosis. J Craniofac Surg 2019;30(6):e514–7.
3. Cornelissen M, Ottelander Bd, Rizopoulos D, et al. Increase of prevalence of craniosynostosis. J Craniomaxillofac Surg 2016;44(9):1273–9.
4. Mathijssen IM. Guideline for care of patients with the diagnoses of craniosynostosis: working group on craniosynostosis. J Craniofac Surg 2015;26(6):1735–807.
5. Johnson D, Wilkie A. Craniosynostosis. Eur J Hum Genet 2011;19(4):369–76.
6. Bir SC, Ambekar S, Notarianni C, et al. Odilon marc lannelongue (1840-1911) and strip craniectomy for craniosynostosis. Neurosurg Focus 2014;36(4):E16.
7. Kaufman BA, Muszynski CA, Matthews A, et al. The circle of sagittal synostosis surgery. Semin Pediatr Neurol 2004;11(4):243–8.
8. Jane JA, Edgerton MT, Futrell JW, et al. Immediate correction of sagittal synostosis. J Neurosurg 1978;49(5):705–10.
9. Jimenez DF, Barone CM. Endoscopic craniectomy for early surgical correction of sagittal craniosynostosis. J Neurosurg 1998;88(1):77–81.
10. Jimenez DF, McGinity MJ, Barone CM. Endoscopy-assisted early correction of single-suture metopic craniosynostosis: a 19-year experience. J Neurosurg Pediatr 2018;23(1):61–74.
11. Jimenez DF, Barone CM. Multiple-suture nonsyndromic craniosynostosis: early and effective management using endoscopic techniques. J Neurosurg Pediatr 2010;5(3):223–31.
12. Lauritzen C, Sugawara Y, Kocabalkan O, et al. Spring mediated dynamic craniofacial reshaping. Case Report. Scand J Plast Reconstr Surg Hand Surg 1998;32(3):331–8.
13. Lauritzen CG, Davis C, Ivarsson A, et al. The evolving role of springs in craniofacial surgery: the first 100 clinical cases. Plast Reconstr Surg 2008;121(2):545–54.
14. Windh P, Davis C, Sanger C, et al. Spring-assisted cranioplasty vs pi-plasty for sagittal synostosis–a long term follow-up study. J Craniofac Surg 2008;19(1):59–64.
15. Salam AA, Khan FA. Cardiac arrest in a child following cranioplasty. J Pak Med Assoc 2013;63(10):1307–8.
16. Faberowski LW, Black S, Mickle JP. Incidence of venous air embolism during craniectomy for craniosynostosis repair. Anesthesiology 2000;92(1):20–3.
17. Tobias JD, Johnson JO, Jimenez DF, et al. Venous air embolism during endoscopic strip craniectomy for repair of craniosynostosis in infants. Anesthesiology 2001;95(2):340–2.
18. Meier PM, Goobie SM, DiNardo JA, et al. Endoscopic strip craniectomy in early infancy: the initial five years of anesthesia experience. Anesth Analg 2011;112(2):407–14.
19. Rajagopalan S, Mascha E, Na J, et al. The effects of mild perioperative hypothermia on blood loss and transfusion requirement. Anesthesiology 2008;108(1):71–7.

20. Lai LL, See MH, Rampal S, et al. Significant factors influencing inadvertent hypothermia in pediatric anesthesia. J Clin Monit Comput 2019;33(6):1105–12.
21. Renier D, Sainte-Rose C, Marchac D, et al. Intracranial pressure in craniostenosis. J Neurosurg 1982;57(3):370–7.
22. Swanson JW, Xu W, Ying GS, et al. Intracranial pressure patterns in children with craniosynostosis utilizing optical coherence tomography. Childs Nerv Syst 2020; 36(3):535–44.
23. Chow I, Purnell CA, Gosain AK. Assessing the impact of blood loss in cranial vault remodeling: a risk assessment model using the 2012 to 2013 pediatric national surgical quality improvement program data sets. Plast Reconstr Surg 2015; 136:1249–60.
24. Bonfield CM, Sharma J, Cochrane DD, et al. Minimizing blood transfusions in the surgical correction of craniosynostosis: a 10-year single-center experience. Childs Nerv Syst 2016;32:143–51.
25. Steinbok P, Heran N, Hicdonmez T, et al. Minimizing blood transfusions in the surgical correction of coronal and metopic craniosynostosis. Childs Nerv Syst 2004; 20:445–52.
26. Stricker PA, Shaw TL, Desouza DG, et al. Blood loss, replacement, and associated morbidity in infants and children undergoing craniofacial surgery. Paediatr Anaesth 2010;20(2):150–9.
27. Pereira de Souza Neto E, Grousson S, Duflo F, et al. Predicting fluid responsiveness in mechanically ventilated children under general anaesthesia using dynamic parameters and transthoracic echocardiography. Br J Anaesth 2011; 106(6):856–64.
28. Gan H, Cannesson M, Chandler JR, et al. Predicting fluid responsiveness in children: a systematic review. Anesth Analg 2013;117(6):1380–92.
29. Marik PE, Baram M, Vahid B. Does central venous pressure predict fluid responsiveness? A systematic review of the literature and the tale of seven mares. Chest 2008;134(1):172–8.
30. Marik PE, Cavallazzi R. Does the central venous pressure predict fluid responsiveness? An updated meta-analysis and a plea for some common sense. Crit Care Med 2013;41(7):1774–81.
31. Stricker PA, Lin EE, Fiadjoe JE, et al. Evaluation of central venous pressure monitoring in children undergoing craniofacial reconstruction surgery. Anesth Analg 2013;116(2):411–9.
32. Stricker PA, Cladis FP, Fiadjoe JE, et al. Perioperative management of children undergoing craniofacial reconstruction surgery: a practice survey. Paediatr Anaesth 2011;21(10):1026–35.
33. Hoffman GM, Ghanayem NS, Berens RJ, et al. Reduction in critical indicators of shock by routine use of two-site NIRS in pediatric ICU patients. Anesthesiology 2006;105:A803.
34. Lee YS, Kim WY, Yoo JW, et al. Correlation between regional tissue perfusion saturation and lactate level during cardiopulmonary bypass. Korean J Anesthesiol 2018;71(5):361–7.
35. Martini M, Röhrig A, Wenghoefer M, et al. Cerebral oxygenation and hemodynamic measurements during craniosynostosis surgery with near-infrared spectroscopy. Childs Nerv Syst 2014;30(8):1367–74.
36. Fernandez PG, Taicher BM, Goobie SM, et al. Pediatric craniofacial collaborative group. Predictors of transfusion outcomes in pediatric complex cranial vault reconstruction: a multicentre observational study from the pediatric craniofacial collaborative group. Can J Anaesth 2019;66(5):512–26.

37. Haas T, Goobie S, Spielmann N, et al. Improvements in patient blood management for pediatric craniosynostosis surgery using a ROTEM(®) -assisted strategy - feasibility and costs. Paediatr Anaesth 2014;24(7):774–80.

38. Bolliger D, Gorlinger K, Tanaka KA. Pathophysiology and treatment of coagulopathy in massive hemorrhage and hemodilution. Anesthesiology 2010;113: 1205–19.

39. Hiippala ST, Myllylä GJ, Vahtera EM. Hemostatic factors and replacement of major blood loss with plasma-poor red cell concentrates. Anesth Analg 1995;81(2): 360–5.

40. Murray DJ, Pennell BJ, Weinstein SL, et al. Packed red cells in acute blood loss: dilutional coagulopathy as a cause of surgical bleeding. Anesth Analg 1995; 80(2):336–42.

41. Stricker PA, Fiadjoe JE, Davis AR, et al. Reconstituted blood reduces blood donor exposures in children undergoing craniofacial reconstruction surgery. Paediatr Anaesth 2011;21:54–61.

42. Brown KA, Bissonnette B, McIntyre B. Hyperkalaemia during rapid blood transfusion and hypovolaemic cardiac arrest in children. Can J Anaesth 1990;37(7): 747–54.

43. Bhananker SM, Ramamoorthy C, Geiduschek JM, et al. Anesthesia-related cardiac arrest in children: update from the pediatric perioperative cardiac arrest registry. Anesth Analg 2007;105:344–50.

44. Lee AC, Reduque LL, Luban NL, et al. Transfusion-associated hyperkalemic cardiac arrest in pediatric patients receiving massive transfusion. Transfusion 2014; 54(1):244–54.

45. Brugnara C, Churchill WH. Effect of irradiation on red cell cation content and transport. Transfusion 1992;32(3):246–52.

46. Hillyer CD, Tiegerman KO, Berkman EM. Evaluation of the red cell storage lesion after irradiation in filtered packed red cell units. Transfusion 1991;31(6):497–9.

47. Olivo RA, da Silva MV, Garcia FB, et al. Evaluation of the effectiveness of packed red blood cell irradiation by a linear accelerator. Rev Bras Hematol Hemoter 2015;37(3):153–9.

48. Wake up Safe. January 27, 2015. Available at: http://wakeupsafe.org/wp-content/uploads/2018/10/Hyperkalemia_statement.pdf. Accessed October 5, 2020.

49. Kelley JP, Boville BM, Sterken DJ, et al. Pediatric blood management protocol in cranial vault surgery. J Craniofac Surg 2019;30(6):1734–7.

50. Vega RA, Lyon C, Kierce JF, et al. Minimizing transfusion requirements for children undergoing craniosynostosis repair: the CHoR protocol. J Neurosurg Pediatr 2014;14(2):190–5.

51. Reddy SK, Volpi-Abadie J, Gordish-Dressman H, et al. Optimizing perioperative red blood cell utilization and wastage in pediatric craniofacial surgery. J Craniofac Surg 2020;31(6):1743–6.

52. Nguyen TT, Hill S, Austin TM, et al. Use of blood-sparing surgical techniques and transfusion algorithms: association with decreased blood administration in children undergoing primary open craniosynostosis repair. J Neurosurg Pediatr 2015;16(5):556–63.

53. Escher PJ, Tu AD, Kearney SL, et al. A protocol of situation-dependent transfusion, erythropoietin and tranexamic acid reduces transfusion in fronto-orbital advancement for metopic and coronal craniosynostosis. Childs Nerv Syst 2020. https://doi.org/10.1007/s00381-020-04654-y.

54. Escher PJ, Tu A, Kearney S, et al. Minimizing transfusion in sagittal craniosynostosis surgery: the Children's Hospital of Minnesota Protocol. Childs Nerv Syst 2019;35(8):1357–62.

55. Kurlander DE, Ascha M, Marshall DC, et al. Impact of multidisciplinary engagement in a quality improvement blood conservation protocol for craniosynostosis. J Neurosurg Pediatr 2020;1–9. https://doi.org/10.3171/2020.4.PEDS19633.

56. Basta MN, Stricker PA, Taylor JA. A systematic review of the use of antifibrinolytic agents in pediatric surgery and implications for craniofacial use. Pediatr Surg Int 2012;28(11):1059–69.

57. Ahmed Z, Stricker L, Rozzelle A, et al. Aprotinin and transfusion requirements in pediatric craniofacial surgery. Paediatr Anaesth 2014;24(2):141–5.

58. Hsu G, Taylor JA, Fiadjoe JE, et al. Aminocaproic acid administration is associated with reduced perioperative blood loss and transfusion in pediatric craniofacial surgery. Acta Anaesthesiol Scand 2016;60(2):158–65.

59. Lu VM, Goyal A, Daniels DJ. Tranexamic acid decreases blood transfusion burden in open craniosynostosis surgery without operative compromise. J Craniofac Surg 2019;30(1):120–6.

60. Goobie SM, Cladis FP, Glover CD, et al. Safety of antifibrinolytics in cranial vault reconstructive surgery: a report from the pediatric craniofacial collaborative group [published correction appears in Paediatr Anaesth 2017 Jun;27(6):670. Gries, Heike [added]; Meier, Petra [added]; Haberkern, Charlie [added]; Nguyen, Thanh [added]; Benzon, Hubert [added]]. Paediatr Anaesth 2017; 27(3):271–81.

61. Krajewski K, Ashley RK, Pung N, et al. Successful blood conservation during craniosynostotic correction with dual therapy using procrit and cell saver. J Craniofac Surg 2008;19:101–5.

62. Dahmani S, Orliaguet GA, Meyer PG, et al. Perioperative blood salvage during surgical correction of craniosynostosis in infants. Br J Anaesth 2000;85:550–5.

63. Fearon JA. Reducing allogenic blood transfusions during pediatric cranial vault surgical procedures: a prospective analysis of blood recycling. Plast Reconstr Surg 2004;113:1126–30.

64. Jimenez DF, Barone CM. Intraoperative autologous blood transfusion in the surgical correction of craniosynostosis. Neurosurgery 1995;37:1075–9.

65. Orliaguet GA, Bruyere M, Meyer PG, et al. Comparison of perioperative blood salvage and postoperative reinfusion of drained blood during surgical correction of craniosynostosis in infants. Paediatr Anaesth 2003;13:797–804.

66. Duncan C, Richardson D, May P, et al. Reducing blood loss in synostosis surgery: the Liverpool experience. J Craniofac Surg 2008;19(5):1424–30.

67. Meneghini L, Zadra N, Aneloni V, et al. Erythropoeitin therapy and acute preoperative normovolaemic haemodilution in infants undergoing craniosynostosis surgery. Paediatr Anaesth 2003;13:392–6.

68. Fearon JA, Weinthal J. The use of recombinant erythropoietin in the reduction of blood transfusion rates in craniosynostosis repair in infants and children. Plast Reconstr Surg 2002;109:2190–6.

69. Helfaer MA, Carson BS, James CS, et al. Increased hematocrit and decreased transfusion requirements in children given erythropoietin before undergoing craniofacial surgery. J Neurosurg 1998;88:704–8.

70. Aljaaly HA, Aldekhayel SA, Diaz-Abele J, et al. Effect of erythropoietin on transfusion requirements for craniosynostosis surgery in children. J Craniofac Surg 2017;28(5):1315–9.

71. Lammerich A, Balcke P, Bias P, et al. Cardiovascular morbidity and pure red cell aplasia associated with epoetin theta therapy in patients with chronic kidney disease: a prospective, noninterventional, multicenter cohort study. Clin Ther 2016; 38(2):276–87.e4.
72. Iwata S, Hirasaki Y, Nomura M, et al. Thromboelastometric evaluation of coagulation profiles of cold-stored autologous whole blood: a prospective observational study. Medicine (Baltimore) 2019;98(39):e17357.
73. Haas T, Fries D, Velik-Salchner C, et al. Fibrinogen in craniosynostosis surgery. Anesth Analg 2008;106(3):725–31, table of contents.
74. Machotta A, Huisman EJ, Appel IM, et al. Prophylactic fibrinogen concentrate administration in surgical correction of paediatric craniosynostosis. Eur J Anaesthesiol 2020. https://doi.org/10.1097/EJA.0000000000001332.
75. Stricker PA, Petersen C, Fiadjoe JE, et al. Successful treatment of intractable hemorrhage with recombinant factor VIIa during cranial vault reconstruction in an infant. Paediatr Anaesth 2009;19:806–7.
76. Dang CN, Katakam LI, Smith PB, et al. Recombinant activated factor VIIa treatment for refractory hemorrhage in infants. J Perinatol 2011;31(3):188–92.
77. Rajpurkar M, Croteau SE, Boggio L, et al. Thrombotic events with recombinant activated factor VII (rFVIIa) in approved indications are rare and associated with older age, cardiovascular disease, and concomitant use of activated prothrombin complex concentrates (aPCC). J Blood Med 2019;10:335–40.

Anesthetic Management of Asleep and Awake Craniotomy for Supratentorial Tumor Resection

Yifan Xu, MD, PhD*, Kamila Vagnerova, MD

KEYWORDS

- Supratentorial tumor resection • Craniotomy • Awake craniotomy
- Neuroanesthesia • Intracranial perfusion management

KEY POINTS

- Because of compensatory changes within the fixed skull, there is often increased intracranial pressure and decreased cerebral perfusion pressure by the time supratentorial tumors are symptomatic.
- Hemodynamic monitoring and neuromonitoring can help ensure adequate cerebral perfusion; new methods of noninvasive cerebral perfusion monitoring have been developed with variable evidence of benefit.
- For patients who meet criteria, awake craniotomies remain the standard of care for tumor resection near eloquent brain regions.
- Perioperative multimodal pain control and intraoperative anesthetic adjuncts are active areas of investigation toward long-term neuroprotection and decreased mortality.

INTRODUCTION

In the United States, primary brain tumors, arising from components of the central nervous system (CNS), are among the most difficult cancers to treat, with an overall 5-year survival no greater than 35%.[1] Between 2012 and 2016, approximately 30.2% and 69.8% of CNS tumors were malignant and nonmalignant, respectively. Glioblastomas lead as the most common malignant tumor type (14.6% of all tumors and 48.3% of malignant tumors), and meningiomas remained the most common nonmalignant tumor type (37.6% of all tumors and 53.3% of nonmalignant tumors). Demographically, glioblastoma was more common in men, and meningioma was more common in women.[2] CNS tumors had an annual mortality of 4.42 per 100,000, and an average of 18,000 deaths per year, with glioblastoma having the lowest 5-year

Department of Anesthesiology and Perioperative Medicine, Oregon Health and Science University, 3181 Southwest Sam Jackson Park Road, Mail Code UH2, Portland, OR 97239, USA
* Corresponding author.
E-mail address: xyi@ohsu.edu

Anesthesiology Clin 39 (2021) 71–92
https://doi.org/10.1016/j.anclin.2020.11.007
1932-2275/21/© 2020 Elsevier Inc. All rights reserved.
anesthesiology.theclinics.com

survival rate at 6.8%.[2] Most primary CNS tumors are supratentorial and may not be discovered until compensatory mechanisms are compromised.[1]

Understanding how anesthetics impact cerebral physiology, cerebral blood flow, brain metabolism, brain relaxation, and neurologic recovery is crucial for optimizing intraoperative and postoperative care during supratentorial craniotomies. Intraoperative goals for supratentorial tumor resection include maintaining cerebral perfusion pressure (CPP) and cerebral autoregulation, optimizing surgical access and neuromonitoring, and facilitating rapid, cooperative emergence.[3-5] Evidence-based studies increasingly expand the impact of anesthetic care beyond immediate perioperative care into both preoperative optimization and minimizing postoperative consequences. New evidence is needed for the role of neuroanesthesia in neurooncology, to prevent conversion from acute to chronic pain, and to decrease the risk of intraoperative ischemia and postoperative delirium. In this review, the authors use the most recent experimental evidence to discuss neuroanesthesia's role in improving patients' outcome and quality of life after resection of supratentorial tumors.

PATHOPHYSIOLOGY OF CEREBRAL PERFUSION, INTRACRANIAL PRESSURE, AND BLOOD-BRAIN BARRIER

The fixed space of the cranial vault enables neurophysiology and brain homeostasis to be expressed as an elegant set of theoretic equations, upon which traditional neuroanesthesia principles are based.

1. The Monro-Kellie doctrine best summarizes this relationship by stating that the additive volumes of cerebrospinal fluid (CSF), brain matter, and intracranial blood must be constant.[5] Because pressure is inversely correlated with volume in a fixed space, ICP is increased when an expanding supratentorial mass shares the cranium with the brain, cerebral blood, and CSF. Although rapidly enlarging masses (such as expanding hematomas) can cause imminent disaster within the skull and represent neurosurgical emergency, slowly growing masses are accommodated by decreasing the intracranial volume of CSF and blood before ICP elevates significantly. A gradual growth in tumor size in the classic pressure-volume curve shows little ICP change (**Fig. 1**, left of the inflection point). However, once the compensatory limit is reached (see **Fig. 1**, right of inflection point), even a small

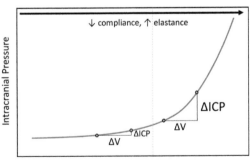

Intracranial Volume

Fig. 1. Hyperbolic ICP-volume curve. Increase in intracranial volume left of the inflection point (*dotted line*) results in small ICP increase. Same increase in intracranial volume right of inflection point results in a large ICP increase. Elastance = ΔPressure/ΔVolume; Compliance = ΔVolume/Δpressure. ΔV, ΔVolume. (*Data from* Bruder N, Ravussin PA. Chapter 11: Supratentorial masses: anesthetic considerations. In: Cottrell JE, Young WL, eds. Cottrell and Young's Neuroanesthesia, 5th ed. Philadelphia: Elsevier; 2010: 184-202.)

increase in volume results in a significant elevation of the ICP.[5] Rapidly growing gliomas surrounded by vasogenic edema can double their volume within weeks, pushing the limits of compensatory mechanisms of brain compliance.

2. CPP equals the difference between mean arterial pressure (MAP) and ICP, or central venous pressure (CVP), whichever is higher. CPP = MAP − ICP (if ICP > CVP), CPP = MAP − CVP (if ICP < CVP).

3. Cushing reflex describes the physiologic response to increased ICP by elevation of systemic MAP to preserve cerebral perfusion. Hemodynamically, this manifests as systolic hypertension with widening pulse pressure, reflexive bradycardia, and decreased, irregular respirations owing to brainstem compression.[5] The presence of Cushing reflex is a neurosurgical emergency. Most strategies in neuroanesthesia revolve around maintaining CPP in the environment of increased ICP, while preventing major changes in MAP that could potentially result in brain edema, bleeding, herniation, or ischemia.

4. Cerebral autoregulation generates a stable cerebral blood flow (CBF) to meet the requirements of cerebral metabolism regardless of changing systemic blood pressure and CPP.[6,7] Indeed, the concept of neurovascular bundling demonstrates the intimate relationship between neuron metabolism and blood supply.[8] Neurons, requiring glucose for metabolic maintenance, are the first to die with prolonged anoxia or decreased energy supply. Functional autoregulation allows for wide CPP range, most commonly 70 to 90 mm Hg, traditionally 50 to 150 mm Hg, with significant variability in the lower limit between individuals and between studies.[6,9] CBF is maintained by the changes in cerebral vasomotor tone (with increasing tone corresponding to increasing cerebrovascular resistance) at the level of the cerebral arteriole (**Fig. 2**). CBF is influenced by Pao_2, $Paco_2$ levels, cerebral metabolic rate (CMR), systemic blood pressure, blood viscosity, and ICP.[10,11] CPP fluctuates with changes in MAP and ICP. If autoregulation is intact, tissue perfusion decreases only once MAP drops to less than 40 or 50 mm Hg.[5] Total brain ischemia is estimated to occur at CBF less than 20 mL/100 g/min.[5]

Is There an Ideal Intraoperative Cerebral Perfusion Pressure?

Optimal intraoperative MAP goal remains a matter of debate. Studies for noncraniotomy surgery have demonstrated that time spent in absolute intraoperative MAP less

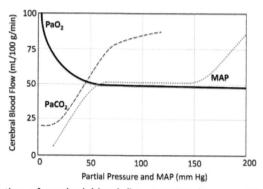

Fig. 2. Autoregulation of cerebral blood flow to MAP between 50 and 150 mm Hg. Decreasing blood flow to increased Pao_2, decreased $Paco_2$, and decreasing MAP. (*Data from* Bruder N, Ravussin PA. Chapter 11: Supratentorial masses: anesthetic considerations. In: Cottrell JE, Young WL, eds. Cottrell and Young's Neuroanesthesia, 5th ed. Philadelphia: Elsevier; 2010: 184-202.)

than 55 to 65 mm Hg or a relative intraoperative MAP less than 20% of baseline has been correlated with increased myocardial infarction and acute kidney injury.[12,13] However, traumatic brain injury literature has shown that, after trauma, a significantly higher MAP is required to maintain CPP because of increased ICP.[14]

Hypertension remodels cerebral artery structure and function. During low perfusion states, vessel lumens accustomed to hypertension mechanically collapse and decrease CBP. Hypertension decreases myogenic reactivity and reduces endothelial response to vasodilatory and vasoconstricting factors, such as nitric oxide and epoxyeicosatrienoic acids.[15] Vascular responses to calcium-activated K+ channels, mechanoreceptor TRPV4, and reactive oxygen species become dysfunctional.[15] Chronic systemic hypertension impairs the renin-angiotensin-aldosterone system and likely impairs cerebral autoregulation by shifting the perfusion curve to the right.[5,16] Autoregulation is thus a complex process, not only with significant study-to-study variability but also with evidence in dramatic contrast to cerebral autoregulation dogma.[9,17]

Intraoperatively, cerebral autoregulation is further impaired by high-dose volatile anesthetics that dilate cerebral vasculature. Intravenous (IV) anesthetics tend to leave autoregulation and $Paco_2$ reactivity intact.[5] Aside from global brain dysregulation from increased ICP and chronic hypertension, the local tumor environment impairs the blood-brain barrier (BBB) by inflammation, oxidative stress, and vasoactive circulating molecules, resulting in loss of autoregulation by $Paco_2$ and MAP.[16] To maintain a continuous energy and oxygen supply that matches the delicate needs of neurons, neuroanesthesia has evolved to optimize CPP, ICP, and CBF. More evidence is needed to see if such intraoperative management offers long-term neuroprotection.

SURGICAL CONSIDERATIONS

Supratentorial brain tumors are often diagnosed after onset of symptoms, such as headaches, vision changes, sensorimotor deficits, or seizures. The symptoms arise from local tumor growth and invasion, increased local pressure, and increased pressure on the brain tissue. Neuroimaging studies, such as computed tomography MRI, will demonstrate a mass frequently surrounded by a halo of vasogenic edema.

Surgical Field Optimization

The role of the anesthesiologist is to optimize conditions for surgical exposure while preventing secondary intracranial and systemic insults (**Table 1**). Hemodynamic stability is of utmost importance during the stimulating events of induction, intubation, surgical head pinning, craniotomy, and dural opening. There may be some prolonged nonstimulating episodes as well, such as correlation of navigational probes between the patient's head and prior volumetric imaging. Brain relaxation should be achieved before dural opening to facilitate surgical access. Emergence and extubation should be ideally smooth, minimizing ICP elevation and allowing for early neurologic assessment.

Brain Relaxation, Blood-Brain Barrier, and Edema

Reducing brain volume through "brain relaxation" facilitates surgical access by neurosurgeons and decreases the amount of retraction needed.

1. The most commonly used osmodiuretic agents are mannitol and hypertonic saline. Mannitol has been used in practice for more than 50 years.[18] Dosing varies from 0.25 to 1 g/kg; 0.5 g/kg has been shown to provide sufficient surgical brain relaxation during supratentorial tumors resection for about 2 to 3 hours.[19] Furthermore, the rheologic effect of mannitol facilitates tissue perfusion. However, massive diuresis can lead

Table 1 Preventable secondary insults to compromised brain tissue		
Secondary Brain Damage	Increased Intracranial Pressure	*Midline shift*: cerebral vessel tearing, hemorrhage *Herniation*: subfalcine, transtentorial, uncal, tonsillar, extracranial
	Inflammation and bleeding:	Epilepsy Vasospasm
Secondary hemodynamic changes:	Hypercapnia Hypoxemia Blood pressure changes: hypotension or hypertension Blood electrolyte changes: hypoosmolality or hyperosmolality Blood glucose changes: hypoglycemia or hyperglycemia Cardiac: decreased output, conduction changes, decreased ejection fraction Hyperthermia	

Data from Bruder N, Ravussin PA. Chapter 11: Supratentorial masses: anesthetic considerations. In: Cottrell JE, Young WL, eds. Cottrell and Young's Neuroanesthesia, 5th ed. Philadelphia: Elsevier; 2010: 184-202.

to impaired tissue perfusion and even to hypoperfusion-related organ injury. Adequate fluid resuscitation guided by goal-directed therapy may help optimize intravascular volume replacement.

Multiple studies demonstrated that hypertonic saline may achieve similar, if not better, brain relaxation without the danger of hypoperfusion.[20,21] There is also increasing evidence that hypertonic saline offers better ICP control than mannitol.[22] One metaanalysis of 9 randomized clinical trials (RCTs) confirmed the superiority of equiosmolar hypertonic saline compared with mannitol for surgical brain relaxation.[23]

Contrary to popular belief, 3% hypertonic saline can be safely administered via peripheral IV in incremental boluses of 100 to 150 mL as well as continuous infusions up to 50 mL/h[24,25] Interestingly, in a recent prospective randomized study, a large dose of 3% NaCl (5 mL/kg) was not more effective than the lower dose of 3 mL/kg for brain relaxation.[26] Adding furosemide to potentiate osmotic diuresis with hypertonic saline has marginal benefit that is not present in combination with mannitol.[27]

2. Hyperventilation is routinely used to achieve surgical brain relaxation.[10] Cerebral vasculature changes tone in response to $Paco_2$ levels. This property is independent of adrenergic stimulation despite copious vascular innervation by the autonomic nervous system.[28] There is an approximately linear relationship between CBF and acute $Paco_2$ change, 1% to 6% alteration in CBF for every 1 mm Hg of $Paco_2$ within the range of 20 to 80 mm Hg (see **Fig. 2**).[28] Extracellular pH, as well as changes in intracellular pH, plays a role in the vasomotor reactivity to $Paco_2$.[29] However, severe hyperventilation can lower jugular venous oxygen saturation and needs to be used with caution.[30] In addition, although the lower limit $Paco_2$ is yet to be established, $Paco_2$ less than 30 mm Hg can result in drastic cerebral vasoconstriction and decreased cerebral perfusion, which has correlated with global ischemia using indirect cerebral oximetry monitors.[31]

3. Optimal hemoglobin (Hgb) or hematocrit levels for blood rheology and O_2 carrying capacity are a topic outside the scope of this article. In terms of maintaining blood osmolarity and brain metabolism, normoglycemia should be maintained because both hypoglycemia and hyperglycemia are correlated with detrimental neurologic outcomes. The NICE-SUGAR trial set a reasonable goal for blood glucose at less than

180 mg/dL in critically ill patients.[32] More studies are needed to determine optimal glucose control.

Steroids for Vasogenic Edema

Systemic steroids are frequently administered for vasogenic edema in the preoperative and intraoperative period.[33] The onset of action is slow, and administration should start 24 to 48 hours before an elective surgical procedure to reduce vasogenic edema by the time of the resection.[33] Standard steroid regimen starts with a 10-mg dose of dexamethasone followed by 4 mg every 6 hours, although some studies showed good efficacy and less adverse effects with lower dose of dexamethasone at only 4 mg a day.[33] The benefits of steroid use should always be balanced against their adverse effects, such as increased delirium, agitation, immunologic depression, and endocrine changes.

Cerebrospinal Fluid Drainage

CSF production and circulation are active processes. Intracranial stasis of the CSF caused by obstruction in CSF circulation or absorption can lead to ventriculomegaly and ICP elevation. Placement of an external ventricular drain directly into the lateral ventricle allows for CSF drainage and alleviates pressure. CSF drainage through a lumbar puncture carries the risk of brain herniation with sudden pressure decrease below the foramen magnum.[5]

ANESTHETIC CONSIDERATIONS
Preanesthetic Optimization and Evaluation

In the anesthesia preoperative assessment, a thorough history and physical examination, including a detailed systems review, should be taken to elicit any concerns or comorbidities. All neurologic signs and symptoms should be noted and documented. Preoperative administration of antiepileptic and steroid therapy needs to be communicated with the surgeon. Some patients will benefit from multimodal pain control, such as initiation of gabapentin and acetaminophen, before surgery. As a precaution, providers should review advanced directives with the patient and their family.

Assessment of Risk Factors

Assessment of cardiopulmonary function is important given the fluid shifts that will occur with osmotic diuresis and blood loss, the risk of air embolism, and dysautonomia from surgical manipulation. Pulmonary comorbidities, such as chronic obstructive pulmonary disease and asthma, may interfere with hyperventilation for brain relaxation. In case of neurosurgery for brain metastases, the location and treatment of the primary tumor may have a detrimental effect on cardiopulmonary function.[34] Forty percent of brain tumors originate from primary lung tumors.[35] Chemotherapy, radiation, and prior lung surgery may decrease lung function before brain surgery.

Vascular atherosclerotic disease can predispose the patient to intraoperative myocardial ischemia as well as ischemic stroke, especially if hyperventilation results in cerebrovascular vasoconstriction. High-grade gliomas carry a clinically significant risk of venous thromboembolic event despite perioperative chemoprophylaxis.[36]

Osmotic diuresis with mannitol can lead to acute kidney injury,[37] and using hypertonic saline for brain relaxation instead of mannitol should be highly considered if renal function is compromised.[38] If any preoperative factors suggest the patient is not optimized for elective surgery, a discussion with the surgeon about additional evaluation and medical optimization may improve patient outcome.

Antiepileptics

The surgery exposes brain to surgical trauma, causing localized inflammation and stress, and increases risk of seizures. Administration of prophylactic antiepileptics (AEDs) in seizure-free patients is generally not advised.[39] Lesions with highest risk of seizures are glioneuronal tumors in the frontotemporal or insular regions.[40,41] Low-grade gliomas are surprisingly more likely to present with seizure symptoms compared with high-grade gliomas.[39] Up to 50% of patients with tumor-related seizures respond well to a single AED,[40] and studies on the use of valproic acid and levetiracetam as first-line monotherapies in tumor-related seizures suggest that preoperative AEDs should be continued throughout perioperative period.[39]

INTRAOPERATIVE MANAGEMENT
Vascular Access

Well-running, large-bore, peripheral IVs should be placed for intraoperative infusion of high-osmolarity solutions, fluids, and pressors, and to ensure good flow of IV anesthetics. Central venous access is generally not required, except for procedures with high risk of significant bleeding, pressor requirement, or air embolism.[5]

Induction of Anesthesia

The goal of induction is to avoid increases in ICP by preventing hypoxia, hypercapnia, sympathetic stimulation, and blood pressure changes.[5] The IV agents propofol and etomidate in combination with local anesthetic (lidocaine) and opioid, either in divided doses or as an infusion, are commonly used to induce anesthesia. Nondepolarizing neuromuscular blocking agents, such as rocuronium, vecuronium, and cisatracurium, are considered safe for intracranial procedures as long as they are fully metabolized or reversed prior to the start of evoked potential monitoring.[42] Beta-blockade may be considered an additional adjunct.

Airway Management

A secured airway using endotracheal intubation is preferred for supratentorial craniotomies under general anesthesia. Oropharyngeal access is likely partially obstructed by surgical positioning and head pins, and any potential kinking or dislodging of the endotracheal tube (ETT) should be preemptively prevented before surgical draping.

Fluid Management

Along with volume resuscitation using isoosmolar crystalloid solutions, transfusion threshold is a debated question in neuroanesthesia and beyond the content of this article. A restrictive transfusion threshold (Hgb < 7.4 g/dL; <8 g/dL) had no worse outcomes than liberal transfusion threshold (average Hgb > 8.7, 8–10) in a retrospective study in craniotomies.[43] Indeed, the FOCUS study provided evidence for the overall transfusion guideline to restrict transfusion threshold to Hgb less than 7.[44]

CHOICE OF ANESTHETIC FOR IMPROVED POSTOPERATIVE OUTCOMES AND NEUROPROTECTION

Current perioperative practice is moving toward enhanced recovery after surgery (ERAS) protocols. Unfortunately, because of the diversity of tumor locations and institutional protocols, Hagan and colleagues[45] stated that the "current body of evidence is insufficient to establish a standardized protocol at this time."[4] The first RCT of use of an ERAS protocol included propofol and sufentanil for induction of anesthesia and propofol, fentanyl, and sevoflurane for maintenance. The protocol included goal-directed fluid restriction with cardiac output guidance for hemodynamic management.[46] However, the study did not seek to measure either anesthetic depth or long-term outcomes.

Neuroprotection and Neurotoxicity

Anesthetic-related neurotoxicity has been demonstrated in vulnerable, developing brains of animal models repeatedly exposed to general anesthesia.[47] However, large human clinical trials, such as PANDA and MASK, showed that only successive, prolonged exposures before 3 years of age could possibly be associated with moderate behavioral and learning difficulties.[48,49] Currently, an active area of investigation focuses on the correlation between the anesthetic exposure (especially volatiles), and postoperative cognitive dysfunction (POCD) and delirium in the elderly.[50] Findings in human trials have been contradictory, although a major metaanalysis suggests there is weak evidence that propofol anesthesia results in less POCD than volatile anesthetic in the elderly noncardiac surgery population.[15,51–53]

In young animals, volatile anesthetics provide the most evidence for neurotoxicity. Such putative neurotoxicity may be especially relevant in the supratentorial tumor population: the BBB breakdown from tumor infiltration may render brain tissue to be as vulnerable to volatile anesthetics as the neonate brain before mature BBB formation.[51] Animal studies also showed enduring learning deficits in aged rodents after volatile anesthesia exposure (potentially from chemical toxicity).[51,52]

Delirium

There is strong motivation to decrease postoperative delirium and improve neuroprotection through perioperative protocols. Currently, the choice for total intravenous anesthesia (TIVA), volatile, or a combination of both depends on the anesthesiologist, surgeon, neuromonitoring technique, and patient factors (see **Table 1**).[3,54] Studies have shown that propofol-based anesthesia maintains lower ICP and higher CPP in comparison to anesthesia maintained by volatile agents, and propofol anesthesia is also superior in the reduction of postoperative nausea and vomiting (PONV), patient satisfaction, reduction of postoperative pain, and postanesthesia care unit length of stay, which may be factors confounding the incidence of delirium.[3,54–57] More trials are being done to assess whether intraoperative protocols lead to changes in long-term quality of life, morbidity, and mortality.[58]

Pain Control

The ongoing opioid epidemic, fueled by decades of inappropriate postoperative opioid prescription,[58] has led to increasing overdose, and death by opioid abuse.[59] There has been strong evidence that, in the craniotomy population, inadequate analgesia in the early perioperative period can lead to the conversion of acute postsurgical pain to chronic pain.[60,61] Opioids are associated with hypoventilation and hypercarbia through their sedation effect and are also tied to increases in postoperative nausea and vomiting as well as postoperative delirium.[62] Although current guidelines recommend using multimodal analgesics, opioids still remain a mainstay of postcraniotomy pain treatment.[61,63]

Anesthetic Management of Emergence

Emergence is just as critical as induction and anesthetic maintenance, and a smooth and rapid recovery without increases in MAP or ICP is critical to prevent intracranial hemorrhage and brain compression.[4] Coughing, pain, nausea, shivering, and uncontrolled blood pressure can all increase ICP, and anesthetic management should minimize these symptoms. Current RCTs on whether IV or volatile agents are the best anesthetic for emergence have been equivocal.[4,64,65] Dexmedetomidine has become increasingly popular in nonawake craniotomy anesthetics. However, it is likely that the "manner in which anesthetic is adjusted contributes more to the quality of emergence than the specific agent used."[4] Target-controlled infusion is commonly used for conceptual modeling of infusion rate adjustments to achieve target plasma concentrations and has evidence that it may facilitate rapid emergence when used in conjunction with a bispectral index (BIS) monitor.[4] However, RCTs on the subject have been contradictory.[64,65]

ROLE OF MULTIMODAL PAIN CONTROL AND ANESTHETIC ADJUNCTS
Benzodiazepines

Administration of benzodiazepines before craniotomy is generally not recommended and should be done cautiously because of the risk of sedation leading to hypoventilation, hypercarbia, and increases in ICP.[5] Benzodiazepines can also unmask neurologic deficits and can exacerbate postoperative delirium, especially in the elderly.[66]

Intraoperative Opioids

Several studies tried and failed to provide evidence for superiority of specific anesthetic and opioid combinations during TIVA (propofol-remifentanil vs sevoflurane-sufentanil or thiopental vs propofol) in terms of time to spontaneous ventilation, time to emergence, and postoperative cognitive recovery.[64,65]

Sufentanil and fentanyl can both blunt physiologic responses to head pins and surgical stimulation, but fentanyl has a long context-sensitive half and potential for delayed awakening if poorly timed after prolonged surgery.[5] Remifentanil, with its ultrafast half-life from plasma esterase metabolism and lack of context-dependent half-life, is frequently used as an opioid adjunct for craniotomy because of its ability to promote rapid emergence. However, its rapid offset makes it the biggest culprit for opioid-induced hyperalgesia.[67]

Currently, the consensus is that multimodal analgesic adjuncts are equally important as intraoperative methods for opioid reduction, delirium prevention, and neuroprotection.[67]

Beta-Blockade

In recent literature, a 0.5 mg/kg bolus of esmolol 10 minutes before induction, followed by 0.2 mg/kg/min esmolol infusion, has been shown to decrease propofol and sevoflurane requirements, allowing for earlier extubation in an RCT.[68] Although the mechanism is not well understood, beta-2 receptor blockade may have an antinociceptive effect and decrease arousal by decreasing beta-adrenergic activation. In addition, using esmolol during a laparoscopic procedure decreases levels of inflammatory markers and may protect against surgery-induced inflammation.[69]

Nonsteroidal Anti-inflammatory Drugs

Nonsteroidal anti-inflammatory drugs (NSAIDs) can mitigate hyperalgesic response from opioid-induced hyperalgesia by regulating glutamate release, spinal cord neurotransmitters, and NMDA receptors.[67] However, nonselective NSAIDs are associated with impaired renal function and gastric ulcers, and may be especially unfavorable in craniotomies because of its platelet inhibition effects and subsequent potential for increased postoperative hematomas.[69]

Acetaminophen

Acetaminophen is a COX inhibitor without a known exact mechanism. It is thought to work centrally without NSAID risk profiles.[67] As an opioid-sparing adjunct, it is recommended to start the night before surgery and continue throughout the postoperative course. Current studies do not show an IV versus oral dosing difference.[67,70,71]

Dexmedetomidine

Dexmedetomidine is a highly selective alpha-2 agonist. In the last 10 years, its numerous benefits have led to its increased use intraoperatively. Hemodynamically, it can cause transient hypertension via alpha-1 receptor stimulation if a loading dose is administered too quickly. As a sympatholytic, it promotes hypotension and bradycardia, which can be attenuated with a slow infusion and anticholinergic agents. As an adjunctive analgesia, it can decrease intraoperative and postoperative opioid use and pain intensity, providing an excellent transitional analgesic bridge between intraoperative and postoperative care.[67] In addition, it has anxiolytic effects and decreases emergence delirium, so it can decrease benzodiazepine requirements. Other benefits include reducing the risk of postoperative bleeding from its antihypertensive properties, its antiemetic properties, and its compatibility with intraoperative neuromonitoring. Although dexmedetomidine does not increase ICP, studies in older animals found a decrease in CBF greater than the decrease in CMR. A decreased CBF velocity has also been found in humans.[72] Although this does not support the use of dexmedetomidine in the tenuous neurosurgical brain, it appeared to decrease CBF and CMR equally in later human studies, mimicking the effect of sleep.[5,73,74] Compared with remifentanil, its intraoperative use does not increase extubation time or time to orientation and allows for a fast postoperative neurocognitive examination because of the preservation of the ability to follow verbal commands.[67,75] Dexmedetomidine has been shown to interact with different CNS biochemical and circuit level pathways to decrease delirium and potentially increase neuroprotection.[52] Furthermore, animal studies described antiapoptotic and anti-inflammatory effects in the setting of anesthesia and surgery.[52]

An RCT of 80 patients receiving supratentorial tumor resection showed that intraoperative dexmedetomidine infusion decreased pain and analgesic needs as well as lessened PONV.[76] In another RCT, dexmedetomidine, compared with a remifentanil infusion, had improved pain scores postoperatively and decreased opioid utilization.[77] In addition, dexmedetomidine may offer adjunctive properties to local anesthetic by prolonging the duration of scalp block.[78] The dexmedetomidine infusion can be continued throughout the postoperative period in the intensive care unit (ICU) and help to treat pain, agitation, and delirium.[67] As a "cooperative sedative," it provides anxiolysis and acts as an antihypertensive while preserving the ability to follow verbal commands and is particularly helpful in the context of awake craniotomies.[79]

Gabapentinoids

Pregabalin and gabapentin are GABA derivatives that bind and inhibit the alpha2delta subunit of the voltage-gated calcium channel, not the GABA receptor itself. They have been used in treatment of chronic neuropathic pain, nociceptive pain, and epilepsy.[80,81] In the neurosurgical population, they have been demonstrated to improve pain scores, decrease postoperative nausea, and decrease opioid consumption,[61,82] with strong indication for continued postoperative use.[67] One protocol showed that preoperative and postoperative administration of pregabalin (150 mg the evening before surgery, 1.5 hours preoperatively, and postoperatively twice daily for 72 hours) reduced postoperative pain without adverse effects, such as oversedation.[82]

Local Anesthetic

Lidocaine is an amide local anesthetic that blocks voltage-gated sodium channels, but may also have off-target effects on potassium and calcium channels, neurotransmitter receptors such as NMDA and 5-HT (serotonin), and opioid receptors.[67,83] It can be used for a rapid-onset nerve block or for a local skin infiltration. Its use as an IV infusion for pain control has been described.[84] An RCT showed that a 1.5-mg/kg bolus of lidocaine after induction followed by an infusion of 2 mg/kg/h reduced postoperative pain.[4] However, it did not improve postoperative cognitive decline after supratentorial tumor surgery and may decrease seizure threshold.[85]

Dissociative Anesthetics

Ketamine is a dissociative anesthetic commonly used as an analgesic adjuvant in both intraoperative and postoperative care for noncraniotomy surgeries.[63,86] Historically regarded as having a poor neuroprotection profile because of its increase of CMR and CBF,[5] it is now being investigated in the context of improving postcraniotomy depression.[87] Brink and colleagues[86] recommended subanesthetic dosing for pain control in order to avoid hallucinogenic properties and dose-dependent psychogenic effects.

Regional Anesthesia

There is moderate evidence that scalp blocks decrease opioid use after general anesthetic for supratentorial craniotomies.[67,78,88] Scalp block is further discussed later under Awake Craniotomy.

Ongoing Investigations for Opioid Reduction

Recently, because opioids have been linked to postoperative delirium and PONV, many protocols have focused on the concept of an "opioid-free craniotomy." Four RCTs for opioid compared with opioid-free craniotomies were reviewed in a systematic review of literature.[89] Despite heterogenous methods and weak evidence, the investigator concluded that perioperative scalp blocks, dexmedetomidine infusion, and acetaminophen were effective toward postoperative opioid-sparing by increasing time to opioid request and potentially decreasing PONV.

Additional nonpharmacologic adjuncts for opioid reduction have been explored. For instance, studies on transcutaneous electroacupuncture stimulation have suggested this may be a useful tool in reduction of postoperative opioids.[90]

INTRAOPERATIVE MONITORING: MAINTAINING ADEQUATE PERFUSION AND ASSESSING NEURAL DAMAGE

Close cardiopulmonary monitoring is essential during neurosurgical procedures to monitor and intervene on acid-base changes from brain relaxation maneuvers, assess the effect of hyperventilation, establish CO_2 gradient, assess the effect of osmotic diuresis, and quantify ongoing blood loss. An arterial line is thus indicated for supratentorial craniotomies. Standard monitoring includes continuous electrocardiogram, $Etco_2$, noninvasive blood pressure and pulse oximetry, and continuous temperature monitoring, all of which has been described in multiple book chapters.[5]

Monitoring and Optimizing Anesthetic Depth

Neuroanesthesiologists must provide an anesthetic that best matches the metabolic demands of a hyperventilated, relaxed brain and does not interfere with neurophysiologic monitoring, while planning for a smooth emergence and timely recovery for a postoperative neurologic examination. Optimizing intraoperative anesthetic depth now includes increasing evidence that anesthetics may serve neuroprotective roles, improve oncologic outcomes, and improve long-term patient function. Indeed, current prerogatives involve optimizing neuroprotection, decreasing neurotoxic exposure, decreasing long-term impact on cardiopulmonary function, and improving oncologic outcome.[52,91]

Although measuring anesthetic depth is relatively standardized with age-normalized MAC values of volatile anesthetics, the prevalence of TIVA for neuromonitoring argues for the use of processed electroencephalogram (pEEG) (such as the Sedline Monitor, Masimo Corp, Irvine, CA, USA) or bi-spectral index (BIS). However, pEEG and BIS do not reliably measure anesthetic depth. Although retrospective studies have found pEEG to decrease postoperative delirium,[92] the prospective ENGAGES trial did not demonstrate the same benefit of pEEG.[93] Processed EEG may also not reduce intraoperative awareness.[94,95] However, none of these studies were done specifically for craniotomies, and most used volatile anesthetics instead of TIVA. Evidence for hysteresis of anesthetic concentrations between induction and emergence further complicates the idea of "true" anesthetic depth.[96–98] At the authors' institution, if somatosensory evoked potentials and motor evoked potentials are being monitored through scalp electrodes, EEG signals derived from electrode placement can help titrate anesthetics to avoid burst suppression.

AWAKE CRANIOTOMY

The first documented awake brain resection for the treatment of epilepsy was performed by Victor Horsley in London in 1886.[99] Awake craniotomy is now indicated for intraoperative mapping and subsequent resection of tumors, often high-grade gliomas, at or near eloquent brain tissues (particularly the language centers and primary sensorimotor cortex).[100] Other indications include epilepsy surgery, deep-brain stimulation, and most recently, cerebrovascular procedures, such as cerebral aneurysm clipping and arteriovenous malformation obliteration.[101,102]

Because of the lack of pain receptors in the brain, the awake craniotomy can be a surgical option if the patient can psychologically and cognitively tolerate a prolonged procedure, and if the surgical facility has trained the necessary multidisciplinary support staff.[54,103] The awake supratentorial tumor resection allows for a greater extent of tumor resection compared with asleep procedures, with less postoperative pain, fewer postoperative neurologic deficits, a shorter ICU and hospital stay, and improved survival.[3,4,100,104,105]

Patient Selection and Assessment

Awake craniotomy requires a motivated patient as well as a skilled multidisciplinary team, including neurosurgeon, anesthesiologist, neurophysiologist, and a neuropsychologist. The procedure has a low rate of failure regardless of American Society of Anesthesiologists class, body mass index, and comorbidities; case reports tout a successful awake craniotomy in a patient with an cardiac ejection fraction of 10%, in pregnant patients, and even in children.[4,106] Currently, the only absolute contraindication for an awake craniotomy is patient refusal. Thorough preoperative neuropsychologic assessment of the patient is required. If a patient has underlying cognitive disorders or cannot sit still for a prolonged period, they are likely not going to tolerate an awake procedure. Likewise, patients with airway compromising factors, such as morbid obesity and obstructive sleep apnea, will likely be more challenging to manage intraoperatively.[103] In addition, if the tumor is large, vascular, or in the middle cerebral fossa floor with likelihood of high blood loss or dural and positional pain, patients may benefit from a general anesthetic.[107] No trials have been done comparing awake and asleep craniotomies in an RCT.

Choice of Sedation for Awake Craniotomy

Premedication

The consensus is to avoid medications that exacerbate somnolence, impair cognitive function, or potentially contribute to emergence delirium and confusion.[100,108] Prophylactic administration of AEDs differs with institutional practices.[100] In very anxious young patients with minimal risk of airway compromise, low-dose midazolam (1–2 mg) might be acceptable. In elderly patients, cholinergics should not be given because of the risk for confusion or delirium.[107] Acetaminophen with or without gabapentin is frequently the medication of choice at the authors' institution.

Intraoperative Management

The degree of sedation during awake craniotomy ranges from fully awake to alternating between general anesthesia and awake stages to match procedural needs. The method of asleep-awake-asleep (AAA) craniotomy has 3 distinct stages.[109] The first stage consists of scalp block, head pinning, and skull opening, when the patient is under a general anesthetic with their airway supported by a supraglottic airway device or endotracheal tube. The patient is then awake, verbally responsive, and without airway support for mapping and resection (stage 2), before being deeply sedated again with or without laryngeal mask airway (LMA) reinsertion for scalp closure and unpinning (stage 3). Alternatively, the awake craniotomy can be entirely done under monitored anesthesia care (MAC). In addition, there are reports of craniotomies and tumor resections under no chemical sedation with the aid of acupuncture or hypnosis.[110,111] Superiority of any method has not been established.[100,109] A nonrandomized retrospective analysis compared outcomes of AAA and MAC techniques at 1 institution and found that, other than a shorter operative time with the MAC technique, no differences in tumor outcomes, complications such as hypertension or seizure, or conversion to general endotracheal tube anesthesia was observed.[103]

Hemodynamic monitoring should be placed on the side ipsilateral to brain lesion in order to avoid interference with contralateral sensorimotor mapping. For either anesthetic choice, standard monitors, including electrocardiography, noninvasive blood pressure, pulse oximetry, end tidal CO_2, and temperature, should be applied before initiation of sedation.[109] Some may prefer the use of intraarterial blood pressure monitoring.[109] Foley catheter placement for urine output monitoring is indicated for long surgeries or when osmotic diuresis will be used.

The success of the awake craniotomy, regardless of anesthetic choice, largely depends on the quality of the scalp block.[112,113] Blockade of 6 nerves (**Fig. 3**) is done by the neurosurgeon or anesthesiologist using a combination of local anesthetics (lidocaine, and ropivacaine or bupivacaine), with or without epinephrine, often at maximum doses.[103] Additional local anesthetic along the meningeal vessels may also decrease nerve irritation from dura opening.[107]

Awake craniotomy requires an uninterrupted high level of vigilance and attention from the multidisciplinary team that must be ready to manage complications that arise in both an AAA and an MAC technique. Decreasing agitation can be done by

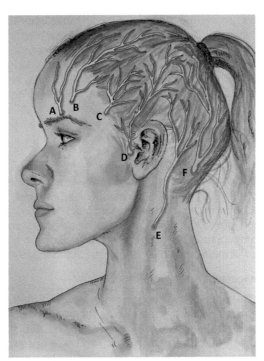

Fig. 3. Targets for scalp block: (A) supraorbital nerve, (B) supratrochlear nerve, (C) zygomaticotemporal nerve, (D) auriculotemporal nerve, (E) lesser occipital nerve, (F) greater occipital nerve. (*Data from* Bruder N, Ravussin PA. Chapter 11: Supratentorial masses: anesthetic considerations. In: Cottrell JE, Young WL, eds. Cottrell and Young's Neuroanesthesia, 5th ed. Philadelphia: Elsevier; 2010: 184-202.)

continued encouragement, positional movement if needed for pressure relief, and distraction. Airway compromise is more likely for the MAC technique leading to desaturation and dangerous hypercarbia; the anesthesiologist should be ready to stop all sedative infusions and conduct airway maneuvers, such as mask ventilation with jaw thrust, placing oral or nasal airways, placing LMA, and even insertion of ETT.

Monitored Anesthesia Care

Infusion medications that can be used for MAC are dexmedetomidine, 0.2 to 0.5 μg/kg/h, propofol, 20 to 100 μg/kg/min, and remifentanil, 0.01 to 0.09 μg/kg/min. Agents and doses vary with different institutional practices.[103,109] Recent literature shows increasing use of dexmedetomidine sedation for its property of maintaining respiratory-drive while providing anxiolysis, analgesia, and antiemesis.[107] In the authors' practice, they currently use the MAC (awake-awake) method. They initiate a dexmedetomidine infusion at the high loading dose of 1 μg/kg/h for 15 to 30 minutes before arrival to the operating room with only acetaminophen premedication. $Etco_2$ and Fio_2 are provided via nasal cannula. A transport monitor continues to assess hemodynamics as the patient is brought to the operating room. The infusion is then decreased to 0.2 to 0.5 μg/kg/h. A remifentanil infusion (0.03–0.05 μg/kg/min) is added and titrated for patient and surgeon's needs. If indicated, a nasal airway can be placed when actively obstructing under moderate sedation; use of a topical vasoconstrictive agent for nasal decongestion (oxymetazoline or phenylephrine) as well as 2% or 5%

lidocaine jelly can facilitate placement.[103] Monitored limbs have to remain accessible by neurophysiologists before the scalp block and head pins are applied. Small incremental boluses of propofol (10–20 mg) or a low-dose infusion is beneficial for stimulating interventions, such as Foley catheter insertion, scalp block placement, and head pinning. Unsedated patient cooperation with the final positioning of the head is important to assure comfort and tolerance of the position. Sedation is then restarted for opening of skin and cranium. It is considered safer to only open the dura once the patient is fully awake in order to prevent herniation or surgical field compromise from wakeup agitation.[103] The patient is required to be fully cooperative for cortical mapping and lesion resection because they will have continuous neurocognitive and sensorimotor assessment via verbal, auditory, and motor cues. Mouth swabs can be given for comfort to decrease thirst. Psychologic techniques, such as conversing with the patient, verbalizing empathy, hand holding, encouragement, giving mouth swabs for thirst, warm blankets, cooling cloths, and positional shifts or cushioning, can greatly increase comfort. The direct visualization between the patient and the provider in both directions is critical.

Asleep-Awake-Asleep

If AAA with general anesthesia is preferred, increased doses of IV sedation are required: propofol (>50 μg/kg/min) along with remifentanil (0.1–0.2 μg/kg/min) and dexmedetomidine (0.2–0.7 μg/kg/h after loading dose) is frequently used; alternatively, volatile anesthetics and opioid can be used.[112] LMA is frequently preferred to an ETT because it causes less airway irritation and is therefore less likely to induce coughing and increased ICP. Once the surgeon is ready for the awake phase, a smooth transition to a cooperative and comfortable state is paramount. All anesthetics are stopped. Supplemental local anesthetic by the surgeon can be given via infiltrating between the dural leaflets around the nerves supplying dura.[103]

After tumor resection, sedation can be restarted with propofol, dexmedetomidine, and remifentanil before the LMA is reinserted for airway support.[103,114]

Neuromonitoring with Awake Craniotomy

Neuromonitoring of the awake patient during mapping and resection period is complex and multidisciplinary. Through neurophysiologic testing, hemodynamic and respiratory status should be kept constant in order to not confound testing variables with cerebral perfusion changes. Close communication of any potential problems, such as intraoperative hypertension, seizures, somnolence, agitation, respiratory compromise, bleeding, lack of brain relaxation, shivering, and nausea, is necessary.

Much feared, seizures occur with a 3% to 16% incidence during cortical and subcortical stimulation mapping.[107] The seizure and postictal state can be unsafe especially if the airway is not protected, and sudden shaking movement against head pins can also result in skull and brain trauma. Studies have also shown that intraoperative seizure activity can lead to longer hospital stays.[115] The surgeon should immediately apply cold crystalloid solution to the surgical field. If that does not abort the seizure, IV propofol in small, divided doses, and antiepileptic medications, such as ativan, levetiracetam, or fosphenytoin, may be given. Prolonged seizure as well as respiratory or hemodynamic instability is a strong indication for conversion to general anesthesia and intubation.

If the patient is especially delirious or agitated when waking up from the asleep stage, potential causes, such as pain, hypercapnia, hypoxia, or bladder distention, should be corrected.

Awake craniotomies are usually associated with a shorter ICU and hospital stay and less delirium risk.[100]

SUMMARY

Understanding how anesthetics impact cerebral physiology, cerebral blood flow, brain metabolism, brain relaxation, and neurologic recovery is crucial for optimizing both intraoperative conditions and postoperative care for supratentorial craniotomies. Using osmodiuretic agents and hyperventilation, the neuroanesthesiologist must balance brain relaxation for surgical exposure while maintaining brain perfusion to prevent primary and secondary insults. Although hemodynamic monitoring is standard of care, consciousness monitoring through processed EEGs and bispectral monitoring has not demonstrated decreased intraoperative awareness or decreased postoperative delirium. As anesthetic care extends the timescale from immediate perioperative care to preoperative optimization and postoperative quality-of-life measurements, anesthesiologists must be increasingly cognizant of how anesthetics and multimodal adjuncts affect postoperative pain control and opioid addiction risk, delirium risk, oncologic outcome, and neurocognitive decline. If tolerated by the patient, awake craniotomies at adequately staffed facilities are an excellent option for resection of brain tumors in eloquent areas and are associated with decreased hospital stays and delirium risk.

CLINICS CARE POINTS

- Brain relaxation is achieved through a combination of hyperventilation and osmodiuretic agents, and must be judicious since decreased cerebral blood flow can result in decreased cerebral perfusion pressure and global ischemia. 3% hypertonic salne can be safely administered via peripheral IV and may control intracranial pressure better than mannitol.
- A patient's baseline MAP will often shift autoregulation limits, and a MAP around 20% of the patient's awake baseline should be maintained intraoperatively to optimize brain perfusion with non-malignant ICP conditions.
- During induction and emergence, maintaining a stable MAP is paramount. If necessary, sympathetic blockade should be given to blunt stimulation, with the goal of a cooperative neurologic exam soon after extubation.
- If SSEP and MEP scalp electrodes allow EEG assessment, anesthetic depth should be titrated to EEG activity that is non-active and non-burst suppressed in order to balance intraoperative reactivity and a short emergence time.

REFERENCES

1. Lapointe S, Perry A, Butowski NA. Primary brain tumours in adults. Lancet 2018; 392(10145):432–46.

2. Ostrom QT, Cioffi G, Gittleman H, et al. CBTRUS statistical report: primary brain and other central nervous system tumors diagnosed in the united states in 2012-2016. Neuro Oncol 2019;21(Suppl 5):v1–100.

3. Flexman AM, Meng L, Gelb AW. Outcomes in neuroanesthesia: what matters most? Can J Anaesth 2015;63:205–2011.

4. Gruenbaum SE, Meng L, Bilotta F. Recent trends in the anesthetic management of craniotomy for supratentorial tumor resection. Curr Opin Anaesthesiol 2016; 29:552–7.

5. Bruder NJ, Ravussin P, Schoettker P. Supratentorial masses: anesthetic considerations. In: Cottrell J, Patel P, editors. Neuroanesthesia. 6th edition. New York (NY): Elsevier; 2016. p. 189–208.
6. Tameem A, Krovvidi H. Cerebral physiology. Cont Ed Anaesth Crit Care & Pain 2013;13(4):113–8.
7. Paulson OB, Strandgaard S, Edvinsson L. Cerebral autoregulation. Cerebrovasc Brain Metab Rev 1990;2(2):161–92.
8. Iadecola C. The neurovascular unit coming of age: a journey through neurovascular coupling in health and disease. Neuron 2017;96(1):17–42.
9. Drummond JC. The lower limit of autoregulation: time to revise our thinking? Anesthesiology 1997;86(6):1431–3.
10. Meng L, Felb AW. Regulation of cerebral autoregulation by carbon dioxide. Anesthesiology 2015;122:196–205.
11. Meng L, Wang Y, Zhang L, et al. Heterogeneity and variability in pressure autoregulation of organ blood flow: lessons learned over 100+ years. Crit Care Med 2019;47:436–48.
12. Salmasi V, Maheshwari K, Yang D, et al. Relationship between intraoperative hypotension, defined by either reduction from baseline or absolute thresholds, and acute kidney and myocardial injury after noncardiac surgery: a retrospective cohort analysis. Anesthesiology 2017;126(1):47–65.
13. Walsh M, Devereaux PJ, Garg AX, et al. Relationship between intraoperative mean arterial pressure and clinical outcomes after noncardiac surgery: toward an empirical definition of hypotension. Anesthesiology 2013;119(3):507–15.
14. Carney N, Totten AM, O'Reilly C, et al. Guidelines for the management of severe traumatic brain injury, fourth edition. Neurosurgery 2017;80(1):6–15.
15. Slupe AM, Kirsch JR. Effects of anesthesia on cerebral blood flow, metabolism, and neuroprotection. J Cereb Blood Flow Metab 2018;38(12):2192–208.
16. Pires PW, Dams Ramos CM, Matin N, et al. The effects of hypertension on the cerebral circulation. Am J Physiol Heart Circ Physiol 2013;304(12):H1598–614.
17. Lucas SJ, Tzeng YC, Galvin SD, et al. Influence of changes in blood pressure on cerebral perfusion and oxygenation. Hypertension 2010;55(3):698–705.
18. Zhang W, Neal J, Lin L, et al. Mannitol in critical care and surgery over 50+ years: a systematic review of randomized controlled trials and complications with meta-analysis. J Neurosurg Anesthesiol 2019;31(3):273–84.
19. Akcil EF, Dilmen OK, Karabulut ES, et al. Effective and safe mannitol administration in patients undergoing supratentorial tumor surgery: a prospective, randomized and double blind study. Clin Neurol Neurosurg 2017;159:55–81.
20. Rozet I, Tontisirin N, Muangman S, et al. Effect of equiosmolar solutions of mannitol versus hypertonic saline on intraoperative brain relaxation and electrolyte balance. Anesthesiology 2007;107(5):697–704.
21. Dostal P, Schreiberova J, Dostalova V, et al. Effects of hypertonic saline and mannitol on cortical cerebral microcirculation in a rabbit craniotomy model. BMC Anesthesiol 2015;15:88.
22. Mortazavi MM, Romeo AK, Deep A, et al. Hypertonic saline for treating raised intracranial pressure: literature review with meta-analysis. J Neurosurg 2012;116(1):210–21.
23. Fang J, Yang Y, Wang W, et al. Comparison of equiosmolar hypertonic saline and mannitol for brain relaxation during craniotomies: a meta-analysis of randomized controlled trials. Neurosurg Rev 2018;41(4):945–56.
24. Ayus JC, Moritz ML. Misconceptions and barriers to the use of hypertonic saline to treat hyponatremic encephalopathy. Front Med (Lausanne) 2019;6:47.

25. Perez CA, Figueroa SA. Complication rates of 3% hypertonic saline infusion through peripheral intravenous access. J Neurosci Nurs 2017;49(3):191–5.

26. Hernández-Palazón J, Fuentes-García D, Doménech-Asensi P, et al. A dose-response relationship study of hypertonic saline on brain relaxation during supratentorial brain tumour craniotomy. Br J Neurosurg 2018;32(6):619–27.

27. Jafari M, Ala S, Haddadi K, et al. Cotreatment with furosemide and hypertonic saline decreases serum neutrophil gelatinase-associated lipocalin (NGAL) and serum creatinine concentrations in traumatic brain injury: a randomized, single-blind clinical trial. Iran J Pharm Res 2018;17(3):1130–40.

28. Willie CK, Macleod DB, Shaw AD, et al. Regional brain blood flow in man during acute changes in arterial blood gases. J Physiol 2012;590(14):3261–75.

29. Boedtkjer E. Acid-base regulation and sensing: accelerators and brakes in metabolic regulation of cerebrovascular tone. J Cereb Blood Flow Metab 2018;38(4):588–602.

30. Schaffranietz L, Heinke W. The effect of different ventilation regimes on jugular venous oxygen saturation in elective neurosurgical patients. Neurol Res 1998; 20(Suppl 1):S66–70.

31. Bagwell TA, Abramo TJ, Albert GW, et al. Cerebral oximetry with blood volume index and capnography in intubated and hyperventilated patients. Am J Emerg Med 2016;34(6):1102–7.

32. NICE-SUGAR Study Investigators, Finfer S, Chittock DR, Steve Yu-Shuo S, et al. Intensive versus conventional glucose control in critically ill patients. N Engl J Med 2009;360(13):1283–97.

33. Dietrich J, Rao K, Pastorino S, et al. Corticosteroids in brain cancer patients: benefits and pitfalls. Expert Rev Clin Pharmacol 2011;4(2):233–42.

34. Bondy ML, Scheurer ME, Malmer B, et al. Brain tumor epidemiology: consensus from the Brain Tumor Epidemiology Consortium. Cancer 2008;113(7 Suppl): 1953–68.

35. D'Antonio C, Passaro A, Gori B, et al. Bone and brain metastasis in lung cancer: recent advances in therapeutic strategies. Ther Adv Med Oncol 2014;6(3): 101–14.

36. Perry JR. Thromboembolic disease in patients with high-grade glioma. Neuro Oncol 2012;14:iv73–80. Suppl 4(Suppl 4).

37. Lin SY, Tang SC, Tsai LK, et al. Incidence and risk factors for acute kidney injury following mannitol infusion in patients with acute stroke: a retrospective cohort study. Medicine (Baltimore) 2015;94(47):e2032.

38. Hays AN, Lazaridis C, Neyens R, et al. Osmotherapy: use among neurointensivists. Neurocrit Care 2011;14(2):222–8.

39. Tremont-Lukats IW, Ratilal BO, Armstrong T, et al. Antiepileptic drugs for preventing seizures in people with brain tumors. Cochrane Database Syst Rev 2008;2:CD004424.

40. van Breemen MS, Rijsman RM, Taphoorn MJ, et al. Efficacy of anti-epileptic drugs in patients with gliomas and seizures. J Neurol 2009;256(9):1519–26.

41. Englot DJ, Magill ST, Han SJ, et al. Seizures in supratentorial meningioma: a systematic review and meta-analysis. J Neurosurg 2016;124(6):1552–61.

42. Bouillon TW, Bruhn J, Radulescu L, et al. Pharmacodynamic interaction between propofol and remifentanil regarding hypnosis, tolerance of laryngoscopy, bispectral index, and electroencephalographic approximate entropy. Anesthesiology 2004;100(6):1353–72.

43. Alkhalid Y, Lagman C, Sheppard JP, et al. Restrictive transfusion threshold is safe in high-risk patients undergoing brain tumor surgery. Clin Neurol Neurosurg 2017;163:103–7.

44. Carson JL, Terrin ML, Noveck H, et al. Liberal or restrictive transfusion in high-risk patients after hip surgery. N Engl J Med 2011;365(26):2453–62.

45. Hagan KB, Bhavsar S, Raza SM, et al. Enhanced recovery after surgery for oncological craniotomies. J Clin Neurosci 2016;24:10–6.

46. Wang Y, Liu B, Zhao T, et al. Safety and efficacy of a novel neurosurgical enhanced recovery after surgery protocol for elective craniotomy: a prospective randomized controlled trial. J Neurosurg 2018;1–12. https://doi.org/10.3171/2018.1.JNS171552.

47. Brambrink AM, Orfanakis A, Kirsch JR. Anesthetic neurotoxicity. Anesthesiol Clin 2012;30(2):207–28.

48. Sun LS, Li G, Miller TL, et al. Association between a single general anesthesia exposure before age 36 months and neurocognitive outcomes in later childhood. JAMA 2016;315(21):2312–20.

49. Warner DO, Shi Y, Flick RP. Anesthesia and neurodevelopment in children: perhaps the end of the beginning. Anesthesiology 2018;128(4):700–3.

50. Deiner S, Silverstein JH. Postoperative delirium and cognitive dysfunction. Br J Anaesth 2009;103:i41–6. Suppl 1(Suppl 1).

51. Culley DJ, Xie Z, Crosby G. General anesthetic-induced neurotoxicity: an emerging problem for the young and old? Curr Opin Anaesthesiol 2007;20:408–19.

52. Wu L, Zhao W, Weng H, et al. Lasting effects of general anesthetics on the brain in the young and elderly: "mixed picture" of neurotoxicity, neuroprotection, and cognitive impairment. J Anesth 2019;33:321–35.

53. Miller D, Lewis SR, Pritchard MW, et al. Intravenous versus inhalational maintenance of anaesthesia for postoperative cognitive outcomes in elderly people undergoing non-cardiac surgery. Cochrane Database Syst Rev 2018;8(8):CD012317.

54. Flexman AM, Wang T, Meng L. Neuroanesthesia and outcomes: evidence, opinions, and speculations on clinically relevant topics. Curr Opin Anaesthesiol 2019;32:539–45.

55. Chui J, Mariappan R, Mehta J, et al. Comparison of propofol and volatile agents for maintenance of anesthesia during elective craniotomy procedures: systematic review and meta-analysis. Can J Anaesth 2014;61(4):347–56.

56. Schraag S, Pradelli L, Alsaleh AJO, et al. Propofol vs. inhalational agents to maintain general anaesthesia in ambulatory and in-patient surgery: a systematic review and meta-analysis. BMC Anesthesiol 2018;18(1):162.

57. Myles PS. More than just morbidity and mortality–quality of recovery and long-term functional recovery after surgery. Anaesthesia 2020;75(S1):e143–50.

58. Neuman MD, Bateman BT, Wunsch H. Inappropriate opioid prescription after surgery. Lancet 2019;393:1547–57.

59. Bohnert ASB, Ilgen MA. Understanding links among opioid use, overdose, and suicide. N Engl J Med 2019;380:71–9 (Ban 2019).

60. Glare P, Aubrey KR, Myles PS. Transition from acute to chronic pain after surgery. Lancet 2019;393:1537–46 (Ban 2019).

61. Tsaousi GG, Logan SW, Bilotta F. Postoperative pain control following craniotomy: a systematic review of recent clinical literature. Pain Prac 2017;17(7):968–81.

62. Benyamin R, Trescot AM, Datta S, et al. Opioid complications and side effects. Pain Physician 2008;11(2 Suppl):S105–20.
63. Chou R, Gordon DB, de Leon-Casasola OA, et al. Management of postoperative pain: a clinical practice guideline from the American Pain Society, the American Society of Regional Anesthesia and Pain Medicine, and the American Society of Anesthesiologists' Committee on Regional Anesthesia. Executive Committee, and Administrative Council. J Pain 2016;17:131–57 (Ban 2019).
64. Necib S, Tubach F, Peuch C, et al. Recovery from anesthesia after craniotomy for supratentorial tumors: comparison of propofol-remifentanil and sevoflurane-sufentanil (the PROMIFLUNIL trial). J Neurosurg Anesthesiol 2014;26:37–44 (Gruenbaum 2016).
65. Rozec B, Floch H, Berlivet P, et al. Propofol versus thiopental by target controlled infusion in patients undergoing craniotomy. Minerva Anestesiol 2014;80:761–8 (Gruenbaum 2016).
66. Radtke FM, Franck M, Hagemann L, et al. Risk factors for inadequate emergence after anesthesia: emergence delirium and hypoactive emergence. Minerva Anestesiol 2010;76(6):394–403.
67. Ban VS, Bhoja R, McDonagh DL. Multimodal analgesia for craniotomy. Curr Opin Anaesthesiol 2019;32:592–9.
68. Asouhidou I, Trikoupi A. Esmolol reduces anesthetic requirements thereby facilitating early extubation: a prospective controlled study in patients undergoing intracranial surgery. BMC Anesthesiol 2015;15:172 (Gruenbaum 2016).
69. Kim Y, Hwang W, Cho ML, et al. The effects of intraoperative esmolol administration on perioperative inflammatory responses in patients undergoing laparoscopic gastrectomy: a dose-response study. Surg Innov 2015;22(2):177–82.
70. Greenberg S, Murphy GS, Avram MJ, et al. Postoperative intravenous acetaminophen for craniotomy patients: a randomized controlled trial. World Neurosurg 2018;109:e554–62.
71. Artime CA, Aijazi H, Zhang H, et al. Scheduled intravenous acetaminophen improves patient satisfaction with postcraniotomy pain management: a prospective, randomized, placebo-controlled double-blind study. J Neurosurg Anesthesiol 2018;30:231–6 (Ban 2019).
72. Zornow MH, Maze M, Dyck JB, et al. Dexmedetomidine decreases cerebral blood flow velocity in humans. J Cereb Blood Flow Metab 1993;13(2):350–3.
73. Drummond JC, Dao AV, Roth DM, et al. Effect of dexmedetomidine on cerebral blood flow velocity, cerebral metabolic rate, and carbon dioxide response in normal humans. Anesthesiology 2008;108(2):225–32.
74. Ma D, Hossain M, Rajakumaraswamy N, et al. Dexmedetomidine produces its neuroprotective effect via the alpha 2A-adrenoceptor subtype. Eur J Pharmacol 2004;502(1–2):87–97.
75. Wang L, Shen J, Ge L, et al. Dexmedetomidine for craniotomy under general anesthesia: a systematic review and meta-analysis of randomized clinical trails. J Clin Anesth 2019;54:114–25 (Ban 2019).
76. Peng K, Jin XH, Liu SL, et al. Effect of intraoperative dexmedetomidine on postcraniotomy pain. Clin Ther 2015;37:1114–21 (Gruenbaum 2016).
77. Rajan S, Hutcherson MT, Sessler DI, et al. The effects of dexmedetomidine and remifentanil on hemodynamic stability and analgesic requirement after craniotomy: a randomized controlled trial. J Neurosurg Anesthesiol 2016;28(4):282–90 (Gruenbaum 2016).
78. Vallapu S, Panda NB, Samagh N, et al. Efficacy of dexmedetomidine as an adjuvant to local anesthetic agent in scalp block and scalp infiltration to control

postcraniotomy pain: a double-blind randomized trial. J Neurosci Rural Pract 2018;9:73–9 (Ban 2019).

79. Prontera A, Baroni S, Marudi A, et al. Awake craniotomy anesthetic management using dexmedetomidine, propofol, and remifentanil. Drug Des Devel Ther 2017;11:593–8.

80. Hu J, Huang D, Li M, et al. Effects of a single dose of preoperative pregabalin and gabapentin for acute postoperative pain: a network meta-analysis of randomized controlled trials. J Pain Res 2018;11:2633–43 (Ban 2019).

81. Zeng M, Dong J, Lin N, et al. Preoperative gabapentin administration improves acute postoperative analgesia in patients undergoing craniotomy: a randomized controlled trial. J Neurosurg Anesthesiol 2019;31(4):392–8 (Ban 2019).

82. Shimony N, Amit U, Minz B, et al. Perioperative pregabalin for reducing pain, analgesic consumption, and anxiety and enhancing sleep quality in elective neurosurgical patients: a prospective, randomized, double-blind, and controlled clinical study. J Neurosurg 2016;125(6):1513–22 (Gruenbaum 2016).

83. Beaussier M, Delbos A, Maurice-Szamburski A, et al. Perioperative use of intravenous lidocaine. Drugs 2018;78:1229–46 (Ban 2019).

84. Kandil E, Melikman E, Adinoff B. Lidocaine infusion: a promising therapeutic approach for chronic pain. J Anesth Clin Res 2017;8(1):697.

85. Peng Y, Zhang W, Kass IS, et al. Lidocaine reduces acute postoperative pain after supratentorial tumor surgery in the PACU: a secondary finding from a randomized, controlled trial. J Neurosurg Anesthesiol 2016;28:309–15 (Ban 2019).

86. Brinck EC, Tiippana E, Heesen M, et al. Perioperative intravenous ketamine for acute postoperative pain in adults. Cochrane Database Syst Rev 2018;12: CD012033 (Ban 2019).

87. Zhou Y, Peng Y, Fang J, et al. Effect of low-dose ketamine on PerioperAtive depreSsive Symptoms in patients undergoing Intracranial tumor resectioN (PASSION): study protocol for a randomized controlled trial. Trials 2018;19: 463 (Ban 2019).

88. Yang X, Ma J, Li K, et al. A comparison of effects of scalp nerve block and local anesthetic infiltration on inflammatory response, hemodynamic response, and postoperative pain in patients undergoing craniotomy for cerebral aneurysms: a randomized controlled trial. BMC Anesthesiol 2019;19:91 (Ban 2019).

89. Darmawikarta D, Sourour M, Couban R, et al. Opioid-free analgesia for supratentorial craniotomies: a systematic review. Can J Neurol Sci 2019;46:415–22.

90. Liu X, Li S, Wang B, et al. Intraoperative and postoperative anaesthetic and analgesic effect of multipoint transcutaneous electrical acupuncture stimulation combined with sufentanil anaesthesia in patients undergoing supratentorial craniotomy. Acupunct Med 2015;33:270–6 (Gruenbaum 2016).

91. Wigmore TJ, Mohammed K, Jhanji S. Long-term survival for patients undergoing volatile versus IV anesthesia for cancer surgery: a retrospective analysis. Anesthesiology 2016;124:69–79.

92. MacKenzie KK, Britt-Spells AM, Sands LP, et al. Processed electroencephalogram monitoring and postoperative delirium: a systematic review and meta-analysis. Anesthesiology 2018;129(3):417–27.

93. Wildes TS, Mickle AM, Ben Abdallah A, et al. Effect of electroencephalography-guided anesthetic administration on postoperative delirium among older adults undergoing major surgery: the ENGAGES randomized clinical trial. JAMA 2019; 321:473–83.

94. Avidan MS, Zhang L, Burnside BA, et al. Anesthesia awareness and the bispectral index. N Engl J Med 2008;358:1097–108.

95. Avidan MS, Jacobsohn E, Glick D, et al. Prevention of intraoperative awareness in a high-risk surgical population. N Engl J Med 2011;365:591–600.
96. Vlisides PE, Li D, Zierau M, et al. Dynamic cortical connectivity during general anesthesia in surgical patients. Anesthesiology 2019;130:885–97.
97. Proekt A, Hudson AE. A stochastic basis for neural inertia in emergence from general anaesthesia. Br J Anaesth 2018;121(1):86–94.
98. Tarnal V, Vlisides PE, Mashour GA. The neurobiology of anesthetic emergence. J Neurosurg Anesthesiol 2016;28(3):250–5.
99. Horsley V. Remarks on ten consecutive cases of operations upon the brain and cranial cavity to illustrate the details and safety of the method employed. Br Med J 1887;1(1373):863–5.
100. Meng L, Berger MS, Gelb AW. The potential benefits of awake craniotomy for brain tumor resection: an anesthesiologist's perspective. J Neurosurg Anesthesiol 2015;27:310–7.
101. Abdulrauf SI, Vuong P, Patel R, et al. Awake" clipping of cerebral aneurysms: report of initial series [published correction appears in J Neurosurg. 2017 Aug;127(2):445]. J Neurosurg 2017;127(2):311–8.
102. Chan DYC, Chan DTM, Zhu CXL, et al. Awake craniotomy for excision of arteriovenous malformations? A qualitative comparison study with stereotactic radiosurgery. J Clin Neurosci 2018;51:52–6.
103. Eseonu CI, ReFaey K, Garcia O, et al. Awake craniotomy anesthesia: a comparison of the monitored anesthesia care and asleep-awake-asleep techniques. World Neurosurg 2017;104:679–86.
104. Hervey-Jumper SL, Li J, Lau D, et al. Awake craniotomy to maximize glioma resection: methods and technical nuances over a 27 year period. J Neurosurg 2015;123:325–39.
105. Serletis D, Bernstein M. Prospective study of awake craniotomy used routinely and nonselectively for supratentorial tumors. J Neurosurg 2007;107:1–6.
106. Klimek M, Verbrugge SJ, Roubos S, et al. Awake craniotomy for glioblastoma in a 9-year-old child. Anaesthesia 2004;59(6):607–9.
107. Zhang K, Gelb AW. Awake craniotomy: indications, benefits, and techniques. Colom J Anesth 2018;46(2S):46–51.
108. Manninen PH, Balki M, Lukitto K, et al. Patient satisfaction with awake craniotomy for tumor surgery: a comparison of remifentanil and fentanyl in conjunction with propofol. Anesth Analg 2006;102(1):237–42.
109. Meng L, McDonagh DL, Berger MS, et al. Anesthesia for awake craniotomy: a how-to guide for the occasional practitioner. Can J Anaesth 2017;64(5):517–29.
110. Chen GB, Zhao YD, Xiao HR, et al. A study of acupuncture anesthesia in surgery on the anterior cranial fossa. J Tradit Chin Med 1984;4:189–96.
111. Frati A, Pesce A, Palmieri M, et al. Hypnosis-aided awake surgery for the management of intrinsic brain tumors versus standard awake-asleep-awake protocol: a preliminary, promising experience. World Neurosurg 2019;121:e882–91.
112. Sewell D, Smith M. Awake craniotomy: anesthetic considerations based on outcome evidence. Curr Opin Anaesthesiol 2019;32(5):546–52.
113. Kulikov A, Bilotta F, Borsellino B, et al. Xenon anesthesia for awake craniotomy: safety and efficacy. Minerva Anestesiol 2019;85(2):148–55.
114. Lobo FA, Wagemakers M, Absalom AR. Anaesthesia for awake craniotomy. Br J Anaesth 2016;116(6):740–4.
115. Dewan MC, White-Dzuro GA, Brinson PR, et al. Perioperative seizure in patients with glioma is associated with longer hospitalization, higher readmission, and decreased overall survival. J Neurosurg 2016;125(4):1033–41.

Anesthetic Management of Patients Undergoing Open Suboccipital Surgery

Kelsey Serfozo, MD, Vijay Tarnal, MBBS, FRCA*

KEYWORDS

- Posterior cranial fossa • Brainstem • Suboccipital craniotomy • Intracranial pressure
- Positioning • Venous air embolism • Patent foramen ovale • Pneumocephalus

KEY POINTS

- The posterior cranial fossa houses key pathways regulating consciousness, autonomic functions, motor and sensory pathways, and cerebellar centers regulating balance and gait.
- The posterior fossa can be accessed from variations of the supine, lateral, park-bench, prone, and sitting positions.
- Suboccipital craniotomies have a high risk of venous air embolism, particularly in the sitting position.
- Improved outcome from suboccipital craniotomy is possible with careful planning and a multidisciplinary team approach to surgical management that includes neurosurgeons, neuroanesthesiologists, nurses, the neurophysiologists responsible for intraoperative neuromonitoring and neurocritical care intensivists.

INTRODUCTION

The posterior cranial fossa with its complex intracranial anatomy is the deepest cranial fossa. It is a compact, rigid compartment with poor compliance that houses key structures such as the brainstem and cerebellum. Small changes to intracranial volume (tumors, hemorrhage) in a poorly compliant fossa is frequently associated with hydrocephalus and significant elevations of intracranial pressure (ICP). This may result in life-threatening brainstem compression and herniation. Cardiorespiratory complications from surgical procedures of posterior cranial fossa can be associated with severe morbidity and mortality. This may include hemodynamic and rhythm disturbances, delayed emergence from anesthesia, inability to protect the airway, and venous air embolism (VAE). Surgical procedures of the posterior cranial fossa, therefore, pose unique challenges and require special considerations for

Department of Anesthesiology, University Hospital, University of Michigan Medical School, 1500 East Medical Center Drive, Ann Arbor, MI 48109-5048, USA
* Corresponding author.
E-mail address: vtarnal@med.umich.edu

Anesthesiology Clin 39 (2021) 93–111
https://doi.org/10.1016/j.anclin.2020.11.001   anesthesiology.theclinics.com
1932-2275/21/© 2020 Elsevier Inc. All rights reserved.

management. Advancements in neuroimaging, microsurgical techniques, and a multi-disciplinary team approach that includes neurosurgeons, neuroanesthesiologists, neuromonitoring, and neurointensive care have made it possible to operate on posterior cranial fossa lesions with improved patient outcomes.

ANATOMY

The posterior cranial fossa occupies one-eighth of the intracranial space and houses key pathways regulating consciousness, autonomic functions, motor and sensory pathways, and cerebellar centers regulating balance and gait.

The posterior fossa extends from the tentorial notch to the foramen magnum in the occipital bone through which it communicates with the spinal canal. It is bounded anteromedially by the dorsum sellae of the sphenoid bone, anterolaterally by the petrosal and mastoid components of the temporal bone, posteriorly by the occipital bone, superiorly by the tentorium cerebelli, and inferiorly by the mastoid part of the temporal bone and occipital bone.

The brainstem occupies the anterior portion of the posterior cranial fossa and comprises the midbrain, pons, and medulla oblongata. The brainstem is composed of the following structures: (i) cerebellum, (ii) cranial nerve nuclei (cranial nerves III–XII), (iii) respiratory and cardiovascular centers, (iv) centers for consciousness and reticular formation, and (v) ascending and descending neural pathways connecting the spinal cord and forebrain. This space contains the cerebral aqueduct, which is a narrow passage for cerebrospinal fluid (CSF) to pass into the fourth ventricle. The vascular system within the posterior cranial fossa is complex and contains deep and relatively inaccessible segments of basilar and vertebral arteries and major cerebellar vessels coursing in relation to cranial nerves. Three dural venous sinuses namely transverse, sigmoid, and occipital sinuses traverse the fossa.[1–3]

SURGICAL INDICATIONS

The most common posterior fossa pathologies for which neurosurgical intervention may be necessary include cerebellopontine angle tumors (acoustic neuromas), aneurysms, arachnoid or epidermoid cysts, hemifacial spasms, and craniofacial abnormalities such as Arnold–Chiari malformations (types I and II). Typical pathologies requiring surgical intervention are listed in **Table 1**.

PREOPERATIVE EVALUATION

The preoperative evaluation for patients undergoing open suboccipital surgery begins with a standard history and physical examination. General medical comorbidities should be evaluated and optimized to minimize risks. Careful assessment of the neurologic, cardiovascular, and pulmonary systems is especially important owing to pathology to associated structures and potential intraoperative positioning requirements.

Patients have a wide-ranging presentation owing to the densely contained neural structures and pathways described elsewhere in this article. **Table 2** shows common symptoms associated with various locations of pathology. Documentation should include a full account of preoperative symptoms and deficits on examination. Elevated ICP is common due to mass effect and involvement of the cerebral aqueduct and fourth ventricle leading to obstructive hydrocephalus. Children with primary posterior fossa tumors commonly present with nausea, vomiting, headaches, and incoordination. Other common symptoms include altered mental status, lethargy, cranial nerve

Table 1 Pathology requiring open suboccipital surgery	
Tumors	Axial tumors Medulloblastoma Metastatic lesions Ependymoma Hemangioblastoma Ependymoma Astrocytoma Gangliocytoma Cerebellopontine angle tumors Acoustic neuroma Meningioma Glomus jugulare tumors
Vascular malformations	Aneurysms of posterior circulation of circle of Willis, posterior cerebellar artery, vertebral and vertebrobasilar arterial system Arteriovenous malformations
Cranial nerve lesions	Hemifacial spasm (CN VII) Trigeminal neuralgia (CN V)
Craniocervical abnormalities	Arnold–Chiari malformation (types I and II)
Cystic lesions	Epidermoid cysts Arachnoid cysts

Abbreviation: CN, cranial nerve.
 Data from Refs.[4–6]

palsies, and diplopia.[7] Presentation in adults is similar but highly variable based on specific pathology.[8,9]

Decreases in acute intracranial hypertension to an ICP of less than 20 mm Hg before surgery should be considered if possible. Patients may be managed with an external ventricular drain, endoscopic third ventriculostomy, or creation of a ventriculoperitoneal shunt system. These systems help measure and treat elevated ICPs throughout the perioperative period so that cerebral perfusion can be maintained.[10,11] Mass effect involving edema is frequently treated with high-dose steroids, often with dexamethasone. The steroids should be continued throughout the perioperative period for this and to avoid refractory hypotension from iatrogenic adrenal suppression.[12]

Suboccipital craniotomies have a high risk of VAE, especially in the sitting position. Because of the risk of paradoxic air embolism (PAE), which can be fatal, a preoperative echocardiogram should be considered to evaluate for intracardiac shunts. Significant carotid disease should also be evaluated as it can impact cerebral blood flow (CBF) and can be worsened when significant head and neck flexion is used during surgical exposure.[13]

Pulmonary status and airway should be examined closely preoperatively. Posterior fossa tumors are commonly associated with disordered respiratory patterns owing to the involvement of the respiratory centers in the medulla oblongata and possibly the cerebellum.[14] Pathology of the glossopharyngeal and vagal nerves may lead to dysphagia, impaired gag reflex, and glottic insufficiency that can predispose patients to aspiration events. In turn, these risks should be taken into consideration when deciding if the patient will tolerate extubation.

Table 2
Neurologic symptoms associated with posterior cranial fossa pathology

Affected Structure	Symptoms	Examination Findings
Cerebellum	Imbalance Dysarthria/scanning speech	Tremor Ataxia Dysmetria Nystagmus Dysdiadochokinesia Hypotonia
Fourth ventricle/CSF outflow tract	Headache Nausea/vomiting Blurry Vision	Macrocephaly (children) Papilledema

Brainstem Structures	Symptoms	Examination Findings
CN III, IV, VI	Blurry vision	Strabismus Pupillary asymmetry
CN V	Facial numbness Weakness in muscles of mastication	
CN VII	Ageusia	Facial asymmetry, droop
CN VIII	Vertigo	Deafness
CN IX	Dysphasia	Loss of gag reflex
CN X	Dysphasia	Autonomic dysfunction
CN XI		Sternocleidomastoid muscle or trapezius weakness
CN XII	Dysarthria	Asymmetric tongue protrusion

Abbreviation: CN, cranial nerve.
Data from Refs.[7–9]

Blood panels and volume status should be evaluated and optimized before surgery because symptoms often predispose patients to hypovolemia, electrolyte disturbances, and malnutrition.

INTRAOPERATIVE CONSIDERATIONS
Neuromonitoring

The use of intraoperative neuromonitoring for suboccipital surgery is highly variable and will depend on pathology, surgical approach, and surgeon preferences. Brainstem auditory evoked potentials, direct nerve stimulation, and free-running electromyography of the facial and pharyngeal muscles are frequently used to monitor cranial nerve integrity. Monitoring motor evoked potentials and somatosensory evoked potentials can be used to help identify ischemia and physical damage to the motor and sensory tracts traveling within the brainstem, but are less commonly used in suboccipital surgeries.[15] Continuous electroencephalographic monitoring may help to identify subclinical brain injury and detect early ischemia during neurosurgical procedures.[16]

Slotty and colleagues[15] performed a multicenter study to evaluate the incidence of alterations in intraoperative neuromonitoring during open suboccipital surgery for various posterior fossa pathologies. Changes were seen in about half of the cases and were correlated with postoperative neurologic deficits. Overall, the usefulness of monitoring was found to be variable based on anatomic location and pathology.[15]

The use of intraoperative neuromonitoring is variably impacted by different anesthetic agents as well as nondepolarizing muscle relaxants. This will need to be considered by the neuroanesthesiologist and discussed with the neuromonitoring team so that ideal conditions for neuromonitoring can be obtained.

Positioning

The posterior fossa can be accessed from variations of supine, lateral/park-bench, prone, and sitting positions. Common positions are shown in **Figs. 1–4**. Midline lesions of the posterior fossa are more likely to require prone or sitting positions, whereas lateral lesions are more likely to require access from a lateral or supine approach. Associated risks and benefits with each position should be considered and determination of the best position for a suboccipital surgical procedure should be based on an interdisciplinary discussion between the neurosurgeon and the neuroanesthesiologist. Specific preoperative testing discussed elsewhere in this article may be necessary to determine safety of different patient positions. All positions require great attention to detail to padding to protect peripheral nerves and pressure points to decrease the risk of postoperative peripheral nerve injury and skin ulcerations.

Owing to the surgical site and significant neck flexion required for open suboccipital craniotomy in any position, there are numerous complications associated with positioning, which includes VAE, PAE, tension pneumocephalus, nerve injuries, quadriplegia, and macroglossia.[13,17–19] The details of these complications are discussed in this section and elsewhere in the article.

Although there are some major advantages to the sitting position, it has historically been controversial owing to a presumed increased risk of adverse events, particularly VAE. Its use is highly variable by institution and country. Recent studies evaluating the incidence of these risks have suggested that this position can be performed safely if a proper preoperative evaluation and intraoperative monitoring are conducted.[13,20,21]

Advantages to the sitting position (see **Fig. 4**) include better surgical access and anatomic orientation while improving gravitational venous and CSF drainage away from the surgical field. This position improves exposure, decreased the need for retraction, and allows better visualization of the interface between tumor and neural tissues. Anesthesiologists typically have good access to the airway, extremities, and various invasive lines. Typically, respiratory dynamics and compliance are not negatively impacted because the chest wall remains free.[13,17]

Sitting positions for any procedure are typically associated with hemodynamic instability. Significant hypotension and decrease cardiac output may result from a

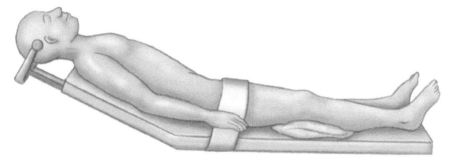

Fig. 1. Supine position. (*From* Kim I, Strom RG, Golfinos JG. Positioning in Cranial Surgery. In: Couldwell WT, Misra BK, Seifert V, et al., editors. Youmans and Winn Neurological surgery, 7th Ed. Philadelphia: Elsevier; 2017. P. 240; with permission.)

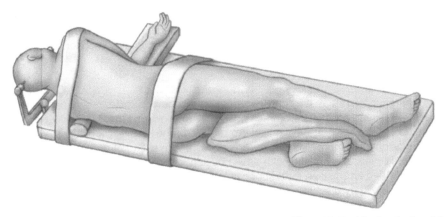

Fig. 2. Lateral decubitus position. (*From* Kim I, Strom RG, Golfinos JG. Positioning in Cranial Surgery. In: Couldwell WT, Misra BK, Seifert V, et al., editors. Youmans and Winn Neurological surgery, 7th Ed. Philadelphia: Elsevier; 2017. P. 240; with permission.)

combination of anesthetic induced vasodilation and gravitationally induced venous pooling. A decreased mean arterial pressure (MAP) may lead to severely reduced CBF and cerebral perfusion pressure (CPP).[22–24] Similarly, ischemic injury can be seen in other organ systems, including the heart and kidneys.

Several studies have documented potential methods to mitigate some of the risks seen in the sitting position during craniotomy. Preoperative cardiovascular screening can help to identify patients with poor cardiac function, intracardiac shunts, and carotid artery disease. Findings may preclude the use of a sitting position for some patients because they may not be able to tolerate the hemodynamic changes caused by this positioning. Intraoperatively, hyperventilation should be used cautiously because it can further decrease CBF. Monitoring for VAE with precordial doppler is generally considered standard of care for patients in the sitting position for posterior fossa craniotomy. Patients may also be monitored for VAE and PAE with transesophageal echocardiography if necessary. Laryngeal dysfunction, dysphagia, swelling and necrosis of the tongue may result from flexion of the head in the sitting position.[25,26] Modified semisitting positions have been developed in an attempt to achieve some of the benefits of sitting while decreasing the likelihood of adverse events.[27]

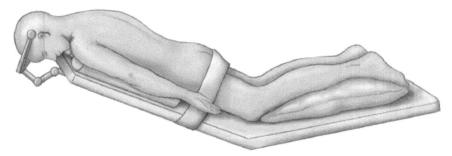

Fig. 3. Prone position. (*From* Kim I, Strom RG, Golfinos JG. Positioning in Cranial Surgery. In: Couldwell WT, Misra BK, Seifert V, et al., editors. Youmans and Winn Neurological surgery, 7th Ed. Philadelphia: Elsevier; 2017. P. 240; with permission.)

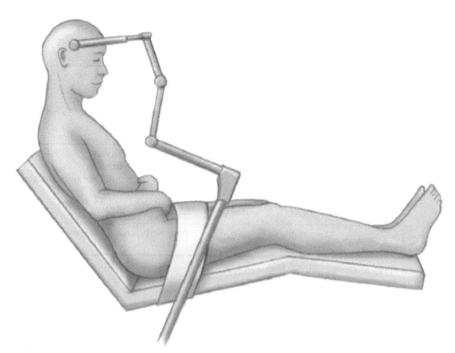

Fig. 4. Sitting position. (*From* Kim I, Strom RG, Golfinos JG. Positioning in Cranial Surgery. In: Couldwell WT, Misra BK, Seifert V, et al., editors. Youmans and Winn Neurological surgery, 7th Ed. Philadelphia: Elsevier; 2017. P. 240; with permission.)

Horizontal positions include various forms of prone, lateral, park bench, and supine. Frequently, these positions require extensive rotation or flexion of the neck to facilitate surgical access, which can lead to complications described elsewhere in this article. However, when compared with the sitting position, the horizontal positions offer improved hemodynamic stability.

Supine positioning (see **Fig. 1**) often modified with lateral head rotation can be performed for cerebellopontine angle tumors and acoustic neuroma resections. The lateral position (see **Fig. 2**) is feasible for unilateral pathology. The park-bench position is a modification of the typical lateral position that includes elevation and rotation of the head. Typically, significant neck flexion is required.[27] This position can provide better access and orientation to midline lesions compared with standard lateral positioning with better hemodynamics and gravitational drainage of venous blood and CSF away from the surgical field.

The prone position (see **Fig. 3**) can provide good access to midline suboccipital lesions. Intracranial procedures performed in prone positions may be associated with increased blood loss and difficulties in creating optimal surgical access. The prone position can be associated with difficulty in ventilation and oxygenation and provides limited access to the airway, monitors, and lines.[27]

Table 3 outlines the major risks and benefits associated with different positioning techniques.

Intraoperative Management

Intraoperative anesthetic management for open suboccipital procedures can be complex. The neuroanesthesiologist needs to account for patient-specific risk factors in

Table 3
Considerations for patient positioning

Position	Advantages	Disadvantages
Sitting	CSF drainage Venous sinus drainage Anatomic orientation Access to airway Ventilatory dynamics preserved	Increased head elevation- increased incidence to VAE Hemodynamic instability Requires extensive neck flexion
Prone	More stable hemodynamics	Poor access to airway Poor access to lines May require significant neck rotation Airway edema Possible ventilatory difficulty owing to chest wall restriction
Lateral and park bench	More stable hemodynamics	Possible brachial plexus injury

Data from Perks A, Chakravarti S, Manninen P. Preoperative anxiety in neurosurgical patients. J Neurosurg Anesthesiol. Apr 2009;21(2):127-30.)

addition to providing an anesthetic that maintains hemodynamic stability and CPP while allowing for appropriate neuromonitoring and optimization of surgical exposure. Patient positioning and associated complications will also impact intraoperative management strategies as discussed elsewhere in this article.

Preinduction anxiolytics with benzodiazepines are not commonly given in this patient population because of the risk of respiratory depression resulting in an elevated partial pressure of carbon dioxide in arterial blood ($Paco_2$) and subsequent increase in the ICP. However, because some patients may benefit from the administration of anxiolytics, the decision as to whether or not administer them should be considered on a patient-by-patient basis.[28]

Invasive arterial blood pressure monitors can be placed preoperatively or intraoperatively to closely monitor MAP. Patients with elevated ICP require a higher MAP to maintain CPP. Some studies have found that these patients may also have impaired CBF autoregulation, making CBF increasingly sensitive to small changes in blood pressure.[29] Similarly, patients with chronic hypertension, especially when uncontrolled, have also been shown to have dysfunctional cerebral autoregulation.[30] Thus, it is important to evaluate each patient's baseline blood pressure and attempt to maintain this throughout the perioperative period. Further cardiovascular dysregulation may also be seen in patients with pathology involving the brainstem.

Induction of general anesthesia should be planned to avoid significant hemodynamic variability. Anesthetic agents typically cause pharmacologic vasodilation which reduces MAP. However, stimulation from direct laryngoscopy, endotracheal tube placement, head-pinning, and surgical incision can cause rapid increases in sympathetic tone, cardiac output, and elevated MAPs. These changes can be problematic as the rapid increases in CBF or cerebral blood volume can worsen intracranial hypertension and contribute to edema. A balanced induction using sedative hypnotics and opioids in addition to lidocaine and or beta-blockers should be considered to mitigate the hemodynamic effects of induction agents. Intravenous vasopressors may be needed to increase MAP and maintain adequate CPP. Prolonged periods of apnea should be avoided because of the associated transient increases in $Paco_2$, which increase CBF and ICP.

Medications that elevate ICP should be avoided when patients have known hydro-cephalus or intracranial hypertension. Safe induction agents include propofol, etomidate, benzodiazepines, barbiturates, and opioids. Ketamine is commonly associated with causing ICP elevation through increasing CBF and metabolism. Recent analyses suggest that ketamine may not increase the ICP and might be ideal for induction, because it generally does not cause vasodilation and decreases in MAP.[31–34] Studies have also suggested there may be some protective effect from ketamine's NMDA antagonism specifically in patients with traumatic brain injuries. Thus, there may be a use for its use in these cases.[35] Succinylcholine is contraindicated in patients with baseline motor deficits owing to the risk of an exaggerated hyperkalemic response.[36,37]

After induction of general anesthesia and intubation, adequate peripheral intravenous access should be established, central venous access and additional monitoring should be considered based on the surgical plan, patient comorbidities, and provider preferences. Beyond standard monitors (electrocardiogram, pulse oximetry, capnography, noninvasive blood pressure, and temperature), invasive arterial blood pressure monitoring with the transducer at the level of the tragus helps assure adequate MAP at the level of the brain and assess CPP. This can also be used to measure volume status parameters such as stroke volume variation and pulse pressure variation, as well as blood gas analysis that can monitor acid–base status, $Paco_2$, electrolytes, and blood hemoglobin.

Central venous access should be considered in any case where there is not adequate peripheral access, a high likelihood of using central vasopressors, a need for monitoring of the central venous pressure, or where a significant risk of VAE is anticipated. Central venous access via the right internal jugular vein may be particularly important if the risk of VAE is high, because it can be used to aspirate venous air in the superior vena cava and right atrium.

Intraoperative Complications

As mentioned elsewhere in this article, cardiovascular instability and collapse can occur from multiple causes during open suboccipital procedures. Sinus arrhythmia, bradycardia, supraventricular tachycardia, paroxysmal ventricular contractions, ventricular fibrillation, and asystole have all been reported.[38]

Bradycardia and asystole have been specifically described in relation to cranial nerve or brainstem pathology as well as surgical stimulation. Neurogenic bradycardia can occur when there is a sudden increase in ICP causing brainstem compression and vagal nerve stimulation. This has the potential to progress to sudden and severe bradycardia.[39] Similarly, there are numerous case reports of asystole suspected secondary to stimulation of the trigeminocardiac reflex. This can occur any time there is stimulation to the trigeminal nerve branches, ganglia, or nucleus. Activation of the vagus nerve efferent pathways results through a connection between the trigeminal and vagal nuclei located closely within the reticular formation. The resulting parasympathetic output can cause bradycardia, asystole, hypotension, and apnea.[39,40] A vasoglossopharyngeal reflex arc has also been described via stimulation of the glossopharyngeal nerve fibers traveling via the nucleus tractus solitarius of the midbrain. This leads to a similar vagal parasympathetic response, as described elsewhere in this article.[39]

These reflexes often abate with the removal of the surgical stimulus and may help surgeons to identify key areas of the brainstem during resection. The resultant cardiovascular depression or cardiac arrest should be addressed immediately using vasopressors and Advanced Cardiac Life Support algorithms.

Venous air embolism

One of the most feared complications during open suboccipital surgery is the occurrence of a VAE. Any position that puts the surgical site above the level of the heart can increase risk. Head elevation above the level of the heart creates negative venous pressure that promotes entrainment of atmospheric air into the venous system at the surgical site. The reported incidence overall has been widely variable, with some studies reporting detection of VAE in up to 100% of cases at some institutions.[41,42] One study found that there was a statistically significant increased risk of VAE events with the head elevated to 45° compared with 30°.[43] Variability is likely based on differences in intraoperative patient positioning, patient pathology, surgical resection techniques, and detection methods. Resection of vascular tumors, as well as inadvertent damage to diploic veins in the skull or the dural venous sinuses around the brain, can all increase risk.

Clinical severity is related to the volume and speed of air entry as well as the final location of the air bubble. Studies suggest clinical manifestations may develop in adults when 100 mL of air is entrained, with lethal doses estimated at 200 to 500 mL or 3 to 5 mL/kg.[44–46] Pediatric patients may show clinical signs with much lower volumes.

The clinical manifestations of VAE can be seen in every organ system including the cardiovascular, pulmonary, neurologic, and hematologic systems. Air entrained via the venous system enters the right heart causing increased right atrial and central venous pressures. Large volume VAE can cause acute right ventricular outflow tract obstruction from an "air lock," leading to immediate right heart failure. This can quickly spiral into hypotension and cardiovascular collapse. The electrocardiogram may show peaked P waves, tachyarrhythmias, ST or T wave changes, or patterns of right heart strain. Auscultation may reveal a classic mill wheel murmur caused by intracardiac air or wheezing from the lungs. This finding typically correlates with a sudden drop in end-tidal carbon dioxide and hypoxia with a decrease in end-tidal carbon dioxide and an increase in $Paco_2$ owing to increased physiologic dead space.[45,47] A recent case report describes the development of stress-induced cardiomyopathy or Takotsubo cardiomyopathy during posterior fossa surgery that was triggered by a VAE.[48]

Slow entrainment of air or small volume VAE can lead to microbubbles that enter the pulmonary circulation. These can cause pulmonary vasoconstriction, leading to a mechanical obstruction, pulmonary hypertension, increased end-tidal carbon dioxide–$PaCO_2$ gradient, and cardiovascular depression. These microemboli can damage pulmonary endothelial cells and release inflammatory mediators, which may precipitate pulmonary edema.[47]

The presence of an intracardiac shunt may result in air entry into the left side of the heart, resulting in a PAE. PAE is much more common in patients with a patent foramen ovale (PFO). Large volumes of air in the left side of the heart can block the left ventricular outflow tract causing immediate systemic heart failure and loss of cardiac output. Small emboli traveling distally from the left heart can impede blood flow to vital organs including the heart and brain resulting in myocardial and cerebral ischemia respectively. Microemboli may pass from the pulmonary capillaries into the pulmonary veins to enter the left heart, however, this is generally thought to be rare.[47] VAE and PAE have also been rarely linked to the development of coagulation abnormalities including thrombocytopenia and factor VIII dysfunction.[49,50]

Cerebral ischemia resulting from VAE is due to either cardiovascular collapse or cerebral air emboli during PAE in patients with an intracardiac shunt. Cerebral ischemia can increase the risk of postoperative altered mental status, focal neurologic deficits, and seizures.

Owing to its significant incidence, patients undergoing open surgery of the posterior fossa should be monitored for the development of VAE, especially when in a sitting or head-up position. Multiple modalities are available and should be considered preoperatively. Transesophageal echocardiography is considered the most sensitive detection method but is invasive, may be associated with adverse effects and requires special training for appropriate interpretation and use. A precordial doppler is placed on the patient's chest wall and is considered the most sensitive noninvasive monitor. A pulmonary artery catheter, which can detect elevated pulmonary pressures from right ventricular outflow tract obstruction and pulmonary vasoconstriction, is an invasive monitor that is, associated with risks during placement[45,47] and from patient positioning. End-tidal carbon dioxide monitoring is considered less sensitive, but is generally thought to detect almost all clinically significant VAEs resulting from significant hemodynamic compromise. The classic mill wheel murmur of intracardiac air is a late sign of significant VAE.[45,51]

Measures to prevent VAE and PAE are of paramount importance. Patients with intracardiac shunts, especially PFO, are not candidates for the sitting position because of the risk of PAE. Research has estimated the prevalence of PFO to be as high as 40%.[52] Some institutions consider evaluation for PFO closure before surgery, whereas others consider it to be a contraindication to open craniotomy in the sitting or semisitting position. Intravascular hydration is thought to help increase central venous pressure to avoid air entrainment. Nitrous oxide increases the size of entrained air and can exacerbate the adverse effects of air in the vasculature; it should be avoided when there is concern for VAE. Early detection of VAE can allow for more rapid management, preventing entrainment of even larger volumes of air and reducing the severity of morbidity and incidence of mortality associated with VAE.

If suspected, air emboli should be treated immediately with 100% oxygen and increased fresh gas flows, and discontinuation of nitrous oxide if it is being used. The surgeon should be notified so that any potential source of air entry can be identified, the field can be flooded with saline and sealant placed over any open sinuses. If it is safe to do so, the patient's head should be lowered as much as possible, preferably below the level of the heart to increase cerebral venous pressure. Manual compression of the jugular veins can also help increase central venous pressure but can promote the embolization of carotid atheromatous plaques in addition to raising ICP. If a mechanical airlock is suspected, placing the patient in left lateral decubitus can help. Aspiration from a central venous catheter in or near the right atrium may help facilitate air removal. Supportive therapy with fluid, vasopressors, and inotropes should be used as needed and cardiopulmonary resuscitation (CPR) should be initiated if indicated. Chest compressions can help to break up large volumes of air trapped in the heart.[19,45] The use of hyperbaric oxygen could also be considered to promote nitrogen absorption and reduce the air burden.[53] Multiple cognitive aids have been developed to help providers manage patients suffering from intraoperative VAE. **Fig. 5** was developed by the Stanford Anesthesia Cognitive Aid Group and can be found online (visit http://emergencymanual. stanford.edu/).

Intraoperative Cardiopulmonary Resuscitation

Because suboccipital surgery is generally not done in a supine position, providing effective chest compressions can be problematic. Although there do not seem to be clear guidelines, there are case reports describing the approaches for successful CPR when patients are in atypical positions.

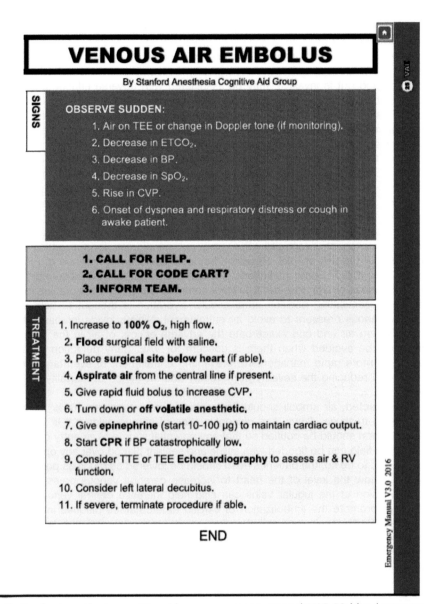

VENOUS AIR EMBOLUS

By Stanford Anesthesia Cognitive Aid Group

SIGNS

OBSERVE SUDDEN:

1. Air on TEE or change in Doppler tone (if monitoring).
2. Decrease in $ETCO_2$.
3. Decrease in BP.
4. Decrease in SpO_2.
5. Rise in CVP.
6. Onset of dyspnea and respiratory distress or cough in awake patient.

1. CALL FOR HELP.
2. CALL FOR CODE CART?
3. INFORM TEAM.

TREATMENT

1. Increase to **100% O_2**, high flow.
2. **Flood** surgical field with saline.
3. Place **surgical site below heart** (if able).
4. **Aspirate air** from the central line if present.
5. Give rapid fluid bolus to increase CVP.
6. Turn down or **off volatile anesthetic.**
7. Give **epinephrine** (start 10-100 μg) to maintain cardiac output.
8. Start **CPR** if BP catastrophically low.
9. Consider TTE or TEE **Echocardiography** to assess air & RV function.
10. Consider left lateral decubitus.
11. If severe, terminate procedure if able.

END

Emergency Manual V3.0 2016

Fig. 5. Stanford anesthesia cognitive aid group emergency manual: VAE. BP, blood pressure; TEE, transesophageal echocardiography; TTE, transthoracic echocardiography. (*From* Howard SK, Chu LF, Goldhaber-Fiebert SN, et al. Emergency Manual: Cognitive aids for perioperative critical events. Stanford Anesthesia Cognitive Aid Group. Available at: https://emergencymanual.stanford.edu/. Reprinted with permission of Steven K. Howard.)

The placement of adhesive defibrillator pads before positioning should be considered in high-risk patients to decrease the time to defibrillation during cardiac arrest. Various placement patterns of defibrillator pads can be used if needed.[54]

Typically, chest compressions in the prone position are not ideal because there is often limited access to the airway and vasculature. However, compressions can be delivered along the thoracic spine so long as there is a hard surface under the sternum to provide counter pressure. This technique is within the 2010 American Heart Association guidelines for CPR when there is an endotracheal tube in place.[55] This is a current topic of discussion in recent articles because of the need for CPR in patients in the intensive care unit who are in the prone position.[56] The 2019 American Heart Association update does not comment on CPR in atypical positions.[57]

Patients undergoing surgery of the posterior fossa should already have a secured airway and vascular access in place. Performing CPR in the prone position may be beneficial to prevent inadvertent loss of airway or vascular access that may occur while attempting to turn supine. Additionally, because the patient's head is often fixated in pins, any change in position will likely take valuable time to accomplish and will also result in loss of access to the surgical field, which may be needed depending on the cause of arrest. Multiple case reports of successful resuscitation in the prone position suggest it is feasible to provide adequate compressions.[54]

There are also case reports of CPR being conducted in the lateral position, all of which describe a technique using a 2-rescuer approach. One person compresses the chest while a second rescuer provides support along the spine to allow for appropriate sternal compression.[54]

If initial attempts are inadequate and not successful, repositioning the patient supine may be indicated.

Postoperative Management

Rapid emergence is desired to allow for an early neurologic examination. Prevention of significant increases in blood pressure, coughing, and straining are also important to minimize worsening of ICP, edema, and hemorrhage at the surgical site. Goals typically include systolic blood pressure goals of less than 160 mm Hg but may need to be adjusted based on preoperative blood pressure. Delayed emergence should be quickly worked through with a high suspicion for neurologic cause and the possible need for imaging.

Safe extubation should consider a number of factors and should be done only after extubation criteria are met. Patients may have edema of the airway or the tongue regardless of positioning used. An endotracheal tube cuff leak test or the use of an airway exchange catheter may be considered. Surgical manipulation of the brainstem and/or cranial nerves may lead to loss of airway reflexes or alterations to the normal respiratory response to oxygen and carbon dioxide. The anesthesia team should be aware of such potential complications.

Historically, postoperative management has varied between early awakening and extubation with a neurologic examination or continued sedation with a routine computed tomography scan of the head and monitoring in an intensive care unit setting. Both approaches were developed to allow early recognition and intervention if there are any neurosurgical complications. Early awakening can minimize unnecessary imaging procedures when a neurologic examination is reassuring.[58] Whether extubated early or not, these patients should be monitored in an intensive care setting postoperatively because swelling or edema at the surgical site may result in rapid neurologic deterioration and should be addressed without delay.

Postoperative pain after craniotomies can be significant, with some studies suggesting that infratentorial and suboccipital procedures are associated with more pain than other craniotomy sites. Higher levels of pain are associated with increased sympathetic output, increased risk of elevated ICP, and systemic hypertension. Opioids, once the mainstay of analgesic therapy, can lead to altered mental status, respiratory depression, and hypercapnia. A wide range of approaches to analgesia should be considered throughout the perioperative period to decrease the risk of both acute complications and the development of chronic pain.[59]

Postoperative Complications

Postoperative complications after open suboccipital surgery are felt occur more frequently than after supratentorial procedures presumably because of the density of neurovascular structures and CSF pathways in the posterior fossa. However, this has not been extensively studied and reviewed. One retrospective study by Dubey and colleagues[60] reported the overall rate of complication to be 31.8% in a group of 500 patients at a single intuition. The most common complications included CSF leak, meningitis, wound infections, and cranial nerve palsies. Additionally, complications like tension pneumocephalus, macroglossia, hemorrhage, and posterior fossa syndrome can cause significant postoperative morbidity and mortality.[60] The incidence of these complications is likely variable between centers and depends on the surgical techniques, pathology, and patient comorbidities.

CSF leaks are common, but the actual incidence is variable and depends on factors including pathology and surgical approach. Patients with a CSF leak may require placement of lumbar drain or surgical repair.[60–62] Similarly, the rate of infection following posterior fossa surgery has been shown to be significantly higher than in supratentorial procedures. This is likely in part owing to the higher rate of CSF leak. Appropriate perioperative antibiotics, sterile technique, and wound management can help reduce this risk of infection.[60]

Pneumocephalus is the presence of any gas within the cranial cavity that can occur any time the dura is interrupted. Entry into the fourth ventricle intraoperatively can lead to air entrainment into the ventricular system and cause ventricular pneumocephalus. Suboccipital craniotomy in the sitting position creates a hydrostatic effect in the CSF causing air to rise and get trapped in dead space. Tension pneumocephalus can occur when high volumes of air in the tightly confined skull cause mass effect and eventual brain herniation.[63]

Clinically, pneumocephalus has variable presentation that is, associated with the amount of air that has been entrapped and the severity of tissue displacement. Patients may show altered mental status, focal neurologic deficits, headaches, and seizures. Tension pneumocephalus may require a surgical intervention such as a burr hole or external ventricular drain to relieve the trapped gas. It should be considered in the event of delayed emergence or acute neurologic change in the postoperative period and can be evaluated with imaging.[63]

Historically, the development of significant tension pneumocephalus has been associated with the use of intraoperative nitrous oxide owing to its rapid diffusion rate compared with nitrogen. However, 100% oxygen is thought to help resolve the accumulation of nitrous oxide.[64] Hong and colleagues studies the use of hyperoxia to treat patients with pneumocephalus. Forty-four patients who developed postoperative supratentorial pneumocephalus following posterior fossa surgery were randomized to treatment group. The authors found that postoperative treatment with 3 hours of 100% fraction of inspired oxygen via an endotracheal tube resulted in significantly increased resorption of the pneumocephalus.[65]

Postoperative swelling involving the tissues of the oropharynx can occur after suboccipital surgery primarily owing to complications with positioning. Any position requiring flexion at the head and neck can cause venous drainage obstruction at the internal jugular veins. Prone positioning has the potential to lead to dependent edema of the nasal, oral, and laryngeal tissues.[66] Airway swelling is also associated with trauma from endotracheal intubation, orogastric tube placement, or biting of the tongue. Significant edema after extubation can lead to hypoxia and hypercapnia and may require reintubation, which can be difficult. Endotracheal tube cuff leak before extubation may help to identify laryngeal or tracheal edema.

Significant neck flexion has also been associated with spinal cord damage from stretch and infarction. Hypoperfusion to the cord caused by hypotension and reduced cardiac output is also associated with spinal cord damage. Rarely, reports of postoperative paraplegia and quadriplegia have been reported in patients undergoing posterior fossa surgery. Intraoperative neuromonitoring of the spinal cord pathways may help identify the risk of spinal cord ischemia early and decrease the resultant morbidity.[67]

Cranial nerve injury can be seen postoperatively in any of nerves III to XII and may result in either transient of permanent dysfunction. This can occur from direct nerve injury or ischemia from retraction or vasospasm. Damage to cranial nerves III, IV, or VI often results in diplopia and may require future corrective surgery. Cranial nerve VIII is particularly sensitive to damage from manipulation, which will result in postoperative hearing loss. Damage to the lower cranial nerves (IX–XII) is less common, but can result in significant loss of airway reflexes and dysphasia, which predisposes patients to aspiration pneumonia and increases the risk of needed postoperative tracheostomy and mechanical ventilation. Intraoperative neuromonitoring of cranial nerves associated with a given lesion has been shown to decrease the incidence of postoperative complications.[60]

Cerebellar mutism or posterior fossa syndrome is a rare occurrence following posterior fossa surgery. This neurologic disorder is often considered a complex of disorders that presents with reduced or absent speech in combination with symptoms such as ataxia, hypotonia, cranial nerve deficits, behavioral changes, and urinary symptoms. Its etiology is unknown. It is primarily seen in children following surgical resection of midline tumors in the posterior fossa. Symptoms often resolve over time; however, it can leave patients with long-term neurologic sequelae.[60,68,69]

Hematoma formation at the surgical site is not common but can be devastating. This typically causes altered mental status or focal neurologic deficits owing to mass effect in the small posterior fossa space. Early recognition and treatment with surgical evacuation is vital to prevent permanent neurologic damage; however, prevention by controlling hypertension and treating any coagulopathy is important.[60]

SUMMARY

The complex intracranial anatomy of the posterior fossa combined with unique positioning for optimal surgical access and management, poses significant challenges to a neuroanesthesiologist. Careful patient selection, thoughtful preoperative planning and discussion with surgical teams, an extensive discussion of relative risks and benefits with patients, a good understanding of the posterior fossa anatomy, physiologic changes associated with positioning and surgery, checklists, cognitive aids, and effective communication among team members may be associated with good outcomes.

REFERENCES

1. Özek MM, Cinalli G, Maixner W, et al. Posterior fossa tumors in children. vol Cham (Switzerland): Springer International Publishing : Springer; 2015.
2. Párraga RG, Possatti LL, Alves RV, et al. Microsurgical anatomy and internal architecture of the brainstem in 3D images: surgical considerations. J Neurosurg 2016;124(5):1377–95.

3. Hardy DG, Peace DA, Rhoton AL Jr. Microsurgical anatomy of the superior cerebellar artery. Neurosurgery 1980;6(1):10–28.

4. Matta BF, Menon DK, Turner JM. Textbook of neuroanaesthesia and critical care. vol London (United Kingdom): Greenwich Medical Media, Ltd.; 2000.

5. Jagannathan S, Krovvidi H. Anaesthetic considerations for posterior fossa surgery. Continuing Education in Anaesthesia Critical Care & Pain 2014;14(5):202–6.

6. Nishikawa M, Sakamoto H, Hakuba A, et al. Pathogenesis of Chiari malformation: a morphometric study of the posterior cranial fossa. J Neurosurg 1997; 86(1):40–7.

7. Kameda-Smith MM, White MA, St George EJ, et al. Time to diagnosis of paediatric posterior fossa tumours: an 11-year West of Scotland experience 2000-2011. Br J Neurosurg 2013;27(3):364–9.

8. Grossman R, Ram Z. Posterior fossa intra-axial tumors in adults. World Neurosurg 2016;88:140–5.

9. Shih RY, Smirniotopoulos JG. Posterior fossa tumors in adult patients. Neuroimaging Clin N Am 2016;26(4):493–510.

10. Marx S, El Damaty A, Manwaring J, et al. Endoscopic third ventriculostomy before posterior fossa tumor surgery in adult patients. J Neurol Surg A Cent Eur Neurosurg 2018;79(2):123–9.

11. Lin CT, Riva-Cambrin JK. Management of posterior fossa tumors and hydrocephalus in children: a review. Childs Nerv Syst 2015;31(10):1781–9.

12. Liu MM, Reidy AB, Saatee S, et al. Perioperative steroid management: approaches based on current evidence. Anesthesiology 2017;127(1):166–72.

13. Rath GP, Bithal PK, Chaturvedi A, et al. Complications related to positioning in posterior fossa craniectomy. J Clin Neurosci 2007;14(6):520–5.

14. Lee A, Chen ML, Abeshaus S, et al. Posterior fossa tumors and their impact on sleep and ventilatory control: a clinical perspective. Respir Physiol Neurobiol 2013;189(2):261–71.

15. Slotty PJ, Abdulazim A, Kodama K, et al. Intraoperative neurophysiological monitoring during resection of infratentorial lesions: the surgeon's view. J Neurosurg 2017;126(1):281–8.

16. Friedman D, Claassen J, Hirsch LJ. Continuous electroencephalogram monitoring in the intensive care unit. Anesth Analg 2009;109(2):506–23.

17. Gupta P, Rath GP, Prabhakar H, et al. Complications related to sitting position during pediatric neurosurgery: an institutional experience and review of literature. Neurol India 2018;66(1):217–22.

18. Leslie K, Kaye AH. The sitting position and the patent foramen ovale. Commentary: "a streamlined protocol for the use of the semi-sitting position in neurosurgery". J Clin Neurosci 2013;20(1):35–6.

19. Ganslandt O, Merkel A, Schmitt H, et al. The sitting position in neurosurgery: indications, complications and results. a single institution experience of 600 cases. Acta Neurochir (Wien) 2013;155(10):1887–93.

20. Feigl GC, Decker K, Wurms M, et al. Neurosurgical procedures in the semisitting position: evaluation of the risk of paradoxical venous air embolism in patients with a patent foramen ovale. World Neurosurg 2014;81(1):159–64.

21. Spektor S, Fraifeld S, Margolin E, et al. Comparison of outcomes following complex posterior fossa surgery performed in the sitting versus lateral position. J Clin Neurosci 2015;22(4):705–12.

22. McCulloch TJ, Liyanagama K, Petchell J. Relative hypotension in the beach-chair position: effects on middle cerebral artery blood velocity. Anaesth Intensive Care 2010;38(3):486–91.

23. Ranjith M, Bidkar PU, Narmadalakshmi K, et al. Effects of crystalloid preloading (20 ml/kg) on Hemodynamics in Relation to Postural Changes in Patients Undergoing Neurosurgical Procedures in Sitting Position. J Neurosci Rural Pract 2018; 9(1):80–5.

24. Schramm P, Tzanova I, Gööck T, et al. Noninvasive hemodynamic measurements during neurosurgical procedures in sitting position. J Neurosurg Anesthesiol 2017;29(3):251–7.

25. Cucchiara RF, Nugent M, Seward JB, et al. Air embolism in upright neurosurgical patients: detection and localization by two-dimensional transesophageal echocardiography. Anesthesiology 1984;60:353–5.

26. Takasaki Y. Transient lingual ischaemia during anaesthesia. Anaesthesia 2003; 58:717.

27. Rozet I, Vavilala MS. Risks and benefits of patient positioning during neurosurgical care. Anesthesiol Clin 2007;25(3):631–53, x.

28. Perks A, Chakravarti S, Manninen P. Preoperative anxiety in neurosurgical patients. J Neurosurg Anesthesiol 2009;21(2):127–30.

29. de-Lima-Oliveira M, Salinet ASM, Nogueira RC, et al. Intracranial hypertension and cerebral autoregulation: a systematic review and meta-analysis. World Neurosurg 2018;113:110–24.

30. Meyer JS, Rogers RL, Mortel KF. Prospective analysis of long term control of mild hypertension on cerebral blood flow. Stroke 1985;16(6):985–90.

31. Wang X, Ding X, Tong Y, et al. Ketamine does not increase intracranial pressure compared with opioids: meta-analysis of randomized controlled trials. J Anesth 2014;28(6):821–7.

32. Mayberg TS, Lam AM, Matta BF, et al. Ketamine does not increase cerebral blood flow velocity or intracranial pressure during isoflurane/nitrous oxide anesthesia in patients undergoing craniotomy. Anesth Analg 1995;81(1):84–9.

33. Farrell D, Bendo AA. Perioperative management of severe traumatic brain injury: what is new? Curr Anesthesiol Rep 2018;8(3):279–89.

34. Zeiler FA, Teitelbaum J, West M, et al. The ketamine effect on ICP in traumatic brain injury. Neurocrit Care 2014;21(1):163–73.

35. Hertle DN, Dreier JP, Woitzik J, et al. Effect of analgesics and sedatives on the occurrence of spreading depolarizations accompanying acute brain injury. Brain 2012;135(Pt 8):2390–8.

36. Cottrell JE. Succinylcholine and intracranial pressure. Anesthesiology 2018; 129(6):1159–62.

37. Patanwala AE, Erstad BL, Roe DJ, et al. Succinylcholine is associated with increased mortality when used for rapid sequence intubation of severely brain injured patients in the emergency department. Pharmacotherapy 2016;36(1): 57–63.

38. Rath GP, Chaturvedi A, Chouhan RS, et al. Transient cardiac asystole in transsphenoidal pituitary surgery: a case report. J Neurosurg Anesthesiol 2004; 16(4):299–301.

39. Goyal K, Philip FA, Rath GP, et al. Asystole during posterior fossa surgery: report of two cases. Asian J Neurosurg 2012;2:87–9.

40. Schaller B. Trigeminocardiac reflex. A clinical phenomenon or a new physiological entity? J Neurol 2004;251(6):658–65.

41. Bithal PK, Pandia MP, Dash HH, et al. Comparative incidence of venous air embolism and associated hypotension in adults and children operated for neurosurgery in the sitting position. Eur J Anaesthesiol 2004;21(7):517–22.

42. Leslie K, Hui R, Kaye AH. Venous air embolism and the sitting position: a case series. J Clin Neurosci 2006;13(4):419–22.
43. Türe H, Harput MV, Bekiroğlu N, et al. Effect of the degree of head elevation on the incidence and severity of venous air embolism in cranial neurosurgical procedures with patients in the semisitting position. J Neurosurg 2018;128(5): 1560–9.
44. Toung TJ, Rossberg MI, Hutchins GM. Volume of air in a lethal venous air embolism. Anesthesiology 2001;94(2):360–1.
45. Mirski MA, Lele AV, Fitzsimmons L, et al. Diagnosis and treatment of vascular air embolism. Anesthesiology 2007;106(1):164–77.
46. Gordy S, Rowell S. Vascular air embolism. Int J Crit Illn Inj Sci 2013;3(1):73–6.
47. Brull SJ, Prielipp RC. Vascular air embolism: a silent hazard to patient safety. J Crit Care 2017;42:255–63.
48. Raimann F, Senft C, Honold J, et al. Takotsubo cardiomyopathy triggered by venous air embolism during craniotomy in the sitting position. World Neurosurg 2017;107:1045.e1–4.
49. Schäfer ST, Sandalcioglu IE, Stegen B, et al. Venous air embolism during semi-sitting craniotomy evokes thrombocytopenia. Anaesthesia 2011;66(1):25–30.
50. Moningi S, Kulkarni D, Bhattacharjee S. Coagulopathy following venous air embolism: a disastrous consequence -a case report. Korean J Anesthesiol 2013;65(4): 349–52.
51. Kapurch CJ, Abcejo AS, Pasternak JJ. The relationship between end-expired carbon dioxide tension and severity of venous air embolism during sitting neurosurgical procedures - A contemporary analysis. J Clin Anesth 2018;51:49–54.
52. Koutroulou I, Tsivgoulis G, Tsalikakis D, et al. Epidemiology of patent foramen ovale in general population and in stroke patients: a narrative review. Front Neurol 2020;11:281.
53. Brodbeck A, Bothma P, Pease J. Venous air embolism: ultrasonographic diagnosis and treatment with hyperbaric oxygen therapy. Br J Anaesth 2018;121(6): 1215–7.
54. Bhatnagar V, Jinjil K, Dwivedi D, et al. Cardiopulmonary resuscitation: unusual techniques for unusual situations. J Emerg Trauma Shock 2018;11(1):31–7.
55. Cave DM, Gazmuri RJ, Otto CW, et al. Part 7: CPR techniques and devices: 2010 American heart association guidelines for cardiopulmonary resuscitation and emergency cardiovascular care. Circulation 2010;122(18 Suppl 3):S720–8.
56. Barker J, Koeckerling D, West R. A need for prone position CPR guidance for intubated and non-intubated patients during the COVID-19 pandemic. Resuscitation 2020;151:135–6.
57. Panchal AR, Berg KM, Hirsch KG, et al. 2019 American heart association focused update on advanced cardiovascular life support: use of advanced airways, vasopressors, and extracorporeal cardiopulmonary resuscitation during cardiac arrest: an update to the American heart association guidelines for cardiopulmonary resuscitation and emergency cardiovascular care. Circulation 2019;140(24):e881–94.
58. Schär RT, Fiechter M, Z'Graggen WJ, et al. No routine postoperative head CT following elective craniotomy–a paradigm shift? PLoS One 2016;11(4):e0153499.
59. Vacas S, Van de Wiele B. Designing a pain management protocol for craniotomy: a narrative review and consideration of promising practices. Surg Neurol Int 2017;8:291.
60. Dubey A, Sung WS, Shaya M, et al. Complications of posterior cranial fossa surgery–an institutional experience of 500 patients. Surg Neurol 2009;72(4):369–75.

61. Altaf I, Vohra AH, Shams S. Management of cerebrospinal fluid leak following posterior cranial fossa surgery. Pak J Med Sci 2016;32(6):1439-43.

62. Bayazit YA, Celenk F, Duzlu M, et al. Management of cerebrospinal fluid leak following retrosigmoid posterior cranial fossa surgery. ORL J Otorhinolaryngol Relat Spec 2009;71(6):329-33.

63. Sachkova A, Schemmerling T, Goldberg M, et al. Predictors of ventricular tension pneumocephalus after posterior fossa surgery in the sitting position. Acta Neurochir (Wien) 2018;160(3):525-38.

64. MacGillivray RG. Pneumocephalus as a complication of posterior fossa surgery in the sitting position. Anaesthesia 1982;37(7):722-5.

65. Hong B, Biertz F, Raab P, et al. Normobaric hyperoxia for treatment of pneumocephalus after posterior fossa surgery in the semisitting position: a prospective randomized controlled trial. PLoS One 2015;10(5):e0125710.

66. Edgcombe H, Carter K, Yarrow S. Anaesthesia in the prone position. Br J Anaesth 2008;100(2):165-83.

67. Yahanda AT, Chicoine MR. Paralysis caused by spinal cord injury after posterior fossa surgery: a systematic review. World Neurosurg 2020;139:151-7.

68. Patay Z. Postoperative posterior fossa syndrome: unraveling the etiology and underlying pathophysiology by using magnetic resonance imaging. Childs Nerv Syst 2015;31(10):1853-8.

69. Wibroe M, Cappelen J, Castor C, et al. Cerebellar mutism syndrome in children with brain tumours of the posterior fossa. BMC Cancer 2017;17(1):439.

Acute Ischemic Stroke

Kate Petty, MD[a], Brian P. Lemkuil, MD[b], Brian Gierl, MD[c],*

KEYWORDS

- Ischemic stroke • Thrombolysis • Thrombectomy
- Tissue plasminogen activator (tPA) • Alteplase • Tenectaplase
- Hemorrhagic transformation • Decompressive hemicraniectomy

KEY POINTS

- tPA is a viable treatment for ischemic stroke patients but its benefits must be balanced against the its increased risk of intraparenchymal hemorrhage.
- Perioperative strokes may occur in as many as 7% of older patients having major surgery. Perioperative strokes are most likely to be thromboembolic in origin and occur on postoperative days 1-4.
- Patients with prior strokes are at increased risk for future strokes. Recommendations are mixed as to delay an elective surgery for 3 or 9 months after an AIS. Maintaining the hemoglobin above 9 g/dL may reduce the rate of stroke in patients at high risk for stroke.

Glossary	
Afib	Atrial Fibrillation
AnStroke	General Anesthesia vs Conscious Sedation for Endovascular Treatment of Acute Ischemic Stroke
AVM	Arteriovenous Malformation
BRIDGE	Perioperative Bridging Anticoagulation in Patients with Atrial Fibrillation
CHADS2	Stroke Risk score of CHF, HTN, Age ≥75 y, Diabetes Mellitus, Prior Stroke or Tia
CS	Conscious sedation
DAWN	Clinical Mismatch in the Triage of Wake Up and Late Presenting Strokes Undergoing Neurointervention With Trevo
DEFUSE 3	Endovascular Therapy Following Imaging Evaluation for Ischemic Stroke 3
ECASS	European Cooperative Acute Stroke Study
EVT	Endovascular Thrombectomy
ECASS	European Cooperative Acute Stroke Study
GA	General Anesthesia
GOLIATH	General Or Local Anaestesia in Intra Arterial Therapy
HTN	Hypertension
HT	Hemorrhagic transformation

[a] University of Pittsburgh Medical Center, 3550 Terrace Street, Scaife Hall, Suite 600, Pittsburgh, PA 15213, USA; [b] 200 West Arbor Drive, San Diego, CA 92103, USA; [c] University of Pittsburgh Medical Center, 200 Lothrop Street, Suite C-200, Pittsburgh, PA 15213, USA
* Corresponding author.
E-mail address: Gierlbt2@upmc.edu

Anesthesiology Clin 39 (2021) 113–125
https://doi.org/10.1016/j.anclin.2020.11.002
1932-2275/21/© 2020 Elsevier Inc. All rights reserved.
anesthesiology.theclinics.com

ICH	Intracranial hemorrhage
INR	International Normalized Units
IS	Ischemic stroke
IV	Intravenous
LA	Local Anesthesia
LKWT	Last Known Well Time
MAP	Mean arterial pressure
mRS	Modified Rankin scale
MASTERSTROKE	MAnagement of Systolic blood pressure during Thrombectomy by Endovascular Route for acute ischaemic STROKE
MI	Myocardial Infarction
MR CLEAN	Randomized Trial of Intraarterial Treatment for Acute Ischemic Stroke
NeuroVISION	Perioperative covert stroke in patients undergoing non-cardiac surgery: a prospective cohort study
NIHSS	National Institutes of Health Stroke Scale
POISE	Perioperative Ischemic Evaluation Study
PT	Prothrombin Time
RCT	Randomized controlled trial
SIESTA	Sedation vs Intubation for Endovascular Stroke TreAtment
SNACC	Society for Neuroscience in Anesthesiology and Critical Care
tPA	Tissue plasminogen activator
TICI	Thrombolysis in cerebral infarction (TICI) scale

INTRODUCTION

There are more than 9 million cases of ischemic stroke (IS) resulting in approximately 3 million deaths each year. In the United States, IS represents approximately 87% of strokes, is the fifth leading cause of death, and is a leading cause of serious long-term disability. Currently, there are approximately 67 million survivors of IS throughout the world.[1]

Table 1
Ischemic stroke types, etiologies, and risk factors

Categories	Etiology	Risk Factors
Thrombotic	Atherosclerosis—typically large extracranial or intracranial arteries, dissection	HTN, diabetes, hyperlipidemia, obesity, lack of exercise, smoking, carotid stenosis
Embolic	Cardiac >> atheroembolic, dissection	Arrythmias (afib > flutter), cardiomyopathy, bacterial endocarditis, PFO, recent MI, non-native heart valve, carotid stenosis
Small vessel disease	CADASIL, sporadic small vessel disease	Hypertension[a]
Other	Hypercoagulopathy, vasospasm, sickle cell disease, vasculitis, RCVS, moyamoya disease, illicit drug use, radiation-induced vasculopathy	Etiology specific

Abbreviations: CADASIL, cerebral autosomal dominant arteriopathy with subcortical infarcts and leukoencephalopathy; PFO, patent foramen ovale; RCVS, reversible cerebral vasoconstriction syndrome.
 [a] Likely other common CV risk factors as well.

Anesthesiologists provide care to acute and subacute IS patients as well as stroke survivors in the interventional radiology (IR) suite, the intensive care unit, and the operating room. These encounters will become more frequent following recent studies that have extended the treatment window from last known well time (LKWT) for both fibrinolytic thrombectomy and endovascular thrombectomy (EVT). The number of stroke centers that are certified to quickly and effectively initiate treatment of IS patients and the number of patients connected to them by telehealth continue to grow. These advances will increase the number of patients treated as well as survivors.

As such, anesthesiologists can expect increased involvement in the care of acute IS patients and should be familiar with all aspects of care, including initial assessment, treatment, anesthetic management, and postoperative care. This article reviews IS pathophysiology, assessment and treatment, pathology, and complications; anesthetic management during EVT; perioperative stroke management; and how anesthesia has an impact on patients with prior stroke. Much has changed in the management of IS since it was last reviewed in *Anesthesiology Clinics* in 2012.[2]

ACUTE ISCHEMIC STROKE

IS is defined as an episode of neurologic dysfunction caused by focal (or global) cerebral, spinal, or retinal infarction. An IS occurs when blood flow through an artery supplying the central nervous system with oxygen and nutrients becomes severely impaired. **Table 1** delineates various stroke types.

PATHOPHYSIOLOGY

The brain is uniquely sensitive to any reduction in metabolic substrate delivery due to its high metabolic demand and limited storage capacity. Therefore, it is highly dependent on continuous cerebral blood flow, which is maintained at approximately 50 mL per 100 g of brain tissue per minute and is tightly regulated over a broad range of cerebral perfusion pressures.

During IS, arterial flow is impaired, resulting in an ischemic core that undergoes rapid irreversible cell death. The area surrounding the core, known as the ischemic penumbra, has cerebral blood flow in the range of 5 mL/100 g/min to 15 mL/100 g/min. Although electrically dysfunctional, it remains salvageable for a period of time if flow can be restored. In the absence of revascularization, the penumbra gradually is recruited into the ischemic core, hence the adage, time is brain. During a stroke, it is estimated that 1.9 million neurons die each minute. Focal ischemia often is tolerated better than global ischemia (cardiac arrest) due to the potential for collateral blood flow from neighboring vascular territories via the circle of Willis or through leptomeningeal collaterals on the surface of the brain in a manner sufficient to stave off energy failure for a period of time.

Rarely, an aberrant clot forms in a vein and occludes outflow, which then stops arterial blood flow into the effected tissue. This is known as a venous infarct, and typically it is treated with a heparin infusion.

Researchers have investigated several drugs intended to limit ischemic damage during the acute phase of stroke, to limit secondary damage due to edema and inflammation in the second phase of stroke, and to support neuronal regrowth. Many have been successful in animal models of stroke, but none has shown efficacy in humans.

GRADING SEVERITY, IMAGING, TREATMENT

The National Institutes of Health Stroke Scale (NIHSS) is a comprehensive but simple neurologic assessment tool that quantifies clinical impairment and helps identify patients for revascularization therapy. Eleven clinical elements are evaluated, with greater impairment receiving higher scores. Scores range from 0 to 42. A score greater than 16 predicts a high probability of death and a score less than 7 predicts a strong probability of good recovery.

Clinical assessment is rapidly followed by imaging. A noncontrast computed tomography (CT) should be obtained as soon as possible in patients with suspected stroke to rule out intracranial hemorrhage (ICH). Usually, this imaging is sufficient to initiate acute treatment with tissue plasminogen activator (tPA), or alteplase. Patients presenting within 6 hours of LKWT also should have vascular imaging of the head and neck to identify large vessel occlusion for EVT candidacy. The angiogram, however, should not delay initiation of tPA. tPA administration does not alter eligibility for EVT. Given the relatively poor recanalization rate of intravenous (IV) tPA for large vessel occlusion, endovascular therapy should not be delayed to assess for a clinical response to tPA in eligible patients.[3]

IV tPA was the original therapy used for vascular recanalization. Initially, alteplase was shown to improved outcomes when administered within 3 hours of LKWT; this window subsequently was expanded to 4.5 hours for most patients following European Cooperative Acute Stroke Study (ECASS) III.[4] The numbers of patients needed to be treated to have 1 additional patient have a good outcome are 10 and 19, if initiated within 3 hours and 4.5 hours of last LKWT, respectively. The relatively brief treatment window, numerous contraindications, and poor recanalization rates for proximal large vessel occlusion helped drive the development of subsequent endovascular therapies.

Intra-arterial catheter-directed tPA is a means to deliver high concentrations of tPA directly to the occluded site. Although it remains a revascularization tool, it rarely is used due to endovascular technology advances and better supportive data for alternative therapies. This technique is used mainly to reduce the risk of hemorrhage in patients with a contraindication to systemic IV tPA who are within the tPA window and have failed mechanical clot removal.

Patients over 18 years of age within 4.5 hours of LKWT are tPA candidates unless absolute contraindications are present. Contraindications and considerations are numerous, many of which require a risk-benefit assessment that is best determined by a stroke physician. Common contraindications for IV tPA therapy are listed in **Table 2**. A comprehensive list of relative contraindications and considerations are summarized in the 2019 American Heart Association (AHA) guidelines for early acute

Table 2 Tissue plasminogen activator contraindications	
Risk	**Criterion**
Head bleed	Hemorrhage on CT; head trauma, IS, intracranial or intraspinal surgery within 3 mo; intracranial neoplasm, arteriovenous malformation or aneurysm; any prior ICH
Coagulopathy	Platelet count <100 k, international normalized ratio >1.7, prothrombin time >15 s Use of direct thrombin inhibitors or factor Xa antagonists

stroke management.[5] Alteplase is the only tPA currently approved. Alteplase treatment consists of a bolus, followed by an infusion over 1 hour. Tenecteplase is an enzyme that was designed to have a higher fibrin specificity and a longer half-life than alteplase and, therefore, does not require an infusion.[6] Although not approved for IS use in the United States or European Union as of 2020, it appears to be at least as effective and potentially safer than alteplase, but there is not a head-to-head trial.

Advanced imaging technology has expanded the window for reperfusion therapy in patients without a clear LKWT or who are outside the traditional 6-hour EVT window. Two studies, Clinical Mismatch in the Triage of Wake Up and Late Presenting Strokes Undergoing Neurointervention With Trevo (DAWN) and Endovascular Therapy Following Imaging Evaluation for Ischemic Stroke 3 (DEFUSE 3), demonstrated improved outcomes in patients with large vessel occlusion and "imaging mismatch" who received EVT 6 hours to 24 hours after LKWT. CT angiography and CT perfusion and/or multimodal magnetic resonance imaging (MRI) sequences, including diffusion-weighted imaging, were used to identify patients with either "clinical-imaging mismatch" or "penumbral imaging." Clinical imaging mismatch was defined as a mismatch between the severity of stroke symptoms and infarct volume and penumbral imaging defined as mismatch between potentially salvageable ischemic tissue and irreversibly damaged tissues.[7,8]

Table 3
Risk factors associated with hemorrhagic transformation

Risk Factor	Recommendation
Advancing age	—
Higher NIHSS score	—
Alteplase	—
Higher glucose	—
Early CT hypodensity	—
Diabetes mellitus	—
Cardioembolic stroke	Alteplase contraindicated with infective endocarditis
Prior ASA → alteplase	Alteplase not contraindicated[a]
Prior ASA + Plavix → alteplase	Alteplase not contraindicated[a]
Alteplase + ASA <24 h post-thrombolysis[b]	ASA generally delayed 24 h post-tPA
Cardioembolic + early anticoagulation	Delay anticoagulation several days
Prior anticoagulation + alteplase	Alteplase contraindicated
Prolonged interval between stroke and recanalization	Imaging mismatch-based treatment
Hypertension (without tPA or EVT)	Permissive up to systolic blood pressure 220 mm Hg
Hypertension + alteplase	Systolic blood pressure <180/105 mm Hg
Hypertension + EVT	Systolic blood pressure <180/105 mm Hg is reasonable maximum
Fever + alteplase	Normothermia

[a] Increased symptomatic HT, no independent association with worse outcome.[9]
[b] Recently contested.[10]

Data from Luo S, Zhuang M, Zeng W, et al. Intravenous Thrombolysis for Acute Ischemic Stroke in Patients Receiving Antiplatelet Therapy: A Systematic Review and Meta-analysis of 19 Studies. J Am Heart Assoc. 2016;5(5); and Jeong H-G, Kim BJ, Yang MH, et al. Stroke outcomes with use of antithrombotics within 24 hours after recanalization treatment. Neurology. 2016;87(10):996-1002.

> **Box 1**
> **Management of symptomatic intracranial hemorrhage less than 24 hours following intravenous alteplase**
>
> Stop alteplase infusion
>
> Laboratory results: complete blood cell count, prothrombin time/international normalized ratio, partial thromboplastin time, fibrinogen, type and crossmatch blood products
>
> CT head
>
> Cryoprecipitate transfusion: 10 U, repeat dose for fibrinogen level less than 150 mg/dL
>
> Tranexamic Acid 1,000 mg over 10 min OR epsilon-aminocaproic acid 4-5 g over 1 h, followed by 1 g/h for 8 h
>
> Hematology and neurosurgery consults
>
> Manage blood pressure, ICP, CPP, temperature, glucose
>
> *Abbreviations:* CPP, cerebral perfusion pressure; ICP, intracranial pressure.

PATHOLOGY AND HEMORRHAGIC CONVERSION

In addition to cytotoxic edema and subsequent cell death, severe ischemic insult results in breakdown of the blood brain barrier 4 hours to 12 hours after insult, which allows plasma protein leakage into the extracellular space. Hydrostatic and osmotic gradients further increase water content within the ischemic territory, referred to as vasogenic edema. Vasogenic edema can lead to profound mass effect, cerebral compression, increased intracranial pressure/reduced cerebral perfusion pressure, and herniation if it is not treated with medical therapy or decompressive craniotomy in a timely fashion.

Reperfusion of a previously ischemic tissue may result in whole-blood extravasation through the disrupted vasculature, referred to as hemorrhagic transformation (HT). HT, although frequently asymptomatic and often found on routine imaging, may be profound and cause acute clinical deterioration. Various therapeutic interventions, such as thrombolytics, endovascular manipulation, and anticoagulation, are known to increase HT rates and severity. Various risk factors are presented in **Table 3**. Anesthesiologists should be prepared to manage symptomatic ICH that occurs within 24 hours of IV tPA (**Box 1, Table 4**).

ENDOVASCULAR THROMBECTOMY AND ANESTHESIA

Endovascular neurosurgery is a rapidly expanding field with frequent technology advancements that have made mechanical clot removal for large vessel occlusions more effective than enzymatic therapy. EVT can improve neurologic outcome up to

Table 4
Comparative risks and benefits of different anesthesia techniques for thrombectomy

Technique	Risk of Hypotension	Risk of Desaturation	Risk of Aspiration	Neurologic Examination	Groin Puncture Time
LA	—	—	—	—	—
CS	↑	↑↑	↑↑	↓	—
GA	↑↑	↓	↓	↓↓	↑↑

24 hours after LKWT when specific criteria are met. The 2 main technologies currently employed are large-bore aspiration catheters and stent retriever systems.

Many patients undergoing attempted endovascular recanalization require anesthesiologists to ensure patient comfort and immobilization, manage the airway, and manipulate systemic physiology to optimize patient outcomes. The specific anesthetic type depends on the institution, anesthesia provider availability, patient comorbidities, and the neurologic status of the patient. Local anesthetic only (LA), conscious sedation (CS), and general anesthesia (GA) all are used. Each anesthetic confers unique benefits and risks within the angiography suite. See **Table 4**.

The benefits of GA include an immobile patient and a secure airway. These benefits are at the expense of a continuous neurologic examination, risk of hypotension, likely increased time to groin puncture, and need of immediate anesthesia availability. Alternatively, LA and CS have the theoretic advantages of a continuous neurologic examination, reduced hemodynamic compromise, and faster time to groin puncture. These advantages are countered by delays due to patient movement and the absence of a secure airway with the attendant risk of aspiration.

Three randomized controlled trials (RCTs) have evaluated various outcomes in patients who received GA versus CS for EVT in setting of large vessel occlusion. The 2017 AnStroke Trial included 90 patients and employed tight hemodynamic goals and normal Pco_2 levels.[11] They reported no difference in 90-day neurologic outcome (modified Rankin scale [mRS] ≤2; 42.2% vs 40%, respectively). The Siesta trial evaluated 150 patients and found that CS did not improve early neurologic recovery (primary outcome). The secondary outcome of mRS score at 90 days favored the GA group (mRS of 0–2 in 37% vs 18.2%, respectively).[12] The 2018 GOLIATH trial randomized 128 patients.[13] They reported a nonsignificant reduction in infarct growth in the GA group as the primary outcome measure. A secondary outcome measure demonstrated improved 90-day mRS scores in the GA group.

A subsequent meta-analysis of these 3 RCTs (368 patients) found a significant improvement in 90-day mRS score (2.8 vs 3.2, respectively) favoring the GA along with improved recanalization rates (85.2% vs 75.7%, respectively); however, door to groin puncture time was significantly longer. The CS group had an 11.5% rate of urgently conversion to GA, thus delaying treatment and reducing the potential benefit of quicker door to groin puncture time.[14] These results do not establish a best anesthetic for EVT but rather demonstrate that GA can be provided without worsening neurologic outcomes when done expeditiously by specialized anesthesiologists who are likely attentive to the physiologic needs of this patient population.

A nonrandomized retrospective analysis of the MR CLEAN registry recently reported much improved neurologic outcomes associated with LA alone compared with CS and slightly improved outcomes when LA was compared with GA. This result should be considered exploratory due to the selection bias inherent in such a study.[15]

A practical approach for clinicians depends on institutional experience, patient comorbidities, physiologic stability, and the patient's ability to cooperate with immobilization. Regardless of the approach, a premium should be placed on expeditious facilitation of groin puncture and optimal surgical conditions to facilitate recanalization. Current guidelines suggest that the provider choose an anesthetic technique based on a patient's clinical picture. If a patient requires intubation for airway protection or immobilization, GA should not be avoided. GA does require, however, vigilant attention to hemodynamics to avoid significant hypotension, which is associated with poorer functional outcome. In the absence of better data, it also is reasonable to avoid hyperventilation and target normocarbia.

Most clinical trials of EVT have studied anterior circulation large vessel occlusion. Occlusion of the posterior circulation can lead to brainstem ischemia, which can compromise the respiratory center, lower cranial nerve nuclei responsible for airway protection, impair consciousness, and cause hemodynamic instability. Although not all patients with posterior circulation occlusion need to be intubated, clinicians must be aware of the potential for catastrophic neurologic decline when determining a plan of care.[16]

Surprisingly, the prophylactic use of low-dose oxygen supplementation in nonhypoxic patients with acute stroke did not reduce death or disability at 3 months.[17] The 2019 AHA/American Stroke Association (ASA) guidelines recommend against supplemental oxygen for patients with acute myocardial infarction or acute IS in patients with Spo_2 greater than or equal to 94% breathing room air.[5] In the absence of high-quality data, it also is reasonable to avoid profound hyperoxia under GA.

The appropriate blood pressure before, during, and after thrombectomy has been the subject of many trials. The AHA/ASA guidance for early stroke treatment includes a recommendation to correct hypotension and hypovolemia, while also stating that "the usefulness of drug induced hypertension has not been established."[5] The MASTERSTROKE RCT compared a systolic blood pressure of 140 mm Hg to 170 mm Hg immediately prior to mechanical thrombectomy and the results are pending. For now, it is reasonable to maintain blood pressure near preanesthetic levels during EVT. Post-thrombectomy blood pressure targets should be discussed with the neurointerventionalist. It is reasonable to set maximum blood pressure limits based on grade of revascularization, preoperative imaging (infarct size), and postprocedure clinical examination (NIHSS). The authors are more inclined to allow higher pressure limits in patients with incomplete revascularization (Thrombolysis in Cerebral Infarction perfusion scale [TICI] <2b) compared with successful vessel recanalization (TICI 2b and 3).

PERIOPERATIVE STROKE

IS that occurs within 30 days of a procedure is considered a perioperative IS. The Society of Neuroscience in Anesthesia and Critical Care (SNACC) published a consensus statement in 2020 to establish the frequency and patient-associated and procedure-associated risk factors of perioperative IS. This section reviews those guidelines and their underlying evidence. Strokes related to cardiac surgery are covered in this article, because they are considered to have distinct etiologies related to the manipulation of the great vessels and the use of cardiopulmonary bypass.

Reviews of the National Surgical Quality Improvement Program database estimates a covert stroke rate of 0.1% in low-risk adults who were having low-risk procedures and a rate of 0.6% to 0.8% in patients who had noncardiac surgery on their aorta. Perioperative strokes are more common during procedures in which the blood supply to the brain can be compromised due to hypotension—most commonly due to blood loss—or the showering of atherosclerotic debris into the brain. Perioperative strokes carry a higher morbidity and mortality than other strokes. Those worse outcomes may be attributed to perioperative inflammation and hypercoagulability.

The NeuroVISION trial performed MRI 2 days to 9 days after noncardiac surgery in 1100 patients aged greater than 65 years. Surprisingly, 7% of the patients had fresh infarcts whereas only 3% of patients demonstrated stroke symptoms. The primary outcome was that 42% of patients with new infarcts experienced postoperative cognitive decline, versus 29% of patients without new strokes. Cognitive decline was defined as a decrease of 2 points on the Montreal Cognitive Assessment. Prior infarcts were present in 23% of the subjects and prior infarcts were not associated with new infarcts or cognitive decline during the study period. The NeuroVISION trial did not have a nonsurgical control and did not analyze perioperative stroke risk factors such as hemodynamics or arrhythmias.[18]

PREDICTORS OF PERIOPERATIVE STROKE

Many studies have attempted to define patient risk factors for postoperative stroke to identify patients who might benefit from more intense care. The results have varied, but the most consistent risk factors have been age, renal disease, atrial fibrillation, and preexisting patent foramen ovale. Preoperative atrial fibrillation may increase the risk of stroke up to 3-fold. A random-effects model of 35 perioperative stroke studies that included a total of more than 2 million patients showed that new-onset perioperative atrial fibrillation was associated with increased risk of both stroke and mortality in the short term and long term.[19] There are no guidelines for managing these patients.

Recent IS increases the risk of perioperative IS, possibly due to the altered cerebral autoregulation that occurs. SNACC guidelines suggest a 9-month delay based on moderate-quality evidence.[20] Any prior stroke or transient ischemic attack has been associated with an odds ratio of new stroke as high as 2.9, with more recent strokes having a higher association with perioperative stroke. The 23% of patients in the NeuroVISION trial, however, with chronic infarcts were no more likely to have new strokes than those without prior IS.

Intraoperative hypotension is weakly associated with IS. It is intuitive to believe that hypotension would decrease cerebral perfusion and increase the risk of IS; however, the body's ability to shunt blood to the brain during periods of hypotension may avoid infarction in such circumstances.[21] In 1 study of patients undergoing general surgery, cumulative time with a mean arterial pressure (MAP) less than 70 mm Hg was not associated with an increased risk of stroke, although blood pressure in that range for an extended period of time has been associated with end organ dysfunction in other studies. The authors believe that maintaining a minimum MAP of 65 mm Hg for normotensive patients is prudent and that induced hypotension should be used sparingly, if at all. A target within 80% to 110% of the baseline blood pressure is appropriate for a patient with poorly controlled hypertension. The location of the blood pressure cuff or arterial pressure transducer relative to the circle of Willis should be taken into account when setting blood pressure goals.

MALIGNANT STROKE

An infarction of a large cerebral or cerebellar volume can cause necrotic edema with intracranial hypertension, which is termed a malignant stroke. Swelling and intracranial hypertension can present within 24 hours of onset, typically with a peak 3 days to 5 days after infarction. It is well known that younger patients without cerebral atrophy have decreased capacity to accommodate for the increased intracranial volume associated with swelling and often require a decompressive hemicraniectomy to relieve the pressure and prevent herniation. Adults over age 60 years often develop swelling more slowly, but it should be treated when it becomes symptomatic and decompressive hemicraniectomy does improve survival without major disability in all adults. Decompressive craniectomy is most efficacious when it is performed within 48 hours of the onset of the stroke but can be considered later in the course of any stroke. A relatively large cerebellar infarction usually requires urgent-emergent suboccipital craniectomy before edema encroaches on the brainstem and fourth ventricle.

PERIOPERATIVE MEDICATIONS AND STROKE

The POISE trial determined that starting high doses of metoprolol in the preoperative period increased the risk of watershed-type ISs.[22] The 2014 American College of Cardiology/AHA guidelines recommend caution in starting a β-blocker perioperatively and recommend against starting one on the day of surgery.[23] A Cochrane review in 2018 associated β-blocker with an increase in all-cause perioperative mortality.[24] Other studies have determined a survival benefit for patients when β-blocker is initiated more than 30 days or as soon as 1 week prior to their procedure and titrated appropriately. One study found perioperative stroke risk to be inversely proportional to the β_1 specificity of individual β-blockers (specificity: bisoprolol > atenolol > metoprolol), but the way that the drugs are prescribed and dosed may impart a bias into the study result.[25]

The only major study of preoperative clonidine failed to show any protection from major adverse cardiac events. Statins reduce primary strokes in patients who are at high risk for stroke and also limit stroke recurrence. There are few data regarding perioperative statins but they probably should be continued in the perioperative period.[19]

The POISE-2 trial determined that dosing perioperative aspirin for patients having noncardiac surgery increased the rate of complications due to bleeding and did not reduce the risk of major adverse cardiac events, including stroke specifically.[26] The BRIDGE trial found that patients taking warfarin with a $CHADS_2$ score of 2 for a minor indication—for example, atrial fibrillation as opposed to a mechanical heart valve—had the same rate of major adverse cardiac events regardless of heparin bridging.[27] The POISE-3 trial examined whether tranexamic acid would reduce the incidence of major complications in patients after noncardiac surgery; the results will be published in 2022.[28]

Hyperglycemia is associated with a worse outcome in all strokes as well as an increased risk of surgical site infection. Various targets for perioperative blood glucose have been tested, and most guidelines target a blood glucose of 140 mg/dL to 180 mg/dL (7.7–10 mM). Tighter glycemic control has had additional benefits in various settings. Although some centers have conducted trials of tight glycemic control (100–140 mg/dL) without episodes of hypoglycemia, it generally is not recommended due to the risk and morbidity from hypoglycemia.[29]

Stroke survivors who had a significant infarct often experience an exacerbation of their symptoms in the postoperative period, a phenomenon known as recrudescence.[30] The anesthesiologist should consider the patient's prior deficits when assessing the patient during emergence and in the early postoperative period. The use of γ-aminobutyric acid antagonists can unmask symptoms in patients with brain tumors[31] and in the authors' experience it also occurs in patients with a history of stroke. Drugs that meet Beers Criteria for potentially inappropriate medication use in older adults usually are best avoided in stroke patients as well.

SUMMARY

Although many therapies have been developed to treat stroke and its risk factors, IS continues to occur at a high rate and cause considerable morbidity and mortality. The wealth of information provided by clinical trials—mostly over this past decade—will help anesthesiologists to provide care that will help stroke patients live longer lives with fewer impairments.

CLINICS CARE POINTS

- Time is Brain; Ischemic brain cells die at a rate that is inversely proportional to the blood flow and restoring blood flow halts stroke progression.

- Advanced imaging can determine the size of the penumbra and the benefit of endovascular thrombectomy for patients with a LKWT of 6-24 hours.
- Symptomatic ICH within 24 hours of a tPA infusion should be treated with tranexamic acid 1,000 mg over 10 min, and 10 Units of cryoprecipitate. Also consult hematology and neurosurgery.
- The anesthetic for mechanical thrombectomy should be chosen to balance time to reperfusion versus the need to support the patient's airway. In most cases, it can be limited to local anesthesia at the site of groin puncture. Randomized controlled trials have demonstrated that if a general anesthetic is conducted quickly it does not adversely impact patient outcome.

REFERENCES

1. Virani SS, Alonso A, Benjamin EJ, et al. Heart disease and stroke statistics-2020 update: a report from the American Heart Association. Circulation 2020;141(9): e139–596.
2. Flexman AM, Donovan AL, Gelb AW. Anesthetic management of patients with acute stroke. Anesthesiol Clin 2012;30(2):175–90.
3. National Institute of Neurological Disorders and Stroke rt-PA Stroke Study Group. Tissue plasminogen activator for acute ischemic stroke. N Engl J Med 1995; 333(24):1581–7.
4. Hacke W, Kaste M, Bluhmki E, et al. Thrombolysis with alteplase 3 to 4.5 hours after acute ischemic stroke. N Engl J Med 2008;359(13):1317–29.
5. Powers WJ, Rabinstein AA, Ackerson T, et al. Guidelines for the early management of patients with acute ischemic stroke: 2019 update to the 2018 guidelines for the early management of acute ischemic stroke: a guideline for healthcare professionals from the American Heart Association/American Stroke Association. Stroke 2019;50(12):e344–418.
6. Campbell BCV, Mitchell PJ, Churilov L, et al. Tenecteplase versus alteplase before thrombectomy for ischemic stroke. N Engl J Med 2018;378(17):1573–82.
7. Albers GW, Marks MP, Kemp S, et al. Thrombectomy for stroke at 6 to 16 hours with selection by perfusion imaging. N Engl J Med 2018;378(8):708–18.
8. Nogueira RG, Jadhav AP, Haussen DC, et al. Thrombectomy 6 to 24 hours after stroke with a mismatch between deficit and infarct. N Engl J Med 2018;378(1): 11–21.
9. Luo S, Zhuang M, Zeng W, et al. Intravenous thrombolysis for acute ischemic stroke in patients receiving antiplatelet therapy: a systematic review and meta-analysis of 19 studies. J Am Heart Assoc 2016;5(5). https://doi.org/10.1161/ JAHA.116.003242.
10. Jeong H-G, Kim BJ, Yang MH, et al. Stroke outcomes with use of antithrombotics within 24 hours after recanalization treatment. Neurology 2016;87(10): 996–1002.
11. Löwhagen Hendén P, Rentzos A, Karlsson J-E, et al. General anesthesia versus conscious sedation for endovascular treatment of acute ischemic stroke: the An-Stroke trial (anesthesia during stroke). Stroke 2017;48(6):1601–7.
12. Schönenberger S, Möhlenbruch M, Pfaff J, et al. Sedation vs. intubation for endovascular stroke TreAtment (SIESTA) - a randomized monocentric trial. Int J Stroke 2015;10(6):969–78.
13. Sørensen LH, Speiser L, Karabegovic S, et al. Safety and quality of endovascular therapy under general anesthesia and conscious sedation are comparable: results from the GOLIATH trial. J Neurointerv Surg 2019;11(11):1070–2.

14. Zhang Y, Jia L, Fang F, et al. General anesthesia versus conscious sedation for intracranial mechanical thrombectomy: a systematic review and meta-analysis of randomized clinical trials. J Am Heart Assoc 2019;8(12):e011754.

15. Goldhoorn R-JB, Bernsen MLE, Hofmeijer J, et al. Anesthetic management during endovascular treatment of acute ischemic stroke in the MR CLEAN Registry. Neurology 2020;94(1):e97–106.

16. Hassan AE, Akbar U, Chaudhry SA, et al. Rate and prognosis of patients under conscious sedation requiring emergent intubation during neuroendovascular procedures. AJNR Am J Neuroradiol 2013;34(7):1375–9.

17. Roffe C, Nevatte T, Sim J, et al. Effect of routine low-dose oxygen supplementation on death and disability in adults with acute stroke: the stroke oxygen study randomized clinical trial. JAMA 2017;318(12):1125–35.

18. NeuroVISION Investigators. Perioperative covert stroke in patients undergoing non-cardiac surgery (NeuroVISION): a prospective cohort study. Lancet 2019; 394(10203):1022–9.

19. Lin MH, Kamel H, Singer DE, et al. Perioperative/postoperative atrial fibrillation and risk of subsequent stroke and/or mortality: a meta-analysis. Stroke 2019. https://doi.org/10.1161/STROKEAHA.118.023921.

20. Vlisides PE, Moore LE, Whalin MK, et al. Perioperative care of patients at high risk for stroke during or after non-cardiac, non-neurological surgery: 2020 guidelines from the Society for Neuroscience in Anesthesiology and Critical Care. J Neurosurg Anesthesiol 2020. https://doi.org/10.1097/ANA.0000000000000686.

21. Drummond JC. Blood pressure and the brain: how low can you go? Anesth Analg 2019;128(4):759–71.

22. POISE Study Group, Devereaux PJ, Yang H, et al. Effects of extended-release metoprolol succinate in patients undergoing non-cardiac surgery (POISE trial): a randomised controlled trial. Lancet 2008;371(9627):1839–47.

23. Wijeysundera DN, Duncan D, Nkonde-Price C, et al. Perioperative beta blockade in noncardiac surgery: a systematic review for the 2014 ACC/AHA guideline on perioperative cardiovascular evaluation and management of patients undergoing noncardiac surgery: a report of the American College of Cardiology/American Heart Association Task Force on Practice Guidelines. Circulation 2014;130(24): 2246–64.

24. Blessberger H, Lewis SR, Pritchard MW, et al. Perioperative beta-blockers for preventing surgery-related mortality and morbidity in adults undergoing non-cardiac surgery. Cochrane Database Syst Rev 2019;(9):CD013438.

25. Ashes C, Judelman S, Wijeysundera DN, et al. Selective β1-antagonism with bisoprolol is associated with fewer postoperative strokes than atenolol or metoprolol: a single-center cohort study of 44,092 consecutive patients. Anesthesiology 2013;119(4):777–87.

26. Devereaux PJ, Mrkobrada M, Sessler DI, et al. Aspirin in patients undergoing noncardiac surgery. N Engl J Med 2014;370(16):1494–503.

27. Douketis JD, Spyropoulos AC, Kaatz S, et al. Perioperative bridging anticoagulation in patients with atrial fibrillation. N Engl J Med 2015;373(9):823–33.

28. PeriOperative ISchemic Evaluation-3 Trial (POISE-3). Available at: https://clinicaltrials.gov/ct2/show/NCT03505723.

29. Duggan EW, Carlson K, Umpierrez GE. Perioperative hyperglycemia management: an update. Anesthesiology 2017;126(3):547–60.

30. Lin N, Han R, Zhou J, et al. Mild sedation exacerbates or unmasks focal neurologic dysfunction in neurosurgical patients with supratentorial brain mass lesions in a drug-specific manner. Anesthesiology 2016;124(3):598–607.
31. Wijdicks EFM, Sheth KN, Carter BS, et al. Recommendations for the management of cerebral and cerebellar infarction with swelling: a statement for healthcare professionals from the American Heart Association/American Stroke Association. Stroke 2014;45(4):1222–38.

Anesthesia for Acute Spinal Cord Injury

Shilpa Rao, MD[a],*, Miriam M. Treggiari, MD, PhD, MPH[b]

KEYWORDS

- Spinal anatomy • Acute spinal cord injury • Spinal shock • ASIA impairment scale
- Autonomic dysreflexia

KEY POINTS

- Spinal cord blood supply: The main blood supply to the anterior two-thirds of the spinal cord is via the single anterior spinal artery originating from the vertebral arteries, whereas the posterior one-third is supplied by the two posterior spinal arteries branching off the posterior inferior cerebellar artery.
- Spinal shock: Spinal shock refers to a clinical syndrome characterized by the loss of reflex, loss of motor and sensory function below the level of the injury, loss of autonomic tone leading to hypotension, hypothermia, urinary retention, and fecal incontinence.
- American Spinal Injury Association (ASIA) Impairment scale: The ASIA Impairment Scale (AIS) is a score assigning the functional level of the injury and the severity of sensory and motor impairment based on five degrees of severity (A to E).
- Autonomic dysreflexia: Autonomic dysreflexia is a potentially life-threatening emergency characterized by hypertension, bradycardia, headache, flushed face, nasal stuffiness, nausea, and sweating above the level of injury that affects patients with spinal cord injuries typically at the T6 level or higher.

INTRODUCTION

Acute spinal cord injury (SCI) has multiple causes and can lead to significant morbidity and persistent, neurologic deficits, carrying significant long-term economic implications.[1] The annual incidence of acute SCI worldwide is about 15 to 40 cases per million and is predominantly seen in young adults. Trauma is an important cause of acute SCI; other causes of acute spinal cord compression are associated with oncologic conditions as a result of pathologic fractures or direct compression on the spine from mass effect. The most common causes of traumatic SCI (TSCI) include motor vehicle

^a Division of Neuroanesthesia, Department of Anesthesiology, Yale School of Medicine, Yale University, PO Box 208051, 333 Cedar Street, TMP 3, New Haven, CT 06510, USA; ^b Department of Anesthesiology, Yale School of Medicine, Yale University, PO Box 208051, 333 Cedar Street, TMP 3, New Haven, CT 06510, USA
* Corresponding author.
E-mail address: shilpa.rao@yale.edu

Anesthesiology Clin 39 (2021) 127–138
https://doi.org/10.1016/j.anclin.2020.11.011
1932-2275/21/© 2020 Elsevier Inc. All rights reserved.
anesthesiology.theclinics.com

collisions, including whiplash injuries (48%), falls (16%), violent crime including gunshot wounds (12%), sports accidents (10%), and other causes (14%).[2] Nontraumatic acute SCIs can occur because of epidural hematomas, abscesses, degenerative diseases, or tumors causing spinal cord instability and compromised spinal cord perfusion. In this article, we discuss the spinal anatomy, blood supply of the spinal cord, pathogenesis of SCI, and expected complications of acute SCI. The discussion focuses on the perioperative anesthetic management of these patients in the acute setting.

A BRIEF OVERVIEW OF SPINAL ANATOMY AND FUNCTION

Longitudinally, the spinal cord extends from the base of the skull to the first lumbar vertebral body and continues as cauda equine at or below the second lumbar vertebra. The vertebral column is longer than the spinal cord and hence there is a difference in the segmental levels. The cord segments consist of cervical, thoracic, lumbar, and sacral areas.

Key anatomic structures of the cervical spinal cord region include C1 (atlas), which supports the atlantooccipital junction, and the section C3-C5, which forms the phrenic nerve and innervates the diaphragm. Important aspects of the thoracic spinal cord region include the intercostal nerves that arise from the thoracic spinal cord and innervate the accessory muscles of respiration. Importantly, the thoracic section of the spinal cord also provides sympathetic innervation to the heart and abdominal organs. Key aspects of the lumbosacral spinal cord region are the role in motor and sensory innervation of the lower extremity. Lastly, sacral nerves also provide parasympathetic innervation to the pelvis and abdominal organs (**Figs. 1** and **2**).

The cross-sectional anatomy of the spinal cord is comprised of gray matter in the center, surrounded by white matter tracts. The principal white matter tracts include: (1) dorsal columns that carry sensory information pertaining to joint position (proprioception) and vibration, which ascend upwards and cross in the medulla to the contralateral

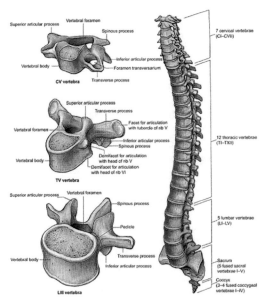

Fig. 1. Vertebral column. (*From* Drake R, Vogl A, Mitchell AWM. Back. In: Drake R, Vogl W, Mitchell AWM, et al, editors. Gray's Atlas of Anatomy, Second Ed. Philadelphia: Elsevier; 2020, P. 22; with permission.)

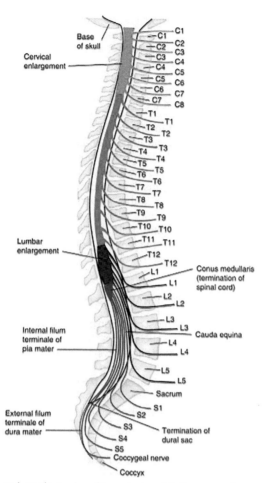

Fig. 2. Spinal cord and cauda equina. (*From* Joshua M. Rosenow. Anatomy of the Nervous system. In: Krames ES, Peckham PH, Rezai AR, Editors. Neuromodulation: Comprehensive Textbook of Principles, Technologies, and Therapies, Second Edition. London: Elsevier; 2018. P. 25-29; with permission. (Figure 7 in original).)

cerebral hemisphere; (2) anterolateral spinothalamic tracts that are ascending pathways carrying sensations of pain, temperature, and touch; and (3) corticospinal tracts that are descending pathways for motor neurons. The fibers of the corticospinal tracts cross cranially at the level of cervicomedullary junction (pyramids). The sympathetic fibers do not have a well-defined tract and lie at the spinal levels between T1 and L3. Noncranial parasympathetic cell bodies originate in the sacral spinal cord at S2-S4.

OVERVIEW OF BLOOD SUPPLY TO THE SPINAL CORD

The chief blood supply of the spinal cord comes from a single anterior spinal artery and two posterior spinal arteries. The anterior spinal artery supplies the anterior two-thirds of the cord, and the two posterior spinal arteries supply the posterior one-third (dorsal columns). Both of these arteries arise from the vertebral arteries at the base of the skull. An important radicular branch arising from the aorta artery of Adamkiewicz enters the spinal cord usually between T9 and T12.

Spinal cord autoregulation is not robust and is more pressure dependent than cerebral autoregulation. In contrast to cerebral tissues, oxygenation of the spinal cord is more sensitive to hypotension and decreases as mean arterial pressure (MAP) decreases less than 60 mm Hg.[3]

MECHANISMS OF SPINAL CORD INJURY

SCIs are often associated with vertebral bone fractures, ligament tears, and/or associated head injury, or as part of a polytrauma scenario. There is often a primary injury that has occurred at the time of initial insult, including complete or partial transection, penetrating injury, and/or contusion to the spinal cord itself. This situation is subsequently exacerbated by a secondary insult caused by ischemia, edema, hypotension, hypoxia, excitotoxicity, apoptosis, or further movement of the spinal cord/vertebral column. The phenomenon of secondary injury is sometimes clinically manifest by neurologic deterioration over the first 8 to 12 hours in patients who initially present with an incomplete cord syndrome.[1] Systemic hypotension is a hallmark physiologic response immediately following SCI.

SIGNS AND SYMPTOMS OF ACUTE SPINAL CORD INJURY

Pain at the site of injury is one of the most common presenting clinical signs of acute SCI. There may be associated injuries, such as fractures, hemothorax, intra-abdominal bleeding, or head injury with associated altered consciousness, which may impair neurologic assessment. There may also be associated acute sensory or motor changes according to the American Spinal Injury Association (ASIA) Impairment Scale (AIS).[1]

American Spinal Injury Association Impairment Scale

Grade A = Complete. No sensory or motor function is preserved in the sacral segments S4-S5.[4]

Grade B = Sensory Incomplete. Sensory but no motor function is preserved below the neurologic level and includes the sacral segments S4-S5 (Light Touch [tests posterior column] or Pin Prick [tests spinothalamic tract] at S4-S5 or Deep Anal Pressure), and no motor function is preserved more than three levels below the motor level on either side of the body.

Grade C = Motor Incomplete. Motor function is preserved at the most caudal sacral segments for voluntary anal contraction or the patient meets the criteria for sensory incomplete status (sensory function preserved at the most caudal sacral segments [S4-S5] by Light Touch [tests posterior column], Pin Prick [tests spinothalamic tract], or Deep Anal Pressure), and has some sparing of motor function more than three levels below the ipsilateral motor level on either side of the body. (This includes key or nonkey muscle functions to determine motor incomplete status.) For AIS C, less than half of key muscle functions below the single neurological level of injury have a muscle grade ≥3.

Grade D = Motor Incomplete. Motor incomplete status as defined previously, with at least half (half or more) of key muscle functions below the single NLI having a muscle grade ≥3.

Grade E = Normal. If sensation and motor function as tested with the International Standards for Neurologic Classification of Spinal Cord Injury are graded as normal in all segments, and the patient had prior deficits, then the AIS grade is E. Someone without an initial SCI does not receive an AIS grade.

For individuals to receive a grade of C or D (ie, motor incomplete status), they must have either voluntary anal sphincter contraction or sacral sensory sparing with sparing of motor function more than three levels below the motor level for that side of the body.

Depicted in **Fig. 3** is the dermatomal distribution of different levels of SCI, and the chart used to determine the level of injury and the severity of impairment.

INITIAL EVALUATION AND TREATMENT OF SPINAL CORD INJURY

Along with the presenting signs and symptoms mentioned previously, imaging can aid in diagnosing associated injuries, such as ligament and/bone fractures. Plain radiographs in the anteroposterior, lateral, and odontoid (in suspected cervical spine injury) views provide information on spinal cord alignment, bony fractures, and other possible displacements of anatomic structures. Computed tomography (CT) has been suggested to be more cost-effective in trauma patients, because often these patients receive thoracic and abdominal CT scans to looks for other injuries. CT imaging is particularly helpful for assessment of bone injury. MRI of the spinal cord provides accurate assessment of the extent of injury. The chief advantage of MRI is that it provides a detailed image of the spinal cord and spinal ligaments, intervertebral disks, and paraspinal soft tissues that is superior to CT and is more sensitive for detecting epidural hematomas or masses.[5]

PRINCIPLES OF MANAGEMENT

The initial assessment of a patient suspected to have acute SCI should always prioritize airway, breathing, and circulatory support. These patients often require transfer to a tertiary care center because of the complexity of injuries.

Patient Monitoring

Large-bore intravenous (IV) lines and/or central venous access may be required for adequate resuscitation. Care must be taken to minimize neck movement when placing central venous access. Ultrasound guidance may help in accurate placement of central lines. Arterial catheter placement aids in monitoring MAPs and drawing frequent blood gas samples to assess adequacy of resuscitation. A Foley catheter is required to monitor urine output and should be placed as early as possible. Patients with traumatic cervical and high thoracic SCI are critically ill and require intensive care unit (ICU) admission, along with continuous monitoring of vitals, and mechanical ventilation. Often, these patients are admitted with "spinal shock" or neurogenic shock. This is a form of distributive shock characterized by hypotension with bradycardia, because of disruption of autonomic sympathetic fibers, causing decreased systemic vascular resistance and lack of compensatory tachycardia. This type of shock may be compounded with hemorrhagic shock because of trauma-induced blood loss. In the resuscitation of patients with SCI, it is critical to maintain adequate perfusion to the spinal cord.

Airway Management

Cervical and high thoracic SCI compromises the primary muscles of respiration, and these patients should be immediately intubated and placed on mechanical ventilator support. Extreme caution must be taken to minimize any movement of the head and neck during laryngoscopy and intubation, to prevent further injury to the spinal cord. Some of the techniques that are used to achieve this include manual in-line axial stabilization and placement of an immobilizing collar on the neck (C-collar). Similar caution must be exercised in the operating room during transfer of patients from

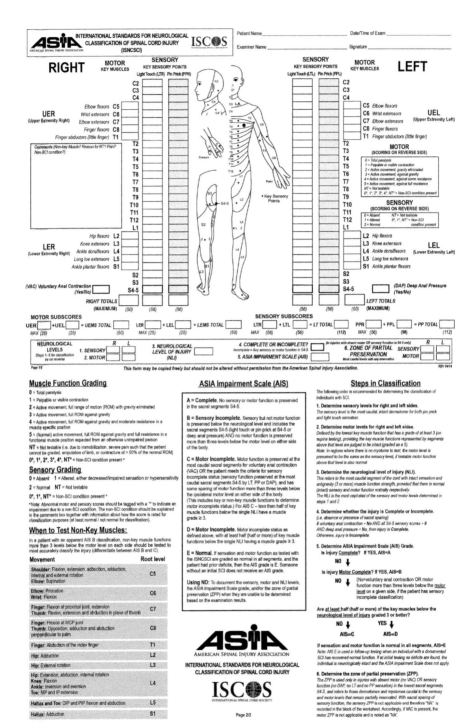

Fig. 3. Dermatomal distribution of different levels of spinal cord injury. (© 2020 American Spinal Injury Association. Reprinted with permission.)

stretcher to operating room table and/or ICU bed. These precautions must be exercised even if there is no obvious visible cervical spine injury, such as in a trauma patient. Rapid sequence induction and intubation is often used as the method of choice in emergent intubations, because of concerns with the possibility of aspiration. If time permits, the authors recommend flexible fiberoptic intubation or use of a videolaryngoscope in the anesthetized and paralyzed patient, to minimize neck movement during intubation, as opposed to traditional laryngoscopy. However, disagreements still exist on the optimal approach to airway management.

Fluid Management and Circulatory Support

Hypotension is an important cause of secondary SCI, and can result from bleeding caused by associated injuries and spinal shock caused by lack of sympathetic tone. The latter can occur because of disruption of sympathetic chain, leading to loss of sympathetic tone and pooling of blood in the lower extremities. Prevention of hypotension (systolic blood pressure <90 mm Hg) is an essential component of the early management of victims of SCI. Although it is well-documented that early aggressive management in an ICU setting involving respiratory and cardiovascular support has been accompanied by considerable improvement in vital and functional outcomes in patients with SCI, the goals of hemodynamic resuscitation have not been investigated in a systematic manner.

Recently, the Consortium for Spinal Cord Medicine released a guideline on the acute management of SCI in adults.[6] These guidelines include standard volume resuscitation to euvolemia and early use of vasopressor agents for the treatment of neurogenic shock (SCI above the level of T6) for the first 72 hours. Resuscitation is performed with crystalloids and/or blood transfusion as indicated.

The Association of Neurologic Surgeons released SCI guidelines in 2013 recommending artificial elevation of an MAP between 85 and 90 mm Hg for the first 7 days following SCI.[7–10] MAP is the average arterial pressure throughout one cardiac cycle, systole, and diastole, and is calculated using the formula:

MAP = Diastolic Pressure + 1/3 (Pulse Pressure).

However, this recommendation is only based on level III evidence from case series, nonexperimental, and noncomparative studies. There is, in theory, a strong rationale for blood pressure manipulation to prevent secondary spinal cord insult. A series of animal-based investigations performed in the 1970s and 1980s suggested that systemic hypotension after SCI was associated with reduced spinal cord perfusion and worsened neurologic outcomes.[11,12] The concept of blood pressure augmentation in neurologic resuscitation assumes that the spinal cord blood flow is pressure passive when there is loss of autoregulation. However, not only is the extent of impairment of spinal cord autoregulation unknown, but potent vasoconstrictors could impair spinal cord blood flow by limiting collateral flow through intercostal anastomosis when increased pressure occurs at the expense of excessive vasoconstriction. The inability to measure or monitor spinal cord blood flow while manipulating blood pressure with potent vasoconstrictors raises concerns regarding the beneficial effects of blood pressure augmentation.

There is substantial debate regarding the optimal vasopressor to induce blood pressure augmentation. Although norepinephrine might have direct toxic effect on myocytes by inducing apoptosis,[13] phenylephrine use might be limited by the occurrence of reflex bradycardia. Treatment of refractory bradycardia is achieved using temporary pacing pads or IV injection of atropine. A recent retrospective cohort study evaluated the short-term effects of vasopressor use on patients with acute SCI.[14] Patients were treated by maintaining an MAP greater than 90 mm Hg (n = 131) and the outcome of interest was complications associated with vasopressors. The authors reported an overall vasopressor-related complication rate of 74% in this patient population with the most common adverse event being cardiac dysrhythmia. Other complications included ST-segment elevation, cardiac troponin elevation, and skin necrosis. A similar study by Martin and colleagues[15] demonstrated that episodes of hypotension and the need for vasopressors did not affect the change in the ASIA motor score during acute hospitalization, regardless of an MAP goal setpoint. With the caveat of lacking long-term follow-up, they concluded that their arbitrarily elevated MAP goals may not be efficacious.

Role of Glucocorticoids

Two blinded, randomized controlled trials have studied the efficacy of glucocorticoid therapy in patients with acute TSCI. The National Acute Spinal Cord Injury Study II compared methylprednisolone, 30 mg/kg IV, followed by 5.4 mg/kg per hour over 23 more hours, naloxone, and placebo in 427 patients with acute TSCI.[16] At 1 year, there was no significant difference in neurologic function among treatment groups. However, within the subset of patients treated within 8 hours, those who received methylprednisolone had a modest improvement in motor recovery compared with those who received placebo. Wound infections, however, were somewhat more common in patients who received methylprednisolone.

National Acute Spinal Cord Injury Study III compared three treatment groups: (1) methylprednisolone administered for 48 hours, (2) methylprednisolone administered for 24 hours, and (3) tirilazad mesylate (a potent lipid peroxidation inhibitor) administered for 48 hours in patients with acute complete or incomplete TSCI.[17] All 499 patients received an initial IV bolus of 30 mg/kg methylprednisolone and were treated within 8 hours of TSCI. For patients treated within 3 hours, there was no difference in outcomes among treatment groups at 1 year. For patients treated between 3 and 8 hours, 48 hours of methylprednisolone was associated with a greater motor but not functional recovery compared with other treatments. Patients who received the longer duration infusion of methylprednisolone had more severe sepsis and severe pneumonia compared with the shorter duration of infusion; mortality was similar in all treatment groups.[18]

More recently, in 2013, based on the available evidence, the American Association of Neurologic Surgeons and Congress of Neurologic Surgeons stated that the use of glucocorticoids in acute SCI is not recommended.[8]

Prevention of Complications from Critical Illness

Concomitant interventions are directed at prevention of potential complications, such as ventilator-associated pneumonia, deep vein thrombosis prevention, pressure ulcers, and gastric stress ulcers. Importantly, attention should be paid to nutritional support with insertion of feeding tube if the patient is incapable of oral intake, and pain control with appropriate evaluation and judicious opioid usage.

ANESTHETIC CONSIDERATIONS FOR EMERGENT SPINAL CORD SURGERY

Patients with acute SCI may present to the operating room for decompression and fixation, in an attempt to stabilize the spinal cord. These patients may arrive on an emergent basis, with a C-collar. All C-spine precautions mentioned previously should be undertaken during laryngoscopy, intubation, positioning, and transport of the patient.

In addition, these patients may have associated orthopedic or soft tissue injuries, which may complicate line placement and positioning. They may also have associated head injuries with increased intracranial pressure, and this has to be kept in mind during anesthetic management. These patients are usually positioned prone for surgical access; hence intubation and lines may have to be performed on a stretcher/hospital bed. Pretreatment with glycopyrrolate is recommended in patients with cervical cord injuries to prevent severe bradycardia, which is associated with intubation in these patients. A rapid sequence induction and intubation with videolaryngoscope is usually preferred to safely secure the airway, if the patient is not already intubated.

In addition to standard American Society of Anesthesiology monitors, which must be used at all times, large-bore venous access and arterial catheter are required for intraoperative fluid resuscitation and monitoring. Most of the surgeries involving cervical and thoracic spinal cord use extensive neuromonitoring, to aid in stabilizing the spinal cord without exacerbating injury. Commonly used modalities include somatosensory evoked potentials and motor evoked potentials (MEPs), which test the integrity of the dorsal columns and motor pathways respectively. Inhaled anesthetic agents, such as sevoflurane, have a dose-dependent depressant effect on somatosensory evoked potentials and MEPs, and are usually avoided.

Intubation with a short-acting or no muscle relaxant technique is preferred to facilitate MEP monitoring. Rocuronium is usually reversible with neostigmine/glycopyrrolate if neuromonitoring will be initiated only after turning prone and final positioning. However, a desire to initiate neuromonitoring before turning the patient prone requires awake intubation, use of succinylcholine, rocuronium/sugammadex, or high-dose remifentanil. The authors recommend maintenance with total IV anesthesia using a balanced combination of propofol infusion and an opioid, such as fentanyl, to facilitate monitoring, and provide anesthesia and analgesia. Vasopressor infusions, such as phenylephrine or norepinephrine, may be required to maintain MAPs, to aid perfusion of the spinal cord, as previously discussed.

Decision to extubate at the end of the surgery depends on multiple factors, such as respiratory muscle involvement in the injury, anticipation of spinal cord swelling during the immediate postsurgical period, associated injuries, and need for multiple subsequent surgeries. Patients with high cervical SCI are usually intubated in the postoperative period with mechanical ventilatory support. These patients may require a tracheostomy for long-term care.

LONG-TERM COMPLICATIONS
Autonomic Hyperreflexia

This phenomenon is seen in SCIs above the level of T6, and is usually seen within the first year of injury, in about 20% to 70% of patients.[19,20] It is characterized by exaggerated and uncoordinated sympathetic responses to noxious stimuli below the level of injury, leading to vasoconstriction and severe hypertension. An insufficient compensatory parasympathetic response occurs because of the SCI, leading to bradycardia and vasodilation above the level of lesion. Inciting stimuli include bladder or bowel distention, attempts to catheterize the bladder, pressure ulcers, and other similar stimuli. Clinical features include bradycardia, flushing, headache, sweating, and increased blood pressure. In severe cases, hypertensive crisis can occur, leading to intracranial hemorrhage, seizures, and cardiac arrest because of severe bradycardia. Anticipation, early recognition, and early treatment is essential for successful management of this medical emergency. Hypertensive crisis can occur in the operating room because these patients frequently present for procedures below the level of lesion.

An inadequate depth of anesthesia for surgical stimulation can trigger intraoperative hypertensive crisis. Treatment involves deepening the anesthetic and lowering the blood pressure with rapid-onset medications, such as nicardipine. An arterial catheter may be required for continuous intraoperative blood pressure monitoring.

Coronary Artery Disease

Studies suggest that the prevalence of coronary artery disease is 3 to 10 times higher in patients with SCI than it is in the general population. Coronary artery disease risk factors, such as adverse lipid profile (low levels of high-density lipoproteins, elevated low-density lipoprotein cholesterol) and abnormal glucose metabolism (impaired glucose tolerance, insulin resistance, and diabetes), are more prevalent in patients with chronic SCI than in the able-bodied population.[21]

Chronic Respiratory Insufficiency and Tracheostomy Dependence

Patients with cervical spinal and high thoracic cord injuries have significant long-term respiratory muscle involvement. Impaired cough and inability to clear lung secretions, along with chronic long-term ventilator care, places them at high risk of acquiring pneumonia. Aggressive chest physical therapy and improving respiratory muscle strength is vital in preventing this condition.

Chronic Urinary Tract Infections

Patients with TSCI are prone to frequent urinary tract infections because of chronic indwelling catheters. The urinary tract is the most frequent source of septicemia in patients with SCI and has a high mortality rate (15%).[22]

Musculoskeletal Contractures

Musculoskeletal contractures can result from chronic immobility and shortening and reorganization of the collagen fibers. Patients with SCI are also prone to bone fractures because of weakened muscles and ligaments. This may prove challenging to place IV lines or to position the patient intraoperatively.

Pressure Ulcers

Pressure ulcers can occur because of chronic immobility and tissue damage on bony prominences.

Chronic Pain

Chronic neuropathic pain is often seen in these patients. The underlying mechanism is poorly understood, and medical treatment involves a combination of antidepressants, gabapentin, and intrathecal morphine/baclofen. Patients with a history of SCI and a combination of one or more long-term complications may present to the operating room for procedures, such as debridement of wound ulcers, suprapubic catheter placement, removal of kidney stones, or any acute abdominal condition, such as appendicitis. As always, the principles of anesthetic management should be guided by airway, breathing, and circulatory support. If the patient has a long-term tracheostomy, appropriate suctioning may be required to clear secretions. If the patient arrives with an uncuffed tracheostomy tube, it may need to be changed to a cuffed tracheostomy tube to facilitate mechanical ventilation in the operating room.

Adequate depth of anesthesia and analgesia is required to prevent autonomic dysfunction from occurring intraoperatively. General anesthesia is used for most procedures, although procedures on the lower torso, such as debridement of sacral pressure ulcer or suprapubic catheter placement, or lower extremity procedures may be performed under spinal anesthesia.

SUMMARY

Patients with acute SCI are typically encountered for decompression in clinical anesthesia practice, often in an emergency setting. There may be insufficient time for a detailed preoperative history and examination. However, it is important to assess the patient's airway and be prepared to use difficult airway equipment, if necessary. It is also important to quickly assess other associated injuries that may influence intraoperative anesthetic management and line placement. The key to successful management is recognition of possible airway difficulty, and providing adequate hemodynamic support to maintain spinal cord perfusion pressure. If neuromonitoring modalities are being used, appropriate anesthetic management needs to be chosen and agents titrated accordingly. Because these patients return for subsequent surgeries or procedures, members of the anesthesia care team have to be cognizant of possible long-term complications, especially autonomic hyperreflexia, and be prepared to treat it.

CLINICS CARE POINTS

- Trauma is one of the most common causes of acute spinal cord injury.
- Delayed resuscitation is associated with worse clinical outcomes and secondary injury after acute high spinal cord injury. The origin of spinal hypoperfusion is typically multifactorial, and includes bleeding, loss of sympathetic tone, and spinal shock. These causes must be promptly recognized and treated.
- Use of high dose glucocorticoids in acute spinal cord injury is no longer recommended.
- It is important to minimize C-spine movement at all times during airway management. Some of the recommended techniques include manual in line axial stabilization, immobilization in a C-collar, and/or use of traction in Halo.
- Autonomic hyperreflexia can develop as a late complication in up to 70% of patients after injuries above T6 level and needs to be immediately recognized and treated.

DISCLOSURE

No conflicts of interest.

REFERENCES

1. Sekhon LH, Fehlings MG. Epidemiology, demographics and pathophysiology of acute spinal cord injury. Spine (Phila Pa 1976) 2001;26(24 Suppl):S2–12.
2. Devivo MJ. Epidemiology of traumatic spinal cord injury: trends and future implications. Spinal Cord 2012;50(5):365–72.
3. Kurita T, Kawashima S, Morita K, et al. Spinal cord autoregulation using near-infrared spectroscopy under normal, hypovolemic, and post-fluid resuscitation conditions in a swine model: a comparison with cerebral autoregulation. J Intensive Care 2020;8:27.
4. Available at: https://asia-spinalinjury.org/wp-content/uploads/2016/02/International_Stds_Diagram_Worksheet.pdf. Accessed November 17, 2020.
5. Demaerel P. Magnetic resonance imaging of spinal cord trauma: a pictorial essay. Neuroradiology 2006;48(4):223–432.

6. Medicine CfSC. Early acute management in adults with spinal cord injury: a clinical practice guideline for health-care professionals. J Spinal Cord Med 2008;31: 403–79.

7. Ryken TC, Hurlbert RJ, Hadley MN, et al. The acute cardiopulmonary management of patients with cervical spinal cord injuries. Neurosurgery 2013;72(Suppl 2):84–92.

8. Hurlbert RJ, Hadley MN, Walters BC, et al. Pharmacological therapy for acute spinal cord injury. Neurosurgery 2013;72(Suppl 2):93–105.

9. Jia X, Kowalski RG, Sciubba DM, et al. Critical care of traumatic spinal cord injury. J Intensive Care Med 2013;28(1):12–23.

10. Hadley MN, Walters BC, Grabb PA, et al. Blood pressure management after acute spinal cord injury. Neurosurgery 2002;50(3 Suppl):S58–62.

11. Smith AJ, McCreery DB, Bloedel JR, et al. Hyperemia, CO2 responsiveness, and autoregulation in the white matter following experimental spinal cord injury. J Neurosurg 1978;48(2):239–51.

12. Fairholm DJ, Turnbull IM. Microangiographic study of experimental spinal cord injuries. J Neurosurg 1971;35(3):277–86.

13. Communal C, Singh K, Pimentel DR, et al. Norepinephrine stimulates apoptosis in adult rat ventricular myocytes by activation of the beta-adrenergic pathway. Circulation 1998;98(13):1329–34.

14. Inoue T, Manley GT, Patel N, et al. Medical and surgical management after spinal cord injury: vasopressor usage, early surgery, and complications. J Neurotrauma 2014;31(3):284–91.

15. Martin ND, Kepler C, Zubair M, et al. Increased mean arterial pressure goals after spinal cord injury and functional outcome. J Emerg Trauma Shock 2015; 8(2):94–8.

16. Bracken MB, Shepard MJ, Collins WF Jr, et al. Methylprednisolone or naloxone treatment after acute spinal cord injury: 1-year follow-up data. Results of the second National Acute Spinal Cord Injury Study. J Neurosurg 1992;76(1):23–31.

17. Bracken MB, Shepard MJ, Holford TR, et al. Methylprednisolone or tirilazad mesylate administration after acute spinal cord injury: 1-year follow up. Results of the third National Acute Spinal Cord Injury randomized controlled trial. J Neurosurg 1998;89(5):699–706.

18. Bracken MB, Shepard MJ, Holford TR, et al. Administration of methylprednisolone for 24 or 48 hours or tirilazad mesylate for 48 hours in the treatment of acute spinal cord injury. Results of the Third National Acute Spinal Cord Injury Randomized Controlled Trial. National Acute Spinal Cord Injury Study. JAMA 1997;277(20): 1597–604.

19. Helkowski WM, Ditunno JF Jr, Boninger M. Autonomic dysreflexia: incidence in persons with neurologically complete and incomplete tetraplegia. J Spinal Cord Med 2003;26(3):244–7.

20. Bycroft J, Shergill IS, Chung EA, et al. Autonomic dysreflexia: a medical emergency. Postgrad Med J 2005;81(954):232–5.

21. Myers J, Lee M, Kiratli J. Cardiovascular disease in spinal cord injury: an overview of prevalence, risk, evaluation, and management. Am J Phys Med Rehabil 2007;86(2):142–52.

22. Siroky MB. Pathogenesis of bacteriuria and infection in the spinal cord injured patient. Am J Med 2002;113(Suppl 1A):67S–79S.

Spinal Cord Tumor Surgery

Sukhbir Walha, MD[a],*, Stacy L. Fairbanks, MD[b]

KEYWORDS

- Spinal cord tumor • Intramedullary tumor • Perioperative visual loss (POVL)
- Context-sensitive half-life • Intraoperative neuromonitoring (IONM)

KEY POINTS

- Unrelenting back pain, especially with nocturnal pain, is the most common presenting symptom of spinal cord tumors.
- Conducting a neurologic examination preoperatively is important to determine any preexisting deficits that may affect intraoperative neuromonitoring signal quality.
- Informed consent may need to include the risk for perioperative visual loss depending on patient risk factors and surgical risk factors.
- A multimodal approach to pain management perioperatively can reduce the incidence of postoperative nausea and vomiting, urinary retention, ileus, and hospital length of stay.
- Understanding the context-sensitive half-lives of common anesthetic infusions helps facilitate a rapid emergence and postoperative neurologic examination.

INTRODUCTION

Spinal cord tumors rarely are present but often require surgical treatment. Although rare, it is important that anesthesiologists recognize the different types of spinal cord tumors and the anesthetic management tools needed to optimize the perioperative care of patients having surgery for spinal cord tumor resection or removal. Spinal cord tumor resection requires a multipronged approach with diligent planning for the preoperative, intraoperative, and postoperative aspects of the surgery. Knowledge of the risks and perioperative complications that may arise prevents postoperative morbidity.

DEFINITION OF SPINAL CORD TUMORS/BACKGROUND/TYPES OF TUMORS

A spinal cord tumor is any tumor involving the spinal cord or immediate surrounding area. Overall, primary tumors of the spinal cord comprise less than 5% of all central nervous system (CNS) tumors.[1] Metastatic tumors of the spinal cord occur 40 times

[a] University of Colorado School of Medicine, 12401 East 17th Avenue, Campus Box B-113, Aurora, CO 80045, USA; [b] Froedtert and Medical College of Wisconsin, 9200 Wisconsin Avenue, PO BOX 26099, Milwaukee, WI 53266, USA
* Corresponding author.
E-mail address: Sukhbir.Walha@cuanschutz.edu

more frequently than primary tumors and are seen much more commonly in the operating room.[1] There are 2 large distinctions that must be made when considering spinal cord tumors: primary tumors versus tumors resulting from metastatic disease; 90% of patients dying of prostate cancer and 75% dying of breast cancer have metastases to the spine.[2]

Tumors typically are classified according to location (extradural vs intradural) and malignant status. **Table 1** describes the types of tumors within each classification and some of the known epidemiology and features.

1. Extradural tumors: this is the most common type of spinal cord tumor. A majority of extradural tumors are secondary to metastases arising from vertebral bodies. A primary tumor in an extradural location is less common. Examples include chordomas and chondrosarcomas. **Fig. 1** depict gross specimens of a resected chondrosarcoma. In this particular patient, the tumor presented with sacral pain and the feeling of constant pressure in the low back.
2. Intradural extramedullary tumors: these tumors occur within the dura but outside of the spinal cord. Examples include meningiomas, nerve sheath tumors, and schwannomas. The typical treatment of most intradural extramedullary tumors is resection (if possible); radiation is used for recurrence not amenable to resection
3. Intramedullary intradural tumors: these are tumors within the dura and within the spinal cord. A majority are subtypes of gliomas, which histologically are similar to normal glial cells. They make up approximately 2% to 4% of all CNS tumors.[4] Examples include astrocytomas and oligodendrogliomas. Typical treatment is preferentially surgical, with en bloc resection attempted; there is a role for radiation therapy and chemotherapy as adjuvants with noncurative resections or recurrence, but adjuvant therapy is not fully established in literature. If resection is curative, then no radiation is necessary.

EVALUATION

Presentation of spinal cord tumors is variable based on tumor location and type. The most common presentations, however, include unrelenting pain near the tumor location that worsens at night or in the supine position.[1,6] Neurologic deficits are possible, and, if present, often are unilateral.[7] Baseline knowledge of neurologic deficits and their corresponding spinal cord lesions aids preoperative neurologic assessment. Although the presenting symptom often is back pain, a spinal cord tumor should be very low in the differential diagnosis of back pain and rarely is the cause of back pain in patients presenting for treatment of chronic back pain.

Primary tumors typically occur in younger populations whereas metastatic disease is, understandably, more likely to occur in aging populations. If a tumor is suspected, negative plain films are not definitive and typically, even with multiple types of imaging, a definitive diagnosis cannot be provided without biopsy. A computed tomography scan provides the best information on cortical bone and tumor calcification. Magnetic resonance imaging is best at delineating soft tissue, paraspinal lesions, neural encroachment, bone marrow infiltration, and epidural extension.[1]

Potential spinal cord tumors should be biopsied only if they cannot be diagnosed via imaging and appear to harbor malignant characteristics (ie, bony destruction). Fine-needle aspiration is the most common type of biopsy, with planned follow-up resection of the biopsy tract at the time of surgery. Of utmost importance with regard to the decision to biopsy is to avoid errors that could result in tumor spread.[1]

Table 1
Spinal cord tumors typically are classified according to their location

Location	Tumor Type Examples	Epidemiology Notes	Treatment Notes	Additional Information
Extradural	• Chordoma, chondrosarcoma	• Rare • Primary chordomas are most common in the 40-year-old to 60-year-old age group. • Males > females[3]	• Mainstay of treatment is en bloc surgical resection. • Poorly sensitive to chemotherapy/radiation	• Sarcomas and lymphomas could be primary or metastases. • Locally invasive • Frequently recur • Lesions arising from vertebral bodies are most commonly metastatic.
	• Ewing sarcoma of spine	• Most common primary spinal column tumor in children	• Treatment variable based on location/timing of diagnosis	• Symptoms usually a result of cord compression and are very slowly progressive, starting with motor symptoms followed by progressive sphincter dysfunction and sensory loss.
	• Benign primary bone lesions			• Examples: osteoid osteomas, osteoblastomas, osteochondromas, chondroblastomas, giant cell tumors, vertebral hemangiomas, and aneurysmal bone cysts
Intradural extramedullary	• Nerve sheath tumors	• Extramedullary tumors are more common in adults.[4]		• Most common location of all spinal cord tumors
	• Meningiomas	• Most common primary spinal cord tumor • Females > males • Incidence increases with age • Highest incidence ages 65–74 • More common in male > female; white > black • Incidence may be increasing?[5]	• Watchful waiting vs surgery/radiation depending on neurologic symptoms	
	• Schwannomas		• Surgical resection often used for larger tumors	
	• Ependymomas			

(continued on next page)

Table 1
(continued)

Location	Tumor Type Examples	Epidemiology Notes	Treatment Notes	Additional Information
Intramedullary intradural		• Intramedullary tumors overall are very rare. • After age 60, intramedullary spinal cord tumors typically are 50% astrocytomas/50% ependymomas. • 2%–4% of all CNS tumors,[4] but more common than extramedullary tumors in children		
	• Ependymomas	• Intramedullary ependymomas are the most common intramedullary tumors in the middle adult years.		
	• Astrocytomas	• Astrocytomas comprise 90% of intramedullary tumors in children <10 y of age and 60% of intramedullary tumors in adolescents.[4]	• Often difficult to achieve full surgical resection • Often radiation used in conjunction with surgery	• Survival rate decreases with increasing age at diagnosis and higher-grade tumor.
	• Oligodendrogliomas			

Data from Refs.[4,5]

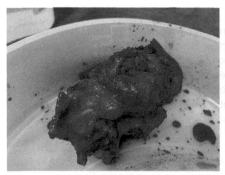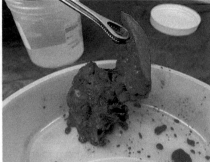

Fig. 1. A 57-year-old woman presented complaining of problems with bowel and bladder function and low back pain. The patient also reported sacral pain and the feeling of constant pressure. She was able to walk and had no evident sensory deficits. This led to imaging, which showed a lesion in the sacrum filling the thecal sac at approximately the S2-3 area downward. Upon resection and biopsy, this was determined to be a chondrosarcoma. (*Photos taken with patient's permission.)

TREATMENT

Once a spinal tumor is characterized, multidisciplinary treatment has been shown to yield the best results. Overall, primary tumors have a 5-year survival rate of greater than 70%, but recurrence is likely.[7] Recommendations for operative management should be made following evaluations from multiple specialties, such as neurology, neuro-oncology, neurosurgery, and neuroradiology.[5] Many tumors are categorized according to responsiveness to chemotherapy or radiation or to lack of response.

Any tumor that progresses to surgical treatment has 2 goals of therapy: resection of the tumor and reconstruction of the load-bearing capacity of the spine. Overall goals aim to improve mortality while also preserving as much function as is safely possible. Typically, non-metastatic tumors that are poorly responsive to adjuvant therapy proceed for aggressive surgical en bloc resection, meaning removal of the tumor in 1 unviolated piece.[1] The decision to do en bloc resection must be based on a tradeoff between expected increased survival and planned surgical morbidity rates. This is one of the most challenging spinal procedures and is relevant only if the tumor has not already spread. If no spread has occurred, en bloc resection offers a survival advantage. The goal is to avoid local and distant seeding that can occur by violating the tumor. There may be planned morbidity because adjacent structures may need to be sacrificed in order to remove the tumor in 1 piece. Spinal stability and reconstruction can be challenging, and patients often need permanent hardware and fusion.

Spinal cord tumors rarely are emergent procedures. Like all neurologic spine surgeries, urgency increases with progressive loss of neurologic function. If cord compromise leads to rapid loss of motor or sensory function, surgery becomes more urgent.

PREOPERATIVE CONSIDERATIONS

A preoperative conversation with a patient's surgeon is vital in order to understand goals of resection, plans for intraoperative neuromonitoring (IONM), and any other specific surgical needs. Continued communication throughout the case is vital in order to appropriately time emergence and plan appropriately for postoperative pain control.

History

When evaluating a patient with a spinal cord tumor to develop an anesthetic plan, it is important to understand the etiology of tumor, tumor location, presenting symptoms, and what treatment the patient has received. A full medical history should be solicited, focusing on any cardiorespiratory illness, renal dysfunction, hepatic dysfunction, coagulopathy, and chronic pain. The specific location of the primary and/or metastatic lesions or a history of chemotherapy or radiation may affect anesthesia care due to limb restrictions, space-occupying lesions of the brain, or organ dysfunction, for example,

Pain

Pain often is the presenting symptom of a spinal cord tumor or metastasis. A detailed history regarding the location of the patient's pain, current medication regimen, and duration of medication is necessary. This allows assessment of the degree of opioid tolerance prior to anesthesia and how it will influence the intraoperative and postoperative plans for pain management. If a patient is on chronic opioids, these should be continued on the morning of surgery, especially if a long operative time is anticipated.

Physical Examination

Neurologic deficits often exist due to the location of the primary tumor or metastatic lesion. A baseline neurologic examination should be conducted, documenting any motor weakness, paresthesia, or bowel/bladder dysfunction. Preexisting neurologic deficits can affect the quality of IONM and should be discussed with the surgical team.

Airway Examination

A full review of imaging and complete airway examination should be completed prior to surgery to address any concerns for cervical spine manipulation during endotracheal intubation. Cervical spine mobility may be affected, depending on the location of the tumor or an associated syrinx, or perhaps by concomitant arthritic changes. Jaw mobility and dentition also could be affected in the setting of prior radiation treatments of the cancer.

Studies

Laboratory work, cardiac testing, and imaging should be driven by the patient's severity of comorbid disease, degree of optimization, and functional capacity. Preoperative crossmatch of blood products may be necessary, depending on the etiology of the tumor to be resected, because metastatic lesions are likely to lead to higher volumes of blood loss intraoperatively than are primary tumors.

Perioperative Visual Loss

Due to required prone positioning for these surgeries, the risk of perioperative visual loss (POVL) should be discussed with the informed consent process for patients who are considered high risk and on a case-by-case basis.

POVL, a devastating complication of spine surgery, can occur by any of several different mechanisms, including anterior of posterior ischemic optic neuropathy, central retinal vein or artery occlusion, direct compression injury, acute angle closure glaucoma, and cortical blindness. POVL occurs in up to 1% of spine surgery, and ischemic optic neuropathy accounts for 89% of POVL cases.[8]

There are several risk factors that increase the likelihood of a patient developing POVL. These include anesthetic duration, hypotension, intraoperative anemia, the use of a Wilson frame, the use of Mayfield pins, and the comorbidities obesity, male sex, vascular disease, smoking, coronary disease, carotid artery disease, and diabetes.[9] Especially for patients with associated comorbidities and those expected to undergo procedures of more than 6 hours' duration or procedures that are likely to have a greater than 1-L blood loss, the risk of POVL should be discussed in the process of obtaining consent for the procedure.[10]

Premedication

Preoperative administration of multimodal adjuncts for pain management, such as acetaminophen, cyclooxygenase-2 inhibitors, and pregabalin, can be effective in reducing perioperative opioid use and postoperative pain.[11,12]

INTRAOPERATIVE CONSIDERATIONS
Induction/Airway

Induction medications and dosage should be tailored to a patient's comorbidities and allow for stable hemodynamics during intubation. The airway plan should account for any concerns regarding the cervical spine, as discussed previously. The use of neuromuscular blockade for intubation also must be reconciled with the IONM plan if monitoring motor evoked potentials (MEPs).

Monitoring and Hemodynamics

In addition to standard American Society of Anesthesiologists monitors, an arterial line allows for close monitoring of blood pressure to consistently maintain stable hemodynamics and adequate spinal cord perfusion pressure. A single anterior spinal artery provides the blood supply to the majority of the spinal cord, leaving the ventral portion of the cord particularly vulnerable to injury secondary to hypotension or anemia. The ventral portion of the spinal cord houses the motor tracts, hence intraoperative monitoring of motor evoked potentials (MEP) is often implemented and can be sensitive to changes in hemodynamics. Processed electroencephalogram, such as bispectral index monitoring, is controversial but can be considered to help taper anesthetic infusions, keeping in mind that it does not predict immobility. A Foley catheter may be needed for longer surgeries and to monitor, in a relatively noninvasive and inexpensive manner, urine output and fluid status.

Venous Access

Patients should have 2 large-bore peripheral lines for administration of medications and intravenous (IV) fluid given that metastatic lesions can be associated with a significant intraoperative blood loss. In contrast, surgery for primary tumors of the spinal cord rarely are associated with a large volume of blood loss. Some patients may have preexisting central access in the form of a port or peripherally inserted central catheter line for chemotherapy infusions. These can be accessed in order to give vasoactive infusions intraoperatively, if needed.

Positioning

Patients need to be positioned prone, with close attention paid to relieving any pressure on the eyes, ears, and lips from the face pillow. Soft bite blocks should be placed on either side of the endotracheal tube between the molars to protect the tongue, lips, and teeth from potential injury during motor stimulation from IONM.

Maintenance of Anesthesia

The choice of anesthetics for the maintenance of anesthesia for spinal cord tumor resection largely depends on the IONM plan, patients' degree of opioid tolerance, and their comorbidities. Generally, the goal is to maintain steady-state anesthetic and hemodynamics to minimize the impact on IONM signals.

- Often, total IV anesthesia (TIVA) using propofol and an opioid infusion is implemented to maintain this steady state. Please refer to the Shilpa Rao and colleagues' article, "Basics of Neuromonitoring and Anesthetic Considerations," in this issue: Neuromonitoring for further information on the effects of specific anesthetics on neuromonitoring signals.
- Context-sensitive half-life is defined as the time it takes for a drug's plasma concentration to decrease by 50% after stopping an infusion set to maintain a specific concentration. The *context* refers to the duration that the drug has been infusing. For example, it takes longer for a patient to awaken from a propofol infusion of 100 μg/kg/min that has been running for 6 hours as opposed to an infusion that has only been running for 1 hour. This pharmacokinetic principle demonstrates that drug activity cannot be predicted solely by its metabolism and elimination but also is dependent on its distribution to, and redistribution from, tissue compartments. Understanding the context-sensitive half-times of the anesthetics being infused facilitates dosing to allow for rapid emergence and the patient's participation in a neurologic examination in the immediate postoperative period.
- Propofol is more favorable than benzodiazepine or barbiturate infusions due to its shorter context-sensitive half-life, allowing it to be more titratable. Processed electroencephalogram monitoring can be used to help taper the infusion rate to help minimize oversedation and the time to emergence.
- Opioid infusions, such as sufentanil, can be titrated to a patient's blood pressure and heart rate.
- Volatile anesthetics can be used at doses less than 0.5 minimum alveolar concentration, although their effects on neuromonitoring signals should be taken into account.
- Neuromuscular blockade should be avoided if the IONM plan includes electromyography or MEPs.
- Maintain normovolemia by replacing urinary output and insensible losses using balanced iso-osmolar fluids. Avoidance of fluid overload is particularly important given the risk of POVL in the prone position.
- A transfusion trigger of 8 g/dL to 10 g/dL should be determined depending on a patient's comorbidities and risk for end-organ dysfunction.

Multimodal Pain Management

The perioperative pain management plan should be tailored to a patient's symptoms and degree of opioid sensitivity. Efforts to reduce opioid consumption perioperatively using nonopioid adjuncts can help reduce the risk of side effects, such as nausea, vomiting, pruritis, urinary retention, ileus, and respiratory depression as well as help reduce the length of hospital stay. If the patient already is taking chronic opioids, these should be continued on the day of surgery. These can be given orally preoperatively, or alternatively, by calculating the patient's daily morphine equivalents and then converting morphine equivalents to an alternate IV form to continue administration while the patient is anesthetized. Ideally, the patient, in conjunction with the prescribing physician, should attempt to taper daily opioid usage in the weeks preceding surgery to help improve opioid sensitivity perioperatively and to minimize the risk of hyperalgesia.[13]

- Dexmedetomidine, a centrally acting α_2-agonist, reduces propofol and opioid requirements but also can cause hypotension, bradycardia, and sedation. It may decrease the amplitude of evoked potentials, especially when used in conjunction with other adjuncts with similar effects, such as lidocaine infusions.[4,13]

- Lidocaine infusions, at 2 mg/kg/h, have been used for their systemic anti-inflammatory properties as well as their ability to reduce opioid requirements and hyperalgesia. The use of lidocaine leads to reduced nausea, vomiting, and hospital length of stay.[14]
- Methadone, an N-methyl-D-aspartate (NMDA) antagonist particularly effective for chronic opioid users, has been shown to reduce opioid requirements by up to 50% at 48 hours as well as postoperative pain scores when given as a 0.2-mg/kg IV bolus prior to incision.[15]
- Ketamine, also an NMDA antagonist, also has been shown to reduce opioid requirements by 30% at 24 hours without increased side effects when given as a 0.5-mg/kg bolus with induction followed by 10-μg/kg/min infusion until wound closure.[16]
- Ketamine also has the added benefit of increasing IONM signal acquisition intraoperatively by increasing signal amplitude.
- Shorter-acting opioid infusions, such as sufentanil and remifentanil, are preferred if opioids are to be used.

Intraoperative Neuromonitoring

There is no gold standard in place for IONM for spinal cord tumor surgery; however, it commonly is used. The location of the tumor may dictate which modalities are monitored intraoperatively. Baseline IONM signals should be acquired prior to positioning and incision. This baseline ideally should be acquired while under whatever anesthetics are planned to be continued throughout the case so anesthetic effects can be accounted for. Please refer to Shilpa Rao and colleagues' article, "Basics of Neuromonitoring and Anesthetic Considerations," in this issue for further information on neuromonitoring.

- MEPs monitor the ventral and lateral corticospinal tracts (efferent and descending), which control voluntary motor function. Perfusion of these tracts consists of a singular anterior spinal artery that supplies the anterior two-thirds of the spinal cord. For this reason, MEPs are very sensitive at detecting ischemic injury to the anterior spinal cord due to hypotension, anemia, or compression, caused by implanted hardware, for example. It is difficult to obtain reproducible MEPs for patients with preoperatively scored 3 out of 5 motor weakness as defined by the Medical Research Council Manual Muscle Testing scale (muscle activation against gravity and full range of motion). MEPs may be almost impossible to obtain if motor weakness scores less than 3 out of 5.[17]
- Electromyography monitors motor activity of specific spinal nerve roots or peripheral nerves.
- Somatosensory evoked potentials monitor the ascending dorsal column sensory pathways.
- It should be kept in mind that physiologic characteristics, such as blood pressure, temperature, anemia, electrolyte disturbances, and acid-base disturbances, all affect can neuromonitoring signals as can the choice of anesthetic agents.

Emergence

Proactive tapering of TIVA with regard to context-sensitive half-lives and organ function allows for a timely emergence and an awake, cooperative patient who can participate in a postoperative neurologic examination. Once IONM has been concluded, conversion to a volatile anesthetic also is a possibility to allow ample time for plasma concentrations of IV anesthetics to decrease. Often, if a dural leak and/or repair is noted during surgery, the patient is required to lie flat for at least 24 hours postoperatively. Avoiding coughing or bucking during emergence can reduce stress on this repair. Consideration for the patient's comorbidities, such as morbid obesity or obstructive sleep apnea, is essential when required to remain flat for emergence and the postoperative period. For prolonged prone procedures, it also is essential to evaluate for potential airway edema prior to moving toward extubation, because this can be a cause of subtle airway compromise, especially when necessary to remain flat postoperatively.

POSTOPERATIVE CONSIDERATIONS

A neurologic examination should be completed soon after emergence to establish if any new deficits are present, especially if changes in IONM signals occurred intraoperatively. Any new sensory or motor deficits should be discussed with the surgeon because these may require further imaging or possibly urgent surgery. Due to prolonged prone positioning, assessment for any pressure injuries to the skin or face should be performed, documented, and followed in the postoperative period. Corneal abrasions also can occur and should be treated promptly per the facility's protocol. Multimodal nonopioid analgesics should be continued into the postoperative period to help reduce opioid administration and its associated side effects. Any chronic pain medications also should be continued postoperatively.

SUMMARY

Although spinal cord tumors overall are rare occurrences, it is important for anesthesiologists to be familiar with the various types of spinal cord tumors. Understanding the most common aspects of spinal cord surgery, such as the use of IONM, context-sensitive half-times, appropriate medications for TIVA, and risks of POVL, is vital in providing the best anesthesia care for patients. The information provided in this article guides anesthesiologists in planning an optimal anesthetic for spinal cord tumor resection.

DISCLOSURE

Neither author has any commercial or financial conflicts of interest or any funding sources outside of their institution of employment.

REFERENCES

1. Clarke MJ, Mendel E, Vrionis FD. Primary spine tumors:diagnosis & treatment. Cancer Control 2014;21(2):114–23.
2. Quraishi NA, Gokaslan ZL, Boriani S. The surgical management of metastatic epidural compression of the spinal cord. J Bone Joint Surg Br 2019;92(8): 1054–60.
3. Tenny S, Varacallo M. Chordoma. In: StatPearls [Internet]. Treasure Island (FL): StatPearls Publishing; 2020. Available at: https://www.ncbi.nlm.nih.gov/books/NBK430846/.
4. Alizada O, Kemerdere R, Onur ulu M, et al. Surgical management of spinal intramedullary tumors: ten-year experience in a single institution. J Clin Neurosci 2020;73:201–8.

5. Tish S, Habboub G, Lang M, et al. The epidemiology of spinal schwannoma in the United States between 2006 and 2014. J Neurosurg 2019;32(5):633–780.
6. Welch WC, Jacobs GB. Surgery for metastatic spinal disease. J Neurooncol 1995;23(2):163–70.
7. Deiner S. Anesthesia for intramedullary spinal cord tumors. In: Mongan PD, Soriano SG, Sloan TB, editors. A practical approach to neuroanesthesia. Philadelphia (PA): Lippincott Williams & Wilkins, Wolters Kluwer; 2013. p. 192–200.
8. Epstein N. Perioperative visual loss following prone spinal surgery: a review. Surg Neurol Int 2016;7(Suppl 13):S347–60.
9. Practice advisory for perioperative visual loss associated with spine surgery 2019: an updated report by the American society of anesthesiologists task force on perioperative visual loss, the north American neuro-ophthalmology society, and the society for neuroscience in anesthesiology and critical care. Anesthesiology 2019;130(1):12–30.
10. Lorie AL, Roth S, Posner KI, et al. The american society of anesthesiologists postoperative visual loss registry: analysis of 93 spine surgery cases with postoperative visual loss. Anesthesiology 2006;105(4):652–9.
11. Raja SDC, Shetty AP, Subramanian B, et al. A prospective randomized study to analyze the efficacy of balanced pre-emptive analgesia in spine surgery. Spine J 2019;19(4):569–77.
12. Jiang HL, Huang S, Song J, et al. Preoperative use of pregabalin for acute pain in spine surgery: a meta-analysis of randomized controlled trials. Medicine 2017;96(11):e6129.
13. Dunn LK, Durieux ME, Nemergut EC. Non-opioid analgesics: novel approaches to perioperative analgesia for major spine surgery. Best Pract Res Clin Anaesthesiol 2016;30(1):79–89.
14. Dunn LK, Durieux ME. Perioperative use of intravenous lidocaine. Anesthesiology 2017;126:729–37.
15. Gottschalk A, Durieux ME, Nemergut EC. Intraoperative methadone improves postoperative pain control in patients undergoing complex spine surgery. Anesth Analg 2011;112(1):218–23.
16. Loftus RW, Yeager MP, Jeffrey AC, et al. Intraoperative ketamine reduces perioperative opiate consumption in opiate-dependent patients with chronic back pain undergoing back surgery. Anesthesiology 2010;113(3):639–46.
17. Guo L, Li Y, Han R, et al. The correlation between recordable MEPs and motor function during spinal surgery for resection of thoracic spinal cord tumor. J Neurosurg Anesthesiol 2018;30(1):39–43.

Anesthetic Management of Patients Undergoing Intravascular Treatment of Cerebral Aneurysms and Arteriovenous Malformations

Magnus Knut Teig, MBChB, MRCP, FRCA, EDIC, FFICM

KEYWORDS

- Anesthesia • Intravascular therapy for cerebral aneurysm
- Intravascular therapy for cerebral arteriovenous malformation

KEY POINTS

- Intravascular therapies for intracerebral vascular pathologic conditions have greatly expanded in scope and capability over the last 30 years.
- Anesthetizing patients scheduled for radiologic treatment of intracerebral vascular lesions is especially challenging.
- Therapies as well as the consideration necessary to plan for and effectively anesthetize patients undergoing them are discussed in this article.

INTRODUCTION

Intravascular therapies for intracerebral vascular pathologic conditions have greatly expanded in scope and capability over the last 30 years. Neurointerventional radiology (NIR) suites now exist throughout the world. In the United States alone, more than 8000 medical practitioners work in all branches of interventional radiology (IR),[1] in large inpatient facilities as well as in approximately 700 ambulatory IR facilities.[2]

Because of the disease being treated, patient comorbidities, the relatively frequent remote location of the interventional neuroradiology (INR) suite from the operating rooms, and the physical layout of the INR suite, anesthetizing patients scheduled for radiologic treatment of intracerebral vascular lesions is especially challenging.

In 1953, the Swedish radiologist, Sven-Ivar Seldinger, described a percutaneous approach to visualize peripheral arteries. The first intravascular IR case was described in 1964 when Dr Charles Dotter performed minimally invasive intraarterial therapy to attempt to restore blood flow to a patient with a critically ischemic left foot.

Department of Anesthesiology, University of Michigan, 1500 East Medical Center Drive, Ann Arbor, MI 48109-5048, USA
E-mail address: mteig@med.umich.edu

Anesthesiology Clin 39 (2021) 151–162
https://doi.org/10.1016/j.anclin.2020.11.008
1932-2275/21/© 2020 Elsevier Inc. All rights reserved.

anesthesiology.theclinics.com

"Interventional Radiology" as a named specialty was coined in 1967 by Dr Alexander Margulis. Techniques rapidly evolved and, as knowledge base grew, interventional radiologists began to treat intracranial vascular disease, leading to the development of the specialty of INR.[3]

Intracranial aneurysms have a lifetime prevalence of approximately 4%[4] and may be found incidentally as part of an evaluation for another medical problem or become apparent after rupture. Treatment of aneurysms depends on aneurysm size, location, and shape in addition to patient age and the site where a patient presents for management. Treatment options include observation, open surgical clipping, and intravascular approaches.

The first known attempted endovascular treatment of intracranial aneurysm using INR imaging was performed in the mid-1970s when Gerard Debrun attempted to use a detachable latex balloon catheter for the treatment of giant intracavernous aneurysms and carotid-cavernous fistulae.[3] The rapid growth in intravascular therapy for intracerebral aneurysms began in 1990 when detachable coils were invented by a neurosurgeon, Guido Guglielmi.[5] Placing coils in the aneurysmal sack eliminates the blood flow into it, causing its obliteration. Widespread adoption of aneurysm coiling began after the International Subarachnoid Aneurysm Trial (ISAT) compared endovascular treatment with open surgical treatment of ruptured intracranial aneurysms. ISAT demonstrated that endovascular coiling resulted in better independent survival at 1 year, with absolute risk reduction of 7.4% and a better outcome that was apparent at least 7 years after treatment.[6] The benefit of endovascular cerebral aneurysm coiling demonstrated in this trial led to the expansion of INR facilities and suggested endovascular coiling as a first-line therapy for intracerebral aneurysm. Newer modalities of intravascular therapies for intracranial aneurysms are constantly being developed, including stenting and stent-coiling techniques.

With the increase in endovascular therapies for the management of intracranial aneurysms, there has been an expansion in INR therapies for treatment of cerebral arteriovenous malformations (AVM). Development of glues to use as embolizing material has allowed for the growth in this area. Intracranial AVMs are rare, usually asymptomatic vascular lesions that are present in 10 to 18 people per 100,000. They may present with spontaneous intracranial hemorrhage (ICH), seizures, or headache, typically in younger adults. Asymptomatic AVMs may be diagnosed after incidental brain imaging. Primary treatment goals are to reduce the risk of spontaneous ICH; options include conservative management, surgical resection, stereotactic radiosurgery, endovascular embolization, or combinations thereof (multimodal therapy).

Studies estimate that AVM rupture risk is 2.3% per year over a 10-year period.[7] This calculation is a complex calculation, and the risks of rupture are influenced by the location and anatomy of the AVM as well as any history of recurrence. Endovascular treatment of AVMs commonly includes embolization using a liquid embolizate of ethyl vinyl alcohol copolymer. The technique has been enhanced by the invention of detachable tip microcatheters. Embolization may be curative or may be used as part of multimodal therapy for AVMs to reduce their size before open or radiosurgery approaches.

These therapies as well as the consideration necessary to plan for and effectively anesthetize patients undergoing them are discussed in this article.

ANESTHESIA FOR INTRAVASCULAR TREATMENT OF CEREBRAL ANEURYSMS

Intracranial aneurysm patients fall into one of 2 broad groups, elective and emergent. Elective patients commonly present after an incidental finding of an aneurysm: either following incidental cerebral imaging or following investigation of a patient who has a family history of symptomatic aneurysm. Occasionally, patients may have a condition that predisposes them to aneurysm formation, such as adult polycystic kidney disease or Ehler-Danlos syndrome.

Emergent, postaneurysm rupture patients may present in extremis and be intubated and ventilated or they may present with recent onset of a severe headache. The Hunt-Hess scale (**Table 1**) and Fisher grade are used to describe the severity of an sub-arachnoid hemorrhage. The Hunt-Hess scale describes how the patient appears to an examiner. Mortality is minimum with grade 1 and maximum with grade 5. The Fisher grade describes how the SAH hemorrhage appears on computed tomographic scan. It is a prognostic tool and is of less immediate relevance to anesthesia providers.

For patients presenting for either elective or emergent management of their intracra-nial aneurysm, blood pressure (BP) control is imperative to reduce the chance of the aneurysm rebleeding. Maintaining BP within 20% of starting BP is recommended. Invasive arterial monitoring is essential for these patients and, when practical, should be in place before induction of anesthesia.

Anesthetic Plan for Endovascular Approach to Intracerebral Aneurysm

The preprocedure evaluation of these patients should, in addition to all the elements included in a preoperative assessment, include specific focus on the patient's likeli-hood of having an allergic reaction to contrast material and their underlying renal func-tion. Reactions to contrast material include nausea, vomiting, and anaphylactoid and anaphylactic reactions. Risk factors for an anaphylactic reaction include previous re-action to contrast material, iodine sensitivity, bronchospasm, or a history of general allergies. Patients at high risk for an allergic reaction should be pretreated with ste-roids and diphenhydramine.[8] Because of the risk of an anaphylactic reaction, every INR suite should have resuscitation medication and equipment available.

There is a risk of contrast-associated acute kidney injury that increases as the de-gree of preexisting renal failure increases. The risk is approximately 5% with an esti-mated glomerular filtration rate (GFR) of ≥ 60 and 30% with a GFR of less than 30 mL/min/1.73 m^2. Prophylaxis is recommended to protect existing renal function in patients who are not being treated with dialysis and who have an estimated GFR of less than 30 mL/min/1.73 m^2.[9] Prophylaxis should include increasing the intravascular volume with an isotonic crystalloid. Typically, fluid administration begins 1 hour before admin-istration of contrast and continues for 3 to 12 hours after administration. Dose recom-mendations range from 500 mL to 1 to 3 mL/kg.[10] N-acetylcysteine is ineffective in prophylaxis.[11]

Table 1 The Hunt Hess scale	
Grade	**Description**
1	Asymptomatic, mild headache, slight nuchal rigidity
2	Moderate to severe headache, nuchal rigidity, no neurologic deficit other than cranial nerve palsy
3	Drowsiness, confusion, mild focal neurologic deficit
4	Stupor, moderate-severe hemiparesis
5	Coma, decerebrate posturing

Data from Hunt WE, Hess RM. Surgical risk as related to time of intervention in the repair of intra-cranial aneurysms. *Journal of Neurosurgery* 1968 Jan;28(1):14-20.

A preinduction anxiolytic, such as midazolam, may be used to reduce patient anxiety. However, often this is avoided, so as not to cloud the postprocedure neurologic examination. Following the preinduction verification process and equipment checks, the anesthesia plan for intracerebral aneurysm embolization is typically general anesthesia with controlled ventilation following induction of general anesthesia. Induction can be accomplished with a GABAergic agent and anesthetic adjuncts, such as opioids, or a beta-blocker to mitigate the hypertensive response to intubation. Neuromuscular blockade is induced to facilitate endotracheal intubation and dosed throughout the procedure to maintain an adequate depth of neuromuscular blockade to stop and allow for rapid and complete recovery of neuromuscular function at the conclusion to the procedure to allow for early assessment of neurologic status. Maintenance of muscle relaxation throughout the procedure improves somatosensory-evoked potential (SSEP) signals for intraoperative neuromonitoring (IONM) and reduces the risk of inadvertent patient movement, which may have catastrophic consequences during an intraarticular procedure.

Total intravenous anesthesia (TIVA), via continuous infusion, is commonly used for maintenance of anesthesia to facilitate IONM signals with or without supplementation with volatile anesthetics. When using TIVA, infusion lines must be inspected regularly for patency and flow, to prevent interruption of drug delivery and to reduce the risk of intraoperative awareness. Short-acting opioid infusions, such as remifentanil, reduce reactivity to procedural stimulation. Other agents that are commonly used for TIVA include sufentanil, propofol, and dexmedetomidine.

The different challenges in caring for patients in the INR suite for treatment of their intracranial aneurysms fall into 3 main categories: procedural concerns, patient positioning and access concerns, and provider environment concerns.

Procedural concerns of aneurysm coiling

Coiling on an intracranial aneurysm is the deployment of a coiled piece of platinum wire into the aneurysmal sack, using an electric current to sever the connection between the catheter and the platinum coil. Once released into the aneurysm, the coil assumes a predetermined shape, reducing blood flow. Deployment of multiple coils is typically necessary. Once the sack of the aneurysm is occluded, blood flow into the aneurysm decreases, and a clot will develop in the sack. Blood flow and shear stress within the aneurysm are immediately reduced with coiling, immediately reducing the chance of aneurysm rupture.

Systemic anticoagulation is required during aneurysm coiling to prevent the formation of clot catheters for aneurysmal access and deployment of the coils. Unless contraindicated, heparin is administered as the anticoagulant, and an activated clotting time (ACT) of greater than 250 seconds during the procedure is the goal of treatment. In addition to clot formation, another risk of intravascular management of intracranial aneurysms includes the migration of coils into the more distal cerebral circulation if they do not nest within an aneurysm sack. The structure of the aneurysm determines in large measure the likelihood of this occurring. Aneurysms that have narrower necks are technically simpler to coil in that the narrower neck tends to hold the coils that have been deployed into the sack. Aneurysms that have a wider neck pose a greater challenge because there is a greater risk of that the coil will migrate out of the aneurysm, causing vessel embolization and a stroke (**Fig. 1**).

Alternative techniques have been developed in recent years to address management aneurysms with wider neck. Although an in-depth discussion of each of these techniques is beyond the scope of this article, they are listed in **Tables 2** and **3** with a brief description.

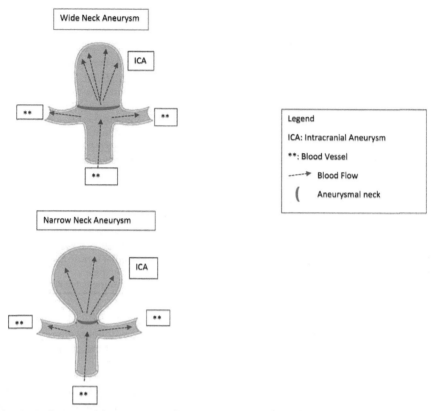

Fig. 1. An intracranial aneurysm with a narrow neck and an intracranial aneurysm with a wide neck. ICA, intracranial aneurysm. **, blood vessel.

Table 2	
Aneurysm management techniques	
Technique of Aneurysm Management	**Brief Description**
Balloon-assisted coiling	A balloon is inflated in the artery adjacent to the site of the aneurysm, to hold coils in place as they are deployed
Intraarterial drug-eluting stent embolization devices	These devices are permanent mesh cylinders (stents). They are similar in function and design to intracoronary arterial stents. Some are impregnated with agents that inhibit endothelization of the stent, aiming to reduce the chance of in-stent *stenosis* occurring. Dual antiplatelet therapy is required to prevent in-stent *thrombosis* from occurring from platelet adherence to the metal of the stent
Pipeline stents	These stents isolate aneurysms from blood flow by covering the entry point like a "sleeve." Following isolation, blood flow stasis within the aneurysm sack leads to thrombosis and aneurysm obliteration

Table 3
Summary of anesthetic management of endovascular coiling of intracranial aneurysms and embolization of arteriovenous malformations

Procedure	Endovascular Coiling of Aneurysms	Embolization of Arteriovenous Malformations
Anesthetic plan	• General anesthetic with an endotracheal tube	• General anesthetic with an endotracheal tube
Intraoperative neuromonitoring	• Somatosensory-evoked potentials • Electroencephalography	• Somatosensory-evoked potentials • Electroencephalography
Arterial access	• Yes, radial artery most proximal to the anesthesia care team	• Yes, radial artery most proximal to the anesthesia care team
Anticoagulation	• Systemic heparinization • Dual antiplatelet therapy	• Systemic heparinization
Unique considerations	• Risk of coil migration • Risk of in-stent thrombosis	• Risk of systemic embolization of occlusive glue
Emergency resources	• External ventricular drain • Protamine • Platelets crossmatched	• External ventricular drain • Protamine • Adenosine 0.4–0.6 mg/kg

Stent embolization devices may be supplemented with conventional aneurysm coiling, either by threading the coiling catheter through the mesh of the stent itself or by placing it adjacent to the stent before deployment.

To successfully isolate very large aneurysms, stents may be deployed one inside another sequentially to "telescope" across a gap longer than any 1 stent. Telescope stenting is a high-risk procedure, but it enables aneurysms that previously could not be treated to be isolated. Complications include stent dislodgement, hemorrhage, distal embolization, and stroke. If it is even technically possible, craniotomy and clipping of massive aneurysms also have a high risk of complications, most notably rupture.

Dual antiplatelet agents, usually aspirin and clopidogrel, must be in place with adequate levels of platelet inhibition before stent embolization. Platelet inhibition should be checked immediately preprocedure and the procedure delayed if levels are inadequate. Redosing of antiplatelet agents may be required during the procedure. It is sensible to secure nasogastric or orogastric access after induction. Although aspirin may be administered rectally and is available as an intravenous (IV) preparation in some countries, clopidogrel is only available as an enteral preparation.

Any inadvertent bleeding will be greatly increased with dual antiplatelet agents on board. Crossmatched platelets should be available for transfusion to reverse platelet inhibition emergently if necessary. Poststent embolization patients may be encountered in a non-NIR setting for incidental surgery. It is important to remember that antiplatelet therapies must be continued, and if interrupted for any reason, restarted as soon as possible afterward. At least 1 antiplatelet agent is required lifelong, with the addition of the second agent, usually clopidogrel, for a minimum of 3 months following stent embolization.

Postaneurysm Isolation

Hemodynamic goals may change after an aneurysm is secured. In patients having an elective procedure, it is reasonable to maintain preoperative BPs. Following intravascular management of a patient with a ruptured aneurysm, pretreatment BP targets aimed at reducing the risk of aneurysm rerupture (conventionally systolic blood pressure [SBP] ≤ 140 mm Hg) are increased to an SBP 180 mm Hg[12] or even higher to reduce the risk of cerebrovascular vasospasm.

Following elective aneurysm management in the INR suite, in order to allow immediate neurologic examination, patients are allowed to emerge from anesthesia right after the procedure. Patients who were treated after aneurysmal rupture and who may have been comatose before the procedure because of a, SAH often are transferred back to a critical care setting, intubated, and ventilated for ongoing therapies. Following femoral arterial puncture for intraarterial access, patients may need to remain supine for up to 6 hours to reduce the risk of puncture site bleeding or pseudoaneurysm formation. This requirement may complicate extubation, particularly in patients with obstructive sleep apnea or obese patients who have respiratory compromise in the supine position. If it is anticipated that a patient will have significant difficulty lying flat following extubation, it may be prudent to delay extubation until 6 hours after the procedure. Precautions also must be taken such that the patient does not bend his knees as emerging from anesthesia or once extubated. The use of a knee splint will help in this regard. Endovascular securing devices to seal the arterial puncture site will also reduce the amount of time that a patient needs to lie flat. Accessing the cerebral circulation through the radial artery will obviate the patient to lie flat.

Treatment of Intracerebral Aneurysm Rupture During Endovascular Therapy

Rupture of an intracranial aneurysm during interventional neuroradiologic procedures is a true emergency. Responses to the emergency include the following:

1. Platelet transfusion to restore platelet function if the patient is on dual antiplatelet therapy: Crossmatched platelets should be immediately available within the INR suite in case of an aneurysm rupture occurring.
2. Reversal of heparin with protamine: Heparin, 100 U, can be reversed with 1 mg protamine, for example, 5000 U IV heparin is antagonized with slow administration of 50 mg protamine (maximum infusion rate 5 mg per minute).
3. BP management: Typically hypertension is treated to maintain SBP less than 140 mm Hg. Avoidance of hypotension is of equal importance, as cerebral blood flow may be impeded by the presence of the intravascular devices themselves or the increase in intracranial pressure (ICP) caused by the hemorrhage.
4. Insertion of an external ventricular drain (EVD) to monitor and treat raised ICP: An EVD should be immediately available in the INR suite. Acute subarachnoid hemorrhage may be rapidly fatal through a catastrophic increase in ICP, causing cerebral compression.
5. Consider burst suppression anesthesia using EEG IONM-targeted dosing.

ICP should not be overtreated during subarachnoid hemorrhage. Overreduction of ICP *increases* the transmural pressure gradient across an aneurysm (SBP minus ICP), increasing the risk of rupture. After placement, an EVD may be clamped to monitor ICP or it may be left open at a relatively high level, for example, at 20 cm above the tragus, to maintain a "high normal" ICP. Similarly, extremes of hyperventilation should be avoided.

Intraoperative Neuromonitoring During Interventional Neuroradiology Procedures

IONM can be used to monitor sufficient cerebral perfusion during the procedure. SSEP and electroencephalography (EEG) are the 2 most commonly used modalities. SSEP allows for indirect monitoring of the adequacy of middle cerebral artery territory perfusion, as this supplies the sensory cortex. EEG allows for assessment of global cerebral metabolic function and indirect perfusion, as well as for targeted dosing of GABAergic anesthetics, including the ability to use intentional burst suppression for neuroprotection, if transient ischemia is anticipated. A sudden 10% change in signal amplitude is a useful warning of relative intravascular insufficiency or reduction in previously adequate BP through vessels impeded by the presence of catheters, coiling, or stenting devices. Any changes in the results of monitoring may be an early warning of significant intracerebral hypoperfusion.

Because perfusion may be compromised to a greater extent during endovascular therapies from the presence of the treatment catheters within the feeding vessels, greater emphasis is put on IONM changes during intravascular therapies than in craniotomies for aneurysm clipping. Because of the potential compromise of blood flow to areas of the brain distal to the treatment catheters, it is important to avoid hypotension during the procedure. Maintaining a patient's BP within 20% of their baseline values or SBP between 110 and 130 mm Hg is empirically recommended to reduce the risk of hypoperfusion and a downstream stroke. It is important to remember that the true BP distal to the deploying devices remains unknown, and periprocedural stroke may still occur even if systolic pressures are maintained in this range.

The IONM signals are optimized with the use of TIVA with an infusion of a sedative hypnotic and one or more analgesics (opioids, dexmedetomidine, ketamine). Administration of supplementary low-dose volatile anesthetics, such as isoflurane or sevoflurane, may be coadministered to reduce the risk of anesthetic awareness. If TIVA alone is used, anesthesia practitioners may wish to be guided on the depth of anesthesia using either a processed commercial EEG monitor or analysis of raw EEG data by the IONM team. Neuromuscular blockade is maintained throughout the procedure with administration of a nondepolarizing neuromuscular blocking agent, the dosing of which is based on the patient's response to quantitative monitoring of depth of neuromuscular blockade.

Positioning and patient access concerns

Patient positioning in the INR suite is a challenge. Often the only access that the anesthesiologist has to the patient is a single hand and wrist. Typically, the IR table is turned 90° from the anesthesia provider, to allow room for the biplane angiography arms to rotate around the patient. Floor space immediately next to the patient is off limits to allow for maneuvering of the biplane apparatus. Infusion lines often require extensions, and airway circuits must be meticulously arranged to prevent entanglement and accidental extubation. There can be variation in INR suite layout even within the same institution; so, review of the physical plant is important, especially if it is the first time caring for a patient in that particular location (**Fig. 2**).

With the location of the patient relative to the anesthesiologist during a procedure, an arterial catheter for invasive BP monitoring is best placed in the left radial artery, with an associated IV line placed in the left upper extremity. The IR table may need to be rotated significantly to allow the anesthesiologist to manage the airway during induction; with it in its position for embolization manual ventilation of the patient may be physically impossible. A radiology technician or nurse may be necessary to rotate the procedure table, and the large amount of equipment adjacent to the patient's head may compound the task of securing the airway. Imaging booms should, if possible, be moved out of the way during airway management, and there should always be someone in the room who has complete knowledge of how to operate the bed if it needs to be adjusted to facilitate emergent anesthesia care. Furthermore,

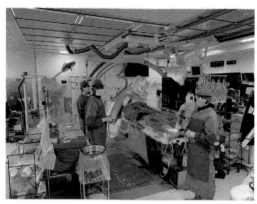

Fig. 2. Typical neuro-NIR setup: note anesthesia provider in limited workspace.

INR procedural areas are often remote from main operating rooms, making it difficult for assisting practitioners to rapidly assist in an emergency.

Because aneurysm coiling and stent embolization can be prolonged procedures, attention should be paid to padding all areas at risk of pressure ulceration (**Fig. 3**).

Provider-centered concerns

Provider safety concerns are always present when working in an environment with exposure to ionizing radiation. Diagnostic cerebral angiography exposes a patient to approximately 10.6 mSv,[13] compared with about 0.1 mSV for a chest radiograph, approximately 106 times the dose during angiography. Treatment cerebral angiography may produce even higher doses of ionizing radiation. Thus, providers should have well-fitting, regularly checked "lead" protection available, complete with a thyroid protection shield. "Lead" glass barriers on wheels should be used as further shielding. It may be appropriate to leave the INR suite briefly during the most intense imaging acquisition runs to reduce radiation exposure. Radiation monitoring badges must be worn correctly, on the outside of any protection if indicated, so that a provider's total exposure to ionizing radiation can be known.

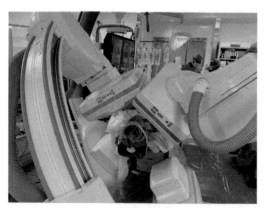

Fig. 3. Imaging boom setup for cranial angiography. Note arrangement of anesthesia circuit.

ANESTHESIA FOR INTRAVASCULAR MANAGEMENT OF ARTERIOVENOUS MALFORMATIONS

AVMs occur when there is an abnormal vascular connection between the arterial and venous plexuses of an organ, bypassing the capillary arcade. Most AVMs are asymptomatic. Symptomatic brain AVMs are rare, occurring in almost 1 per 100,000 person-years.[14]

Morbidity from AVMs may occur in various ways. They can bleed, causing ICH; they may cause chronic hypoperfusion and underdevelopment of brain regions. They may act as a nidus for a seizure, or they may cause a direct mass effect, distorting underlying brain. AVMs may occur as a congenital phenomenon, or they may occur spontaneously, following previous surgery, or as a sequala of head-injury trauma.

Arteriovenous Malformation Treatment Options

Historical treatments for intracranial AVMs were complex open craniotomies associated with significant bleeding and comorbidities. More recently, treatment options have increased, with the addition of effective intraluminal treatments. Initial endovascular attempts to treat AVMs were unsuccessful because of the small diameter of the vascular structures involved, making it difficult to pass even a small catheter. Technologies such as placing coils or directly gluing the AVMs initially proved unsuccessful. The first practical endovascular AVM therapy came with the development of Onyx in 1990.[15] Onyx is an elastic copolymer, ethylene vinyl alcohol copolymer dissolved in dimethyl sulfoxide (DMSO) that functions effectively as a "slow superglue." Onyx is injected via an intraluminal catheter proximal to an AVM and then allowed to drift with blood flow into the AVM, where it sets and occludes it (**Fig. 4**).

Anesthesia for Arteriovenous Malformation Embolization

Anesthesia for embolization of an intracranial AVM is typically a general anesthetic with an endotracheal tube, with invasive arterial BP monitoring in addition to routine monitors. IONM is commonly performed, typically using SSEP to assess for adequacy of perfusion through the vessels in which the embolization catheters are situated. Propofol-based TIVA, with or without supplemental low-dose volatile anesthetics, improves the IONM signals. NMBDs are used to prevent reflex patient movement.

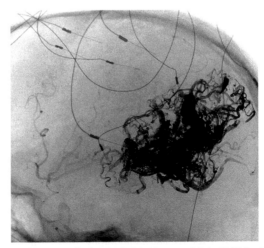

Fig. 4. Successful embolization of a brain AVM. Note multiple IONM wires in place.

Heparinization is necessary for embolization glue to be deployed in order to prevent clot formation on deployment catheters. Heparin is conventionally used, aiming for an ACT of greater than 250 seconds during procedures. Protamine must be on hand in case AVM disruption occurs, to minimize any resultant hemorrhage. AVM endovascular embolization is a delicate procedure with significant interpatient and interprocedure variability. Embolization with gluelike substances has the potential for significant risk. Open communication with INR colleagues is essential to anticipate rare but serious complications, such as hemorrhage or unintended distal embolization of the glue. Unintended distal embolization can result in ischemia to distal vessels or territories, including pulmonary embolism if the embolization material is carried into the systemic venous circulation. If blood flow through the AVM is great enough to increase the likelihood of distal embolization, adenosine can be given in doses of up to 0.4 to 0.6 mg/kg to produce a brief period of circulatory arrest, enabling the glue to set within the targeted AVM[16,17] and not be carried through the AVM to more distant vascular sites. AVMs can be quite large and, in these cases, complete obliteration with a single therapeutic session may not be advisable because of posttreatment cerebral edema and restructuring of cerebral blood flow. In these cases, patients may return to the INR suite for staged embolization of their AVMs.

Even when smaller AVMs are embolized, normal perfusion pressure breakthrough can occur following the occlusion, because brain that had been underperfused may, after treatment, be perfused at a much higher relative pressure than it had seen previously, possibly resulting in localized cerebral edema or hemorrhage, which and is a serious medical emergency. Close BP control minimizes this risk.[18]

Following successful AVM occlusion, the patient should be allowed to emerge from anesthesia and extubated for immediate neurologic assessment. Postprocedure observation in a monitored setting capable of frequent neurologic checks is essential to detect late complications of the embolization, such as normal perfusion pressure breakthrough. Of note, it is normal for patients to have a very peculiar odor, not dissimilar to rotten eggs, for several days after embolization with Onyx, a glue that is used, as the DMSO is released in their breath. Patients and their families should be informed that this is normal.

Endovascular Therapy Summary

Many general anesthesiologists will intermittently have to manage INR cases. The scope of INR therapies has increased steadily over recent years, resulting in less-invasive treatment of intracranial vascular procedures. Anesthetic plans need to accommodate the need for IONM and aim for smooth emergence to allow for early postprocedure neurologic assessment.

INR suites are often cramped with challenging and unfamiliar layouts. It is important to become familiar with the working environment before providing an anesthetic there. Physical patient access is limited, and rotating imaging booms can interfere with monitoring wires, IV lines, and anesthesia circuits. Careful setup and positioning of these patients are essential. In addition, transporting patients to and from the INR suite may be complex and involve vertical as well as horizontal transport from a critical care unit or an emergency department. The anesthesia team and transporters need to be mindful to have sufficient emergency supplies, such as full oxygen cylinders and any necessary medications.

Radiation exposure from these procedures can be significant; it is essential that providers take care of and use personal protective equipment as well as items such as lead glass barriers to limit ionizing radiation exposure.

DECLARATIONS OF INTEREST

The author M.K. Teig, hereby declare that he have no commercial or financial conflicts of interest, or funding sources in relation to this work.

REFERENCES

1. Available at: https://www.sirweb.org/about-sir/. Accessed August 17, 2020.
2. Available at: https://oeisociety.com/. Accessed August 17, 2020.
3. Maingard J, Kok HK, Ranatunga D, et al. The future of interventional and neuro-interventional radiology: learning lessons from the past. Br J Radiol 2017; 90(1080):20170473.
4. Keedy A. An overview of intracranial aneurysms. Mcgill J Med 2006;9(2):141–6.
5. Guglielmi G. History of the genesis of detachable coils. J Neurosurg 2009; 111(1):1–8.
6. Molyneux A. International Subarachnoid Aneurysm Trial (ISAT) of neurosurgical clipping versus endovascular coiling in 2143 patients with ruptured intracranial aneurysms: a randomised trial. Lancet 2002;360(Issue 9342):1267–74.
7. Derdeyn CP, Zipfel GJ, Albuquerque FC, et al. Management of brain arteriovenous malformations: a scientific statement for healthcare professionals from the American Heart Association/American Stroke Association. Stroke 2017;48(8): e200–24.
8. Davenport MS, Parezella MA, Yee J, et al. Use of intravenous iodinated contrast media in patients with kidney disease: consensus statements from the American College of Radiology and the National Kidney Foundation. Radiology 2020;294: 660–8.
9. Greenberger P, Patterson R, Lelly J. Administration of radiographic contrast media in high risk patients. Invest Radiol 1980;15:540–3.
10. Faucon AL, Bobrie G, Clément O. Nephrotoxicity of iodinated contrast media: from pathophysiology to prevention strategies. Eur J Radiol 2019;116:231–41.
11. Weisbord SD, Gallagher M, Jneid H, et al. Outcomes after angiography with sodium bicarbonate and acetylcysteine. N Engl J Med 2018;378(7):603–14.
12. Hunt WE, Hess RM. Surgical risk as related to time of intervention in the repair of intracranial aneurysms. J Neurosurg 1968;28(1):14–20.
13. Feygelman VM, Huda W, Peters KR. Effective dose equivalents to patients undergoing cerebral angiography. AJNR Am J Neuroradiol 1992;13(3):845–9.
14. Berman MF, Sciacca RR, Pile-Spellman J, et al. The epidemiology of brain arteriovenous malformations. Neurosurgery 2000;47(2):389–97.
15. Szajner M, Roman T, Markowicz J, et al. Onyx (®) in endovascular treatment of cerebral arteriovenous malformations - a review. Pol J Radiol 2013;78(3):35–41.
16. Gopal S, Sekar A, Rudrappa S, et al. Adenosine induced cardiac pause in neuro-endovascular management of AVM with fistula. Interdisciplinary Neurosurgery 2020;20:100662. https://doi.org/10.1016/j.inat.2019.100662.
17. Lylyk P, Chudyk J, Bleise C, et al. Endovascular occlusion of pial arteriovenous macrofistulae, using pCANvas1 and adenosine-induced asystole to control nBCA injection. Interv Neuroradiol 2017;23(6):644–9.
18. Day AL, Friedman WA, Sypert GW, et al. Successful treatment of the normal perfusion pressure breakthrough syndrome. Neurosurgery 1982;11(5):625–30.

Decompressive Surgery for Patients with Traumatic Brain Injury

Austin Peters, MD, MCR*, Gabriel Kleinman, MD

KEYWORDS

- Traumatic brain injury • Craniectomy • Biomarkers • Ketamine • Steroids

KEY POINTS

- Males and the elderly experience disproportionately worse outcomes from traumatic brain injury.
- As with all traumas, additional injuries must be considered including cervical instability. A full stomach should be assumed even with appropriate nil per os time.
- Hemodynamic goals include maintaining intracranial pressure of less than 22 mm Hg and maintaining cerebral perfusion pressure between 60 and 70 mm Hg.
- Steroids should be avoided and there is no established benefit to initiating hypothermia.
- Tranexamic acid has been shown to improve survival in mild and moderate traumatic brain injury.

BACKGROUND

Prevalence and Incidence

Traumatic brain injury (TBI) affects more than 2.8 million Americans each year and is one of the leading causes of death and disability of young adults, with an estimated annual cost of $60 billion.[1] Around 80% of TBIs are classified as mild, with the remainder split between 10% moderate TBI and 10% severe TBI.[2] TBI disproportionately affects males, accounting for 60% of these injuries.[3]

DIAGNOSIS

TBI is a clinical diagnosis made based on patient history, bystander reporting, or observation of physical injuries to the patient's head and can be separated into primary and secondary mechanisms of injury. Primary injury should be suspected in all trauma patients, especially those with fractures, intracranial hemorrhage, contusion and traumatic axonal injury. Secondary injury resulting from a disruption of the blood–brain barrier and oxidative injury should be suspected in patients with altered

Oregon Health and Science University, 3181 Southwest Sam Jackson Park Road, Portland, OR 97239, USA
* Corresponding author.
E-mail address: peterau@ohsu.edu

Anesthesiology Clin 39 (2021) 163–178
https://doi.org/10.1016/j.anclin.2020.11.003
1932-2275/21/© 2020 Elsevier Inc. All rights reserved.
anesthesiology.theclinics.com

mental status and in all patients presenting after a loss of consciousness. Patients who are suspected of having a TBI require close monitoring for acute changes that can develop as their injury progresses.

Patients suspected to have had a TBI should be evaluated upon admission to the hospital using the Glasgow Coma Scale (GCS), which assesses a patient's ability to follow commands and respond to stimuli (**Table 1**). The severity of the TBI is stratified according to the patient's GCS score: mild if the GCS is 13 to 15; moderate if the GCS is 9 to 12; and severe if the GCS is 3 to 8.[1] In addition to GCS, length of posttraumatic amnesia and the presence or absence of loss of consciousness at the time of injury should be assessed at the time of patient presentation to the hospital to further assess TBI severity.[2]

Head imaging provides essential information about the presence and extent of injury to the head and should be considered for all patients with TBI. A noncontrast computed tomography (CT) scan of the head should be used for initial triage of the extent of the head injury, including intracranial hemorrhages, fluid collections, edema, bone fractures, and foreign bodies. CT scans of the head can be assessed via the Marshall or Rotterdam Score to grade injury severity (**Table 2**). A noncontrast head CT scan is often sufficient for initial TBI evaluation; additional imaging should be considered with any clinical deterioration in the patient. MRI is generally not indicated for the initial evaluation of TBI, although it is exquisitely sensitive to pathologic changes related to mild TBI and has a demonstrated usefulness for assessing injury severity and prognostication.[4]

An emerging area of interest in the evaluation of TBI is the quantification of circulating biomarkers levels in the peripheral blood stream. These biomarkers are usually proteins native to cells of the central nervous system or inflammatory proteins that are released through cellular injury and disruption of the blood–brain barrier as well as clearance via the brain's glymphatic system. There are multitudes of TBI-related biomarkers being explored and evaluated for their diagnostic potential, with the most commonly evaluated being the neuronally derived UCHL1 and MAP2, and the astrocytic proteins S100 B and glial fibrillary acidic protein (**Table 3**). Biomarker

Table 1
GCS scoring and severity

GCS					
Best Eye Opening Response		**Best Verbal Response**		**Best Motor Response**	
Spontaneously	4	Oriented and conversational	5	Obeys request	6
To verbal request	3	Disoriented and conversational	4	Appropriate withdrawal	5
To pain	2	Inappropriate words	3	Flexion: withdraw	4
No response	1	Incomprehensible sounds	2	Flexion: decorticate	3
		No response	1	Extension	2
				No response	1

GCS Severity	Score Range
Mild	13–15
Moderate	9–12
Severe	3–8

Table 2
Marshall and Rotterdam CT scoring

Score	Marshall Scoring	CT Finding	Rotterdam Scoring	Definition
1	No visible intracranial pathology on CT scan	Basal cistern	0 1 2	Normal Compressed Absent
2	Cisterns are present with 0–5 mm midline shift and/or lesion densities present; no high- or mixed-density lesion >25 mL includes bone fragments or foreign bodies	Midline shift	0 1	≤5 mm ≥5 mm
3	Cisterns compressed or absent with 0–5 mm midline shift; no high- or mixed-density lesion >25 mL	Epidural hematoma	0 1	Present Absent
4	Midline shift >5 mm; no high- or mixed-density lesion >25 mL	Subarachnoid hemorrhage/ intraventricular hemorrhage	0 1	Absent Present
5	Any lesion surgically evacuated			
6	High- or mixed-density lesion >25 mL; not surgically evacuated			

concentrations are usually collected upon admission to the hospital and can provide further detail on the presence and severity of brain injury, complementing the GCS and imaging data (**Fig. 1**).

PROGNOSIS

Long-term outcomes after TBI are often evaluated using the Glasgow Outcomes Scale or the more detailed Glasgow Outcomes Scale Extended version, which provides a numerical score for the presence of death or the extent of disability after a head injury (**Table 4**). Persons age 60 years and older have the highest death rate after TBI,[3] and males have roughly triple the mortality rate as females.[5]

Despite more sophisticated measures available to evaluate the presence or extent of a head injury, the GCS remains a powerful and accurate method of predicting long-term outcomes after TBI, with lower GCS scores correlating with poorer outcomes in a linear fashion.[6] Additional detail in the prognosis can be achieved via trending GCS over time to monitor for clinically significant changes.

Protein Biomarkers for Prognostication

The prognostic usefulness of a single serum biomarker sample drawn on patient admission to the hospital is currently no more accurate than the initial GCS score or Marshall classification,[7] both of which are noninvasive and simple to perform. Trends of these biomarker concentrations, measured longitudinally over a period of days or weeks can improve prediction of long term patient outcomes and can even identify acute, preclinical deterioration in some circumstances.[8]

Table 3
List of common TBI-related biomarkers and their source tissue

Biomarker	Abbreviation	Source Tissue
Neurofilament	NF	Neuronal cytoskeletal protein
Amyloid beta	A	Cleaved product from the neuron-associated amyloid precursor protein
Spectrin breakdown products	SBDP	Cleaved cytoskeletal proteins originally located within both neurons and glial cells
Myelin basic protein	MBP	Oligodendrocytes and Schwann cells
Interleukin-6	IL-6	Inflammatory cytokine
Tau	Tau	A microtubule-associated protein located predominantly within neuronal axons
Tumor necrosis factor alpha	TNF-α	Inflammatory cytokine
S100 calcium binding protein B	S100 B	Astrocytic (primarily) calcium binding protein
Neuron-specific enolase	NSE	Neuronal glycolytic protein; also found in neuroendocrine cells and erythrocytes
Glial fibrillary acidic protein	GFAP	Astrocyte specific cytoskeletal protein
Ubiquitin carboxy-terminal hydrolase L1	UCH-L1	Neuronal enzyme involved in protein ubiquitination and elimination

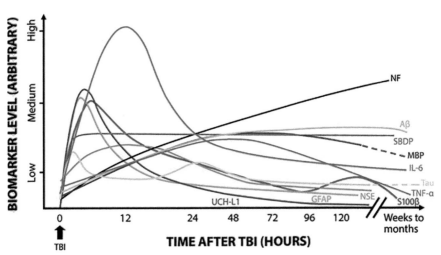

Fig. 1. TBI biomarker concentration time course in serum. Expected relative concentrations of TBI-related biomarkers and their respective time courses. A, amyloid beta; GFAP, glial fibrillary acidic protein; IL-6, interleukin-6; MBP, myelin basic protein; NF, neurofilament; NSE, neuron-specific enolase; S100 B, S100 calcium binding protein B; SBDP, spectrin breakdown products; TBI, traumatic brain injury; TNF-α, tumor necrosis factor alpha; UCH-L1, ubiquitin carboxy-terminal hydrolase L1. (*From* Adrian H, Mårten K, Salla N, et al. Biomarkers of Traumatic Brain Injury: Temporal Changes in Body Fluids. eNeuro 8 December 2016; 3 (6); with permission.)

Table 4
Glasgow outcome scale and Glasgow outcome scale extended

GOS	GOS-E	Interpretation
1 = Dead	1 = Dead	Dead
2 = Vegetative state	2 = Vegetative state	Absence of awareness of self and environment
3 = Severe disability	3 = Lower severe disability	Needs full assistance in ADL
	4 = Upper severe disability	Needs partial assistance in ADL
4 = Moderate disability	5 = Lower moderate disability	Independent, but cannot resume work/school or all previous social activities
	6 = Upper moderate disability	Some disability exists, but can partly resume work or previous activities
5 = Good recovery	7 = Lower good recovery	Minor physical or mental deficits that affect daily life
	8 = Upper good recovery	Fully recovery or minor symptoms that do not affect daily life

Abbreviations: ADL, activities of daily living; GOS, Glasgow outcome scale; GOS-E, Glasgow outcome scale extended.

CLINICAL MANAGEMENT
Airway Protection

The focus of the initial clinical management after a TBI is to provide supportive care to maintain the patient's vital signs and to mitigate secondary brain injury from resulting edema. For patients with a severe TBI (GCS of ≤8), immediate intubation is almost always necessary to prevent hypoxia and hypercapnia and, thus, secondary cerebral injury. Patients with mild or moderate TBI should be assessed on an individual basis for their risk of further decompensation and need for protective intubation.[9]

Intracranial Pressure Monitoring

Patients at risk for worsening brain edema and clinical deterioration should be have their intracranial pressure (ICP) monitored; this goal can be accomplished with either an external ventricular drain (EVD) (**Fig. 2**) or a subdural screw (also known as a bolt). Although both devices can be used to monitor ICP, an EVD can also be used to decrease ICP by the removal of CSF. An EVD accomplishes the external drainage by removing CSF from the lateral ventricles of the brain, or the lumbar space of the spine, into an external collection bag. The right frontal cerebral hemisphere is the preferred site of placement given its nondominance for language function in more than 90% of patients. Complications such as hemorrhage and inadvertent placement into brain tissue are reported in 10% to 40% of cases. Generally in patients with severe TBI requiring intracranial pressure monitoring and cerebrospinal fluid diversion, the height of the transducer is initially set to 0, to quickly decrease the ICP. When positioning an EVD, the pressure transducer is leveled with the Foramen of Monro, which falls at the level of the external auditory meatus of the ear in the supine position. Drainage can be continuous at a set level, fixed volume removal per hour, or as needed to treat increases in the ICP. EVD-associated meningitis or ventriculitis are common complications, with an incidence of up to 22%.[10]

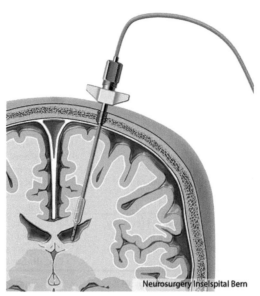

Fig. 2. EVD positioning. Standard placement of an extraventricular drain (EVD) into the lateral ventricle. EVDs will sometimes be placed into the third ventricle as well. (*From* Jens Fichtner, Astrid Jilch, Lennart Henning Stieglitz, et al. Infection rate of emergency bolt-kit vs. non-emergency conventional implanted silver bearing external ventricular drainage catheters. Clinical Neurology and Neurosurgery; July 2014; Volume 122:Pages 70-76 (http://www.sciencedirect.com/science/article/pii/S0303846714001528).)

Hyperosmolar Therapy

Patients with an elevated ICP—a sustained ICP of greater than 22 mm Hg—are at high risk for clinical deterioration and should be monitored closely and aggressively treated to decrease the ICP. Before, or concurrently with, cerebrospinal fluid drainage, hyperosmolar therapy can decrease cerebral swelling and lower the ICP. The 2 options available in the United States are mannitol and hypertonic saline. Both of these agents decrease the ICP through cerebral dehydration and improved microcirculatory flow via decreased blood viscosity. Both mannitol and hypertonic saline can transiently increase the overall total blood volume and should be used judiciously in patients at risk for circulatory overload (eg, heart failure); they are contraindicated in patients with end-stage renal failure. The goal of hyperosmolar therapy is to either increase the serum osmolarity to a target of 300 to 320 mOsm/L with mannitol or increase the serum sodium to 145 to 150 mmol/L, assuming a normal starting sodium (**Box 1**). The decrease in the ICP secondary to mannitol administration is dose dependent, occurring within 10 to 20 minutes with a peak effect seen between 20 and 60 minutes and lasting between 4 and 6 hours. The published literature has found that more significant ICP decreases and sustained responses occur when mannitol is dosed between 0.5 to 1.5 g/kg/dose and may be repeated every 4 hours to maintain the target osmolarity. In patients with a chronically low baseline sodium, a change in 10 mmol/L above their baseline theoretically offers the same benefit while protecting the patient from central pontine myelinolysis.[11]

Hemodynamic Management

Hypotension in patients with TBI is a devastating complication and should be prevented with fluid and vasoconstrictors. The underlying causes for the hypotension

Box 1
Calculating the recommended dose of hypertonic saline
3% NaCl = 513 mEq Na$^+$/L
Sodium (Na$^+$) deficit = 0.6 × weight (kg) × (change in Na$^+$ desired)
Amount needed to increase serum Na$^+$ by 3 mEq/h = 0.6 × weight × 3
Desired rate (L/h): amount needed (mEq/hour) ÷ concentration of saline (mEq/L) × 1000

should be explored, including hypovolemia from ongoing trauma-related blood loss. Optimal blood pressure parameters after TBI are an area of active investigation. Current recommendations are to maintain a systolic blood pressure of at least 100 mm Hg and ideally greater than 110 mm Hg, because a systolic blood pressure of less than 100 mm Hg is associated with increased mortality.[9] The cerebral perfusion pressure (CPP), the driver of blood flow to the brain, calculated as mean arterial pressure minus either the CVP or the ICP, depending on which value is higher, should optimally be maintained between 60 and 70 mm Hg. Both a CPP of less than 60 mm Hg and greater than 70 mm Hg are associated with worse outcomes in patients with TBI.[9]

Hypovolemia from blood loss should be treated with blood transfusions in line with the current trauma literature. Intravascular volume depletion not consistent with blood loss should be treated with isotonic/hypertonic crystalloid replacement owing to the disrupted blood brain barrier.[12] Colloids should be avoided for fluid resuscitation in TBI because albumin has been associated with increased mortality after TBI, and synthetic colloids such as hetastarch are associated with coagulopathy and renal failure.[13] Dextrose-containing fluids should be avoided as well owing to their ability to cross the blood–brain barrier and induce cerebral edema.

Hyperventilation

Carbon dioxide (CO_2) plays an important role in cerebral blood vessel tone, and overall cerebral blood volume. Increased plasma CO_2 levels induces cerebral vasodilation, increasing cerebral blood volume, resulting in increased ICP. Conversely, a decreased CO_2 plasma level in the cerebral circulation induces cerebral vasoconstriction, decreasing the ICP. In the injured edematous brain, this physiologic response can be manipulated to help acutely decrease the ICP. Hyperventilation in the intubated patient should target an arterial CO_2 level of 25 to 30 mm Hg. Ventilation that decreases the arterial CO_2 to less than 25 mm Hg can induce vasoconstriction severe enough to restrict blood flow and induce secondary hypoxic injury to brain tissues and should be avoided.[9] Reduced plasma CO_2 levels maintain their effect on ICP for only approximately 6 hours, after which bicarbonate buffering by the kidneys normalizes the plasma pH. Therefore, hyperventilation is only indicated for temporary, acute correction of an increased ICP.[14]

Anticonvulsants

Patients with TBI are at risk of experiencing both subclinical and gross seizures acutely, and can go on to develop post-traumatic epilepsy, defined as seizure activity persisting for more than 7 days after injury.[9] In the acute injury setting, seizure activity greatly increases metabolic demands in the brain and can result in further increasing of ICP and the risk of cerebral herniation. Phenytoin and levetiracetam are the most commonly used anticonvulsants. The prophylactic use of anticonvulsants after TBI has been found to be beneficial in preventing early seizure activity, but has not been found to prevent the development of post-traumatic epilepsy; in addition, the sedative qualities of anticonvulsants can interfere with neuropsychological testing.[9,11]

Nutrition

TBI is associated with increased metabolic activity and demands, as well as stress-induced hyperglycemia. As in other critical illnesses, enteric nutrition is preferred over parenterally administered nutrition when possible. Regardless of route, basal calorie replacement should be initiated by day 5 after the injury.[9]

DISEASE COMPLICATIONS
Disruption of Cerebral Perfusion Autoregulation

Cerebral perfusion autoregulation (CPA) refers to the brain's intrinsic ability to maintain consistent blood flow through a wide range of CPPs (**Fig. 3**). TBI disrupts the CPA, and as a result blood flow to the brain becomes dependent on the blood pressure provided by the systemic circulation. CPA disruption places patients at higher risk of cerebral ischemia during periods of hypotension and cerebral edema during periods of hypertension, and therefore necessitates strict blood pressure control and ICP monitoring.[15] As mentioned elsewhere in this article, the blood pressure should be maintained at least above 100 mm Hg systolic and ideally at greater than 110 mm Hg systolic, and the ICP should be maintained between 60 and 70 mm Hg.

Coagulopathies and Thrombotic Events

Patients with TBI are at an increased risk of developing coagulopathies as compared with patients who experience other traumatic injuries. TBI-related coagulopathies are poorly understood, but are likely a consequence of disturbances to coagulation-related proteins as opposed to the blood loss–related coagulopathies seen in other major traumas.[16] After a TBI, approximately one-third of patients show evidence of developing coagulopathies, usually within the first 24 hours of injury, and this is a significant predictor of poor outcomes when it occurs.[17] Guidelines for the management of TBI-related coagulopathies do not exist currently.[17] Treatment should be directed toward a primary underlying cause, if discernible, such as administering fresh frozen plasma, platelets, and packed red blood cells to actively bleeding patients, and

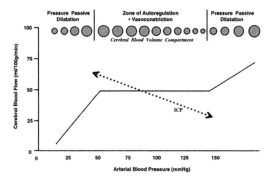

Fig. 3. Normal CPA. Illustration of intact CPA. Within the zone of autoregulation, there is no correlation between cerebral blood flow and ICP. Traumatic brain injury disrupts CPA, causing cerebral blood flow to become dependent on systemic blood pressure. (*From* Yam AT, Lang EW, Lagopoulos J, et al. Cerebral autoregulation and ageing. Journal of Clinical Neuroscience. 2005; 12(6): p.643-646; with permission.)

repleting fibrinogen with cryoprecipitate in patients experiencing disseminated intra-vascular coagulation.[17]

Unlike coagulopathies, patients with TBI are not at increased risk of developing blood clots as compared with other patients who experienced major trauma.[18] Regardless, the incidence of thrombotic events is high, because up to one-half of patients with a TBI conversely develop deep vein thromboses (DVT) during their hospitalization.[9] As such, DVT prophylaxis is warranted, but must be balanced with the risk of inducing or exacerbating intracranial bleeding. Mechanical DVT prophylaxis using compression stockings or intermittent pneumatic compression devices should be initiated if possible because these therapies do not increase the risk of bleeding. Pharmacologic DVT pro-phylaxis is usually achieved with low-molecular-weight heparin or low-dose unfractio-nated heparin; the choice of pharmacologic agent as well as the specific dose and timing remain an area of active investigation without specific consensus guidance.[9]

TECHNIQUES
Surgical Approach

The goal of the surgical decompressive craniectomy is to remove portions of the skull to allow the brain room to expand, thereby decreasing the ICP and improving blood flow and brain oxygenation. Decompression can be accomplished in multiple ways, including through removal of the bilateral frontal portion of the skull (ie, bifrontal cra-niectomy) or through removing portions of the lateral aspect of the skull (ie, frontotem-poroparietal craniectomy) **(Fig. 4)**.

The decision about whether to decompress the brain via unilateral or bilateral cra-niectomy, or a larger versus smaller unilateral craniectomy, has some limited evidence-based guidance. A larger frontotemporoparietal decompressive craniec-tomy (ie, >12 × 15 cm or 15 cm in diameter) is recommended over smaller sized cra-niectomies to decrease mortality and improve neurologic outcomes after a severe TBI; bifrontal craniectomies are not recommended over unilateral craniectomies to improve outcomes.[9] The portion of the skull removed during decompression is often stored for

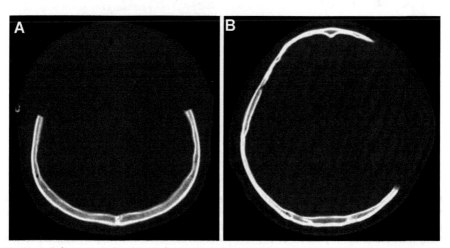

Fig. 4. Axial computed topography images demonstrating postoperative changes after (*A*) bifrontal craniectomy and (*B*) left-sided frontotemporoparietal craniectomy. (*From* Moon JW, Hyun DK. Decompressive Craniectomy in Traumatic Brain Injury: A Review Article. Korean J Neurotrauma. 2017;13(1):1-8; with permission.)

several months and reattached after swelling and other pathologies have subsided; synthetic components are available if the original bone is not able to be used.[19]

Intubation

Patients with acute TBI being intubated for airway protection or surgical intervention should be treated as having a full stomach regardless of safe fasting time owing to the decreased gut motility associated with trauma. As such, intubation, if indicated, should be performed via rapid sequence intubation to protect the patient's airway from aspiration.

Cervical or other spinal injury should be assumed unless formally cleared, because up to 10% of patients with sever TBI have a concurrent cervical spine injury.[20] Methods to decrease any neck motion with intubation should be taken including manual in-line neck stabilization and video or fiberoptic intubation (**Fig. 5**). Likewise, patients with an acute TBI should be assumed to have an increased ICP and precautions should be taken to prevent further ICP increases.

Anesthetics Choices for Induction in Traumatic Brain Injury

Induction agents should be chosen based on the hemodynamic stability of the patient, the experience of the provider, and with consideration to the effects of the

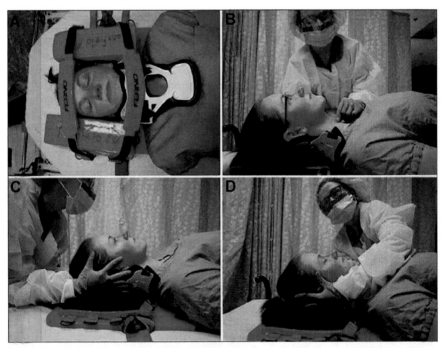

Fig. 5. Neck stabilization and intubation maneuvers in trauma scenarios. Neck stabilization techniques. (A) Heavy sandbags and cervical collar in place to stabilize the head and neck for patient transport. (B) Cricoid pressure being applied, such as during rapid sequence intubation, with the anterior portion of the cervical collar removed and support applied to the rear of the neck. (C) Manual in-line neck stabilization applied from the head of the bed. (D) Manual in-line neck stabilization applied from the side of the bed to facilitate intubation. (From Austin N, Krishnamoorthy V, Dagal A. Airway management in cervical spine injury. Int J Crit Illn Inj Sci. 2014;4(1):50-56; with permission.)

agent on cerebral physiology (**Table 5**). Supplemental opioids blunt the sympathetic response to laryngoscopy, allowing for less of an increase in the ICP with intubation. However, because opioids also lead to hypercapnia and thus an increased ICP, they should be administered cautiously to the spontaneously breathing patient with a TBI until the time of intubation. Rapid sequence induction dosing of paralytics should be used in the trauma setting. Succinylcholine may transiently increase the ICP, but the clinical significance of this increase has not been established. In precarious conditions of a very high ICP, rapid sequence intubation dosing of rocuronium can be used without concern for ICP effects, given the ability to reverse rocuronium with sugammadex administration for neurologic examination.

Anesthetic Choices for Maintenance of Anesthesia

Volatile anesthetics have been shown experimentally to increase cerebral blood flow, but decrease the cerebral metabolic rate of oxygen, resulting in a net increase in ICP. This occurs only at a minimal alveolar concentration of approximately 1.5, and the ICP increase is negligible if volatile agents are kept at less than 1 minimal alveolar concentration.[21] However, even when maintained at less than 1 minimal alveolar concentration, volatile anesthetics have direct vasodilatory effects, which are independent of anesthetic depth and could theoretically affect the ICP[22] (Slupe/Kirsch JCBFM 2018). In contrast, intravenous GABA-ergic anesthetics such as propofol decrease both cerebral blood flow and the cerebral metabolic rate of oxygen, resulting in overall decreased ICP (see **Table 5**). In practice, however, there is no clinical evidence to suggest the benefit of an intravenous anesthetic versus a volatile anesthetic on patient outcomes.[23] It is important to keep in mind that decreased blood flow from hypotension remains very harmful for the patient with TBI and should be avoided, regardless of the method of anesthesia maintenance.

Reduction of the Intracranial Pressure

Patients being emergently brought to the operating room for cranial decompression are already in a state of precariously high ICP. All efforts should focus on efficient

Table 5
Effects of anesthetic choice on neurophysiology

Anesthetic	CBF	CMRO$_2$	ICP
GABA receptor agonists			
Isoflurane, sevoflurane, desflurane	↑	↓	↑/↔
Propofol	↓	↓	↓
Midazolam	↓	↓	↓
Etomidate	↓	↓	↓
Barbiturates	↓	↓	↓
NMDA receptor antagonists			
Nitrous oxide	↑	↑	↑
Ketamine	↑	↑	↑/↔
Opioids	↓	↑	↔

Abbreviations: CBF, cerebral blood flow; CMRO$_2$, cerebral metabolic rate of oxygen; GABA, gamma aminobutyric acid; ICP, intracranial pressure; NMDA, N-Methyl- D-aspartic acid or N-Methyl- D-aspartate.

transport to the operating room, with temporizing measures to decrease the ICP taken simultaneously. As detailed elsewhere in this article, hypertonic saline and/or mannitol, hyperventilation if the patient is intubated, elevating the head, and maintaining venous outflow by avoiding rotation of the neck can all help to relieve an elevated ICP.

Blood Transfusions

Patients with TBI who are anemic from trauma-related bleeding or other causes are at risk of exacerbated hypoxic injury, have worse outcomes, and experience increased mortality. Conversely, there is risk associated with blood transfusions in patients with TBI including lung injury and extended intensive care unit and hospital stays. As is standard in most perioperative patients, the lower limit of hemoglobin should remain at 7 g/dL, and there is no benefit to transfusing beyond a hemoglobin level of 10 g/dL.[24]

Monitors

In addition to standard monitors, given the ongoing bleeding related to trauma and emergent surgical intervention, the need for beat-to-beat blood pressure management as well as frequent laboratory testing, an arterial line is an important monitor of intraoperative anesthetic care in the patient with a TBI undergoing decompressive craniotomy. Although helpful, an arterial line is not absolutely essential to patient care in this situation, and priority should be given to expedient surgical intervention to relieve an elevated ICP and should not delay the start of surgery. An arterial line can be placed after surgical incision or performed in parallel with other procedures once the anesthesia has been induced and the patient has been appropriately positioned for the surgery.

EVIDENCE AND CONTROVERSIES
Evidence Supporting Decompressive Craniectomy

Increasing ICP from accumulating cerebral edema presents a risk for cerebral herniation and death. Although an elevated ICP can be mitigated by therapies such as hyperosmotic therapy, paralysis, hyperventilation, elevation of the patient's head, and EVD placement, if these techniques become insufficient, surgical decompressive craniectomy remains a final option for alleviating ICP and allowing the brain additional room for expansion. The decision about whether to pursue decompressive craniectomy as an early, preventative measure or a last-tier intervention has been examined by clinical trials, finding that decompressive craniectomies resulted in lower mortality but higher rates of vegetative state, and lower severe disability and upper severe disability than with medical care alone. The multiple studies suggest age and comorbidity cutoffs, and a frank discussion with the surgeons and patients' surrogate decision makers must be had before proceeding to this extremely morbid procedure.[19]

Tranexamic Acid

Tranexamic acid (TXA) is a synthetic lysine analogue medication that is most commonly used in the setting of significant hemorrhage for its antifibrinolytic properties (**Fig. 6**). TXA has gained prominence in the setting of TBI for potential benefits in decreasing mortality. The recently completed CRASH-3 study found a survival benefit for patients given TXA early after a mild or moderate TBI, but no survival benefit for severe TBI.[25] Ongoing studies are exploring the benefit of earlier and higher doses of TXA after TBI.[26]

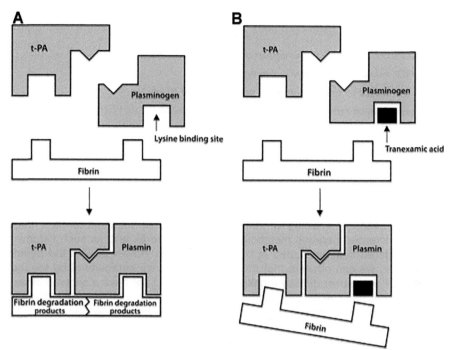

Fig. 6. TXA antifibrinolysis mechanism of action. Illustration of TXA's interaction site and effect. (*A*) Normal interaction in which t-PA and plasminogen bind, leading to breakdown of fibrin clots. (*B*) TXA blocks the lysine binding site in plasminogen, preventing fibrin binding and breakdown. t-PA, tissue plasminogen activator. (*From* Vaněk T, Straka Z. Topical use of tranexamic acid in cardiac surgery—A review and meta-analysis of four randomized controlled trials. Cor et Vasa. 2013; 55(2): p. e184-e189; with permission.)

Hypothermia

Hypothermia decreases cerebral metabolism and ICP, and in theory should be beneficial in the setting of acute TBI. In practice, however, clinical studies remain inconclusive, with no clear evidence of a benefit to patient outcomes or survival; in addition, there are real risks associated with hypothermia including, coagulopathy and pneumonia. Although this area remains under intensive study and conflicting opinion, current recommendations are to avoid hypothermia in the setting of acute TBI.[9]

Steroids

Historically, steroids were frequently used after a TBI for the presumed purpose of decreasing cerebral edema, a benefit that was observed in brain tumor resection surgeries and subsequently translated to TBI. Ensuing studies focusing specifically on patients with an acute TBI failed to find a clear benefit, and eventually large-scale randomized, controlled studies observed a clear deleterious effect on survival in patients with TBI when administered high-dose steroids. As such, steroids should be considered contraindicated in the setting of acute TBI given the propensity for inducing unnecessary patient harm.[9]

Ketamine

Ketamine is a dissociative anesthetic drug that achieves its effects primarily through antagonism of the NMDA receptor. Early studies of its effects on human

> **Box 2**
> **Clinical care points**
>
> - A GCS score of ≤ 8 necessitates intubation for airway protection.
> - The ICP should be kept below 22 mm Hg.
> - The CPP should be strictly maintained between 60 and 70 mm Hg.
> - Hyperventilation reduces ICP for approximately 6 hours and should target an arterial CO_2 level of 25 to 30 mm Hg.
> - Steroids have been shown to be harmful in TBI; hypothermia has not been shown to be beneficial. TXA may improve outcomes after TBI, and ketamine is increasingly being used after TBI but lacks definitive safety studies.

physiology observed it raising ICP, an effect attributed to increased cerebral blood flow and increased cerebral metabolic rate (see **Table 5**), and as such ketamine was considered contraindicated in the setting of TBI. However, with the benefit of hindsight, we can observe that these early trials were confounded by the fact that the ICP was never directly monitored, patients did not have a secured airway (and thus consistent ventilation), and doses much higher than the current standard induction dose of 2 mg/kg were used. Moreover, ketamine was never directly examined in patients with TBI until the 1990s. Experience with ketamine in battlefield scenarios provided favorable anecdotal experiences, because blood pressure and spontaneous ventilation are better preserved as compared with GABA-ergic anesthetic drugs like propofol. These experiences have since been explored in smaller clinical trials, which found ketamine either decreased or minimally increased ICP. Large retrospective, observational studies have since identified no evidence of patient harm associated with the use of ketamine in patients with TBI. Ketamine is increasingly being used for patients with TBI, although a definitive safety trial has not been performed.[27]

SUMMARY

TBI is a leading cause of death and disability in young adults, disproportionately affects males, and mortality greatly increases with patient age and lower initial GCS score. A TBI should be suspected in any trauma or loss of consciousness situation and requires strict monitoring for clinical decompensation because patients are not only at risk from their initial trauma, but also from ongoing secondary injuries. Decompressive craniectomy is a life-saving intervention of last resort when other methods to decrease an elevated ICP have failed. The anesthetic management of decompressive surgery for patients with a TBI must involve rapid transport to the operating room and expedient induction of anesthesia. Perioperative anesthetic management must balance the maintenance of CPP, treatment and reduction of increased ICP, optimization of surgical conditions to allow for minimal harm to healthy tissues, and avoidance of secondary injuries from hypoxia, extreme CO_2 alterations from ventilation strategies, hypotension, and electrolyte disturbances **(Box 2)**.[24]

DISCLOSURE

The authors have nothing to disclose.

REFERENCES

1. Surveillance report of traumatic brain injury-related emergency department visits, hospitalizations, and Deaths—United States, 2014. Cent Dis Control Prev US Dep Heal Hum Serv. Published online 2019. Available at: https://www.cdc.gov/traumaticbraininjury/get_the_facts.html. Accessed June, 2020.

2. Frost RB, Farrer TJ, Primosch M, et al. Prevalence of traumatic brain injury in the general adult population: a meta-analysis. Neuroepidemiology 2013;40(3):154–9.

3. Callahan BP, Rabb CH. Chapter 17 - Traumatic Brain Injury. In: Harken AH, Moore EE, editors. Abernathy's Surgical Secrets (Sixth Edition). Mosby; 2009. p. 99-104. https://doi.org/10.1016/B978-0-323-05711-0.00017-3.

4. Wintermark M, Sanelli PC, Anzai Y, et al. Imaging evidence and recommendations for traumatic brain injury: conventional neuroimaging techniques. J Am Coll Radiol 2015;12(2):e1–14.

5. Centers for Disease Control and Prevention. Report to Congress on Traumatic Brain Injury in the United States: Epidemiology and Rehabilitation. National Center for Injury Prevention and Control; Division of Unintentional Injury Prevention. Atlanta (GA): 2015.

6. Perel PA, Olldashi F, Muzha I, et al. Predicting outcome after traumatic brain injury: practical prognostic models based on large cohort of international patients. BMJ 2008;336(7641):425–9.

7. Takala R, Posti J, Runtti H, et al. Glial fibrillary acidic protein and ubiquitin C-terminal hydrolase-L1 as outcome predictors in traumatic brain injury. World Neurosurg 2016;87(March):8–20.

8. Thelin EP, Nelson DW, Bellander BM. Secondary peaks of S100B in serum relate to subsequent radiological pathology in traumatic brain injury. Neurocrit Care 2014;20(2):217–29.

9. Carney N, Totten AM, O'Reilly C, et al. Guidelines for the management of severe traumatic brain injury, fourth edition.; 2016. Neurosurgery 2017;80(1):6–15.

10. Dey M, Jaffe J, Stadnik A, et al. External ventricular drainage for intraventricular hemorrhage. Curr Neurol Neurosci Rep 2012;12:24–33.

11. Dash HH, Chavali S. Management of traumatic brain injury patients. Korean J Anesthesiol 2018;71(1):12–21.

12. Rowell SE, Fair KA, Barbosa RR, et al. The impact of pre-hospital administration of lactated ringer's solution versus normal saline in patients with traumatic brain injury. J Neurotrauma 2016;33(11):1054–9.

13. Chowdhury T, Cappellani RB, Schaller B, et al. Role of colloids in traumatic brain injury: use or not to be used? J Anaesthesiol Clin Pharmacol 2013;29(3):299–302.

14. Godoy DA, Seifi A, Garza D, et al. Hyperventilation therapy for control of posttraumatic intracranial hypertension. Front Neurol 2017;8(JUL):1–13.

15. Rangel-Castilla L, Gasco J, Nauta HJW, et al. Cerebral pressure autoregulation in traumatic brain injury. Neurosurg Focus 2008;25(4):1–8.

16. Zhang J, Jiang R, Liu L, et al. Traumatic brain injury-associated coagulopathy. J Neurotrauma 2012;29(17):2597–605.

17. Harhangi BS, Kompanje EJO, Leebeek FWG, et al. Coagulation disorders after traumatic brain injury. Acta Neurochir (Wien) 2008;150(2):165–75.

18. Geerts WH, Code KI, Jay RM, et al. A prospective study of venous thromboembolism after major trauma. N Engl J Med 1994;331(24):1601–6.

19. Cooper DJ, Rosenfeld JV, Murray L, et al. Decompressive craniectomy in diffuse traumatic brain injury. N Engl J Med 2011;364(16):1493–502.

20. Demetriades D, Charalambides K, Chahwan S, et al. Nonskeletal cervical spine injuries: epidemiology and diagnostic pitfalls. J Trauma 2000;48(4):724–7.
21. Engelhard K, Werner C. Inhalational or intravenous anesthetics for craniotomies? Pro inhalational. Curr Opin Anaesthesiol 2006;19(5):504–8.
22. Slupe AM, Kirsch JR. Effects of anesthesia on cerebral blood flow, metabolism, and neuroprotection. J Cereb Blood Flow Metab 2018;38(12):2192–208.
23. Wan Hassan WMN, Mohd Nasir Y, Mohamad Zaini RH, et al. Target-controlled infusion propofol versus sevoflurane anaesthesia for emergency traumatic brain surgery: comparison of the outcomes. Malays J Med Sci 2017;24(5):73–82.
24. Curry P, Viernes D, Sharma D. Perioperative management of traumatic brain injury. Int J Crit Illn Inj Sci 2011;1(1):27–35.
25. Collaborators C-3 trial. Effects of tranexamic acid on death, disability, vascular occlusive events and other morbidities in patients with acute traumatic brain injury (CRASH-3): a randomised, placebo-controlled trial. Lancet 2019; 394(10210):1713–23.
26. Rowell SE, Meier EN, McKnight B, et al. Effect of out-of-hospital tranexamic acid vs placebo on 6-month functional neurologic outcomes in patients with moderate or severe traumatic brain injury. JAMA 2020;324(10):961–74. https://doi.org/10. 1001/jama.2020.8958.
27. Chang L, Raty S, Ortiz J, et al. The emerging use of ketamine for anesthesia and sedation in traumatic brain injuries. CNS Neurosci Ther 2013;19(6):390–5.

Pain Management in Neurosurgery

Back and Lower Extremity Pain, Trigeminal Neuralgia

Yifan Xu, MD, PhD[a],*, Kimberly M. Mauer, MD[b], Amit Singh, DO[c]

KEYWORDS

- Chronic back pain • Epidural steroid injection • Facet joint • Sympathetic block
- Radiofrequency ablation • Trigeminal neuralgia • Trigger point injections

KEY POINTS

- Minimally invasive anesthetic techniques for chronic back and head pain treatment are an integral part of a multidisciplinary evaluation for disease diagnosis and treatment.
- Patient selection, with careful attention to the biopsychosocial model of pain, is a crucial component for diagnostic or interventional neural blockade.
- Fluoroscopy-guided and ultrasonography-guided techniques are now standard of care for anesthetic injections; real-time guidance of needle placement around anatomic structures can more specifically target suspected disorders while minimizing complications.
- Epidural steroid injections and facet and sacroiliac joint procedures remain the most commonly performed procedures for back pain and are most effective if combined with a multidisciplinary approach such as physical therapy. Evidence suggests they delay but do not change the eventual need for spine surgery.
- Understanding nervous system anatomy, physiology, and pathology allows pain physicians to customize anesthetic injections and nerve blockades.

INTRODUCTION TO LOW BACK PAIN

Low back pain is one of the most common and burdensome health conditions for which individuals seek care.[1] In addition, it is the cause of the greatest global disability compared with other conditions, primarily because of recurrence of these symptoms within 1 year after recovery from the original episode.[1–3] There are numerous potential

[a] Anesthesiology, Oregon Health and Science University, Portland, OR, USA; [b] Comprehensive Pain Center, Anesthesiology and Perioperative Medicine, Oregon Health and Sciences University, 3303 South West Bond Avenue Suite Ch4p Floor 4, Portland, OR 97239, USA; [c] Anesthesiology, Medical College of Wisconsin, Milwaukee, 959 North Mayfair Road, Wauwatosa, WI 53226, USA
* Corresponding author. 3181 SW Sam Jackson Park Road, Mail Code UH2, Portland, OR 97239.
E-mail address: xyi@ohsu.edu

Anesthesiology Clin 39 (2021) 179–194
https://doi.org/10.1016/j.anclin.2020.11.004
1932-2275/21/© 2020 Elsevier Inc. All rights reserved.

causes of low back pain and various treatment options, including interventional procedures to alleviate pain symptoms and thus increase functionality. It is often helpful to discuss low back pain and the subsequent treatment options based on the acuity and possible sources of low back pain. Acute low back pain is new in onset and less than 4 weeks old. For individuals with pain lasting between 4 and 12 weeks, it is referred to as subacute, and chronic if the pain lasts greater than 12 weeks. Furthermore, 3 distinct sources can be identified: axial, radicular, and referred pain.[4]

Pain originating from the L1-L5 vertebrae or the sacrum is referred to as axial low back pain. Examples of axial low back pain include discogenic pain, lumbar facet joint–mediated pain, and sacroiliac (SI) joint pain. Radicular pain refers to pain that travels along the lower extremity dermatomes because of disorders of the lumbosacral nerve roots or the lumbar dorsal root ganglion. Lumbar and lumbosacral radiculitis secondary to disc protrusions or extrusions can cause radicular pain. In addition, referred pain travels to a location distant from the site of the pain cause and in a non-dermatomal distribution. Most commonly, lumbar or gluteal myofascial trigger points can cause referred pain in the back, hips, or lower extremities. Depending on the cause of the pain, various treatment options may be offered. This article focuses on minimally invasive interventional techniques for low back and extremity pain that can either diagnose indications for spine surgery or delay the need for surgical intervention.

MINIMALLY INVASIVE TECHNIQUES TO DIAGNOSE SPINE DISORDERS

Appropriate diagnosis of the cause of pain is required before any interventional pain procedures. Although physical examination can be diagnostic of neuropathology, diagnostic injections can localize a pain source down to specific nerve roots. Patients should be counseled that any pain benefit from diagnostic injections should be short lived, with the goal of locating the source of pain in order to plan future targeted therapies.[5] Local anesthetic is injected adjacent to the target nerve with image guidance by either fluoroscopy or ultrasonography. The local anesthetic blocks sodium channels in the nerve to decrease transmission of sensory and motor signals. On completion of the diagnostic injection, the patient is sent home with a pain diary in which the numeric pain scores are recorded for 12 to 24 hours. A diagnostic injection is deemed successful if pain significantly improves with the expected temporality and location: the pain relief should be in the distribution of the targeted nerve, and the duration of improvement in pain should match the known pharmacokinetics of the injected local anesthetic. Once the diagnostic injection is determined to be successful, further interventions to therapeutically target diseased areas may include radiofrequency ablation, neurolysis, or open surgery. Examples of diagnostic injections include medial branch blocks for facet joint–mediated pain, and selective nerve root injections to identify neuroforaminal sources for radicular pain.

THERAPEUTIC INJECTIONS THAT TREAT PAIN FROM NEUROLOGIC DISORDERS

Therapeutic injections are performed with the goal of alleviating pain symptoms to improve the patient's functionality and quality of life, while minimizing the need for chronic medications such as opioids. One of the most commonly performed therapeutic injections is the epidural steroid injection (ESI), which can provide short-term and long-term relief of radicular pain in the cervical, thoracic, and lumbar spine.[6] The therapeutic injection cocktails for ESIs are diverse, based on both provider preference and pain cause. Injected solutions may contain only steroid or may include local anesthetic to blunt procedural pain and predict area of steroid action before the slower benefit of injected steroids occurs. Corticosteroids are beneficial based on the principle that they can reduce perineural inflammation, which is often a cause of pain symptoms. In addition, corticosteroids have membrane-stabilizing and antiinflammatory properties, which contribute to symptomatic improvement. In addition, improvement in pain symptoms secondary to systemic uptake of the injected steroids cannot be discounted.[7] Although ESIs are the "bread and butter" of interventional pain procedures, most studies show that they have only short-term benefit, and may delay, but not prevent, the need for spine surgery. Although therapeutic spinal injections tend to include steroids, interventional injections in nonspinal locations, such as sympathetic nerve blocks, may be therapeutic with only local anesthetic.

ENHANCED PAIN TREATMENT BY MULTIMODAL APPROACH

Pain complaints are subjective and this can significantly affect outcomes of injections because of a placebo response or expectation bias as high as 35%.[8–11] Anatomic variation can also result in unexpected responses to injections to include incomplete blocks or blocks of unintended nerves. The therapeutic nature of the physician-patient encounter can often affect patient reporting of benefit from therapeutic interventions, resulting from placebo or nocebo effects.[12]

It is best to approach pain within the biopsychosocial model of chronic disease. Thus, although invasive interventions may be beneficial, the psychosocial factors affecting the patient's pain complaints should be accounted for in a multimodal and ideally interdisciplinary treatment plan. Prospective studies show increased pain improvement with combined therapies, including 1 randomized study showing that the combination of ESIs and physical therapy improved pain more than either treatment alone for cervical spine pain.[13–15]

COMMON MINIMALLY INVASIVE TECHNIQUES FOR BACK PAIN TREATMENT
Epidural and Selective Nerve Root Injections

First described in 1952, the ESI is the most commonly performed injection for back pain.[5,8] Nondiscriminant use of the ESI for back and lower extremity pain has led to questions about its efficacy, with multiple studies critically investigating its long-term efficacy and cost-effectiveness.[5,16–18] In a study by Bicket and colleagues,[19] ESI performed with a placebo in the injectate was as effective as the injection performed with corticosteroid in the injectate. Perhaps not surprisingly, studies by pain practitioners tend to conclude more ESI benefit compared with studies by non–pain practitioners, which may be because of bias on the part of the interventionalists, or better patient selection by expert physicians.[5] There does not exist a prospective, randomized study that conclusively shows long-term benefit with ESIs, even compared with placebo.[20] The Wessex Epidural Steroids Trial (WEST) found that multiple ESIs also did not provide superior results compared with placebo at 35 days postinjection.[21]

As with most therapeutic interventions, the success of the ESI likely depends on strict, accurate diagnosis; good patient selection; and proper injection technique. At present, ESIs are indicated therapeutically for radicular pain, most commonly cervical or lumbar, as part of a multimodal treatment plan focusing on symptomatic and functional improvement. However, there is wide acknowledgment that the procedure does not reduce the long-term risk of neurosurgery. Studies have shown that the ESI is not beneficial for pain symptoms caused by spinal stenosis, nonradicular back pain, or facet joint–mediated pain.[22,23] Despite the numerous caveats to the application of ESI as an isolated treatment option, it remains an important treatment modality for properly selected patients in a multimodal treatment plan.[13,22,24]

Injection technique and anatomic approach

The purpose of the ESI is to deliver steroid, most commonly mixed with local anesthetic or preservative-free saline, adjacent to a single or multiple irritated nerve roots that are presumed to cause radicular pain symptoms.[24] The most common approaches for ESI are the interlaminar (parasagittal or midline) and transforaminal approaches, as illustrated in **Fig. 1**.

The midline technique requires accessing the epidural space with the needle between 2 vertebral laminae. With fluoroscopic guidance, a 17-gauge, 18-gauge, 20-gauge, or 22-gauge Tuohy epidural needle is used, most often in combination with a loss-of-resistance technique to air or saline; saline is used more consistently in the thoracic and cervical regions. On entry into the epidural space, contrast is injected to ensure appropriate placement of the needle tip while simultaneously demonstrating a lack of intravascular or intrathecal injection. With safety being the priority, cervical nerve roots can often be targeted for diagnostic purposes by accessing the epidural space in the lower cervical/upper thoracic spine and then using a Racz catheter to deliver the injectate at the target cervical nerve root.

In the transforaminal injection technique, the space is accessed via the neuroforamen. This approach is advantageous in 2 specific scenarios: first, the interlaminar approach may not be possible because of altered anatomy from previous surgery; second, specific nerve roots must be targeted for diagnostic or therapeutic purposes. With this technique, the needle can be adjusted to achieve contrast spread medially into the epidural space or only along the nerve root at the neuroforamen, the latter resulting in a selective nerve root injection. The landmarks for this approach include the transverse process above the target nerve root, which is the superior border of the foramen. A 7.6-cm to 17.8-cm, 22-gauge or 25-gauge spinal needle is directed toward the neuroforamen with fluoroscopic guidance. The needle is advanced until the tip is seen to be adjacent to or within the neuroforamen, at which point contrast in injected with live fluoroscopy to confirm the desired spread, once again ensuring a

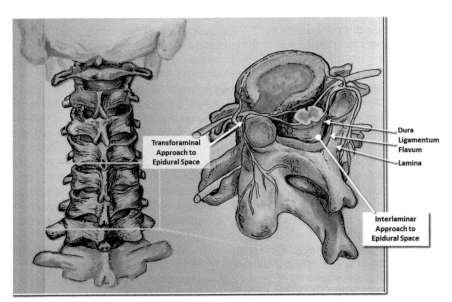

Fig. 1. Cervical spine anatomy with epidural space. (*Courtesy of* Yifan Xu, Oregon Health & Science University, Portland, OR.)

lack of intravascular or intrathecal injection. Of note, there are reported cases of para-plegia from unrecognized injection of particulate steroid solution into the artery of Adamkiewicz.[25,26] The injectates for both approaches typically include steroid with sa-line or local anesthetic for therapeutic injections and local anesthetic only for diag-nostic selective nerve root injections.

Adverse events
Complications of ESIs include new or worsened pain, dural puncture, intravascular local anesthetic injection, adhesive arachnoiditis, epidural hematoma, bleeding, infec-tion, and nerve damage to include paralysis.[27] An important sequela of steroid injec-tions is immunosuppression, which may result in new or recurrent infections, with case reports of meningitis and varicella zoster infections.[28–31]

Facet Joint Injections and Medial Branch Nerve Procedures

Introduction and neuroanatomy
Facet joint injections, including intraarticular and medial branch blocks, are the sec-ond most frequently performed procedure in interventional pain clinics.[5] Bogduk and Long[32] clarified the neuroanatomy of the zygapophyseal, or facet, joint in the late 1970s, allowing nerve targeting in this space to treat facet joint–mediated pain. Fluoroscopic visualization has made it possible to identify and inject medication into the facet joint space, and 1 study showed the potential for ultrasonography-guided in-jection as well.[33] The anatomy of the cervical, thoracic, and lumbar medial branches is shown in **Fig. 2**. Facet joints are synovial joints that begin at C1-C2 and are present down to the L5-S1 spinal levels. The capsule and synovium are extensively innervated with sensory fibers, which derive from the medial branch of the primary posterior rami of 2 segmental spinal nerves, originating from both above and below the interspace. These sensory fibers express mechanoreceptors and multiple nociception-related neurotransmitters such as substance P.[34,35] In addition to the facet joint, this medial nerve branch also provides the only innervation for the multifidus muscle in a segmental manner. Because the multifidus muscle is a dynamic spine stabilizer as well as a significant pain generator, lumbar medial branch blocks and denervations may result in analgesia from both muscle and joint sources.[34]

Multiple placebo-controlled studies have been conducted to evaluate the efficacy of radiofrequency denervation of medial branch nerves.[36] When saline is compared with short-acting or long-acting local anesthetic injectates, facet joint injections have shown false-positive rates as high as 20% to 40%.[23,37–39] According to the FACTS trial, facet joint injections with local anesthetic may also have value as a diagnostic tool in predicting success with radiofrequency ablation to treat low back pain.[36,40] Se-lective radiofrequency denervation of the facet joints through medial branch ablation to reduce pain has gained much support because of an increasingly positive body of evidence in the medical literature. In contrast, there are also contradictory studies showing that psychological variables play a large role in long-term denervation out-comes and that such procedures may not be more beneficial than a placebo procedure.[5]

Indications and techniques for diagnostic medial branch blocks
Lumbar facet arthropathy pain is diagnosed based on an accurate history and physical examination, incorporating facet-loading maneuvers to assess pain distribution and referral pattern (see **Fig. 2**; **Fig. 3**). Patients often have a characteristic localized uni-lateral low back pain that is exacerbated by rotation and extension and eased by flexion, as well as pain caused by unilateral palpation of the facet joint or transverse process. There is also a lack of radicular features, although referred pain located

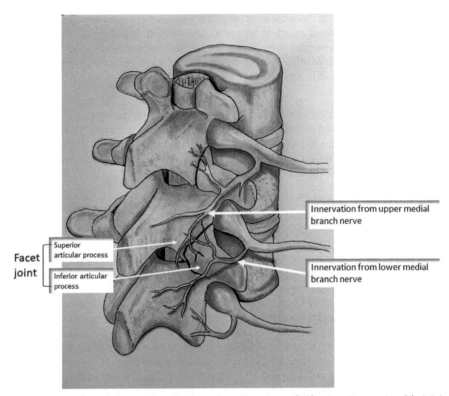

Fig. 2. Lumbar facet joints and medial branches. (*Courtesy of* Yifan Xu, Oregon Health & Science University, Portland, OR.)

above the knee is often present.[41] If facet pain is suspected, diagnostic injections of the medial branches will help secure the diagnosis. The patient often experiences 2 sets of patient-blinded, unsedated diagnostic medial branch injections under fluoroscopic guidance, with each set containing either a short-acting (2% lidocaine) or long-acting (0.5% bupivacaine) local anesthetic. Postprocedure, the patient completes a pain diary, scoring numeric pain ratings. If temporally concordant pain relief for each of the 2 blocks occurs, the clinician can evaluate the patient for radiofrequency denervation as a longer-term analgesic.

Indications and technique for radiofrequency denervation

Although neurolysis can be achieved using many techniques, radiofrequency energy has emerged as the method of choice for medial branch denervation because of the precision of lesion size and the ability to assess proximity and prevent damage to surroundings structures.[42] Recent technical improvements include small-diameter (22 gauge) and curved probes, which both decrease tissue trauma and guide navigation. The probe can stimulate adjacent structures with preset electrical wattage, which allows motor and sensory testing with harmless stimulation before denervation to rule out contact with nerve roots. In addition to being used for low back pain in the lumbar space, head and neck pain can be treated with radiofrequency denervation of cervical medial branches. The evidence for radiofrequency ablation indicates that it may be best in the cervical space, with most studies showing prolonged benefit.[43–45]

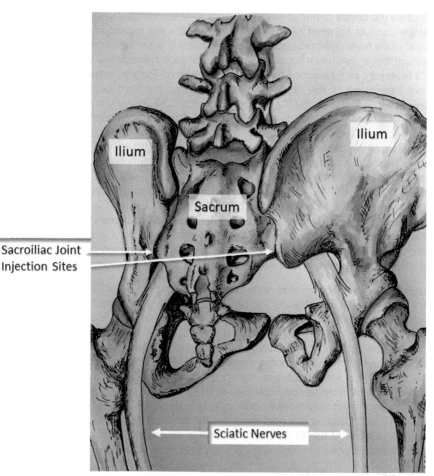

Fig. 3. Lumbar spine, sacrum, and ilium, showing the sacroiliac joint. (*Courtesy of* Yifan Xu, Oregon Health & Science University, Portland, OR.)

In 1 study, McDonald and colleagues[46] reported significant pain relief after radiofrequency cervical medial branch denervation in 71% of treated patients, with a median relief duration of 422 days. Recurrent pain from nerve regrowth can also be treated by repeating the denervation procedure. Although this diagnostic paradigm can have false-positive rates ranging from 15% to 67%, no other single model has been validated to replace it.[47]

Probe placement is critical for accurate neurolysis and varies by spinal level. Identical to the target for diagnostic facet joint injections, the medial branches of 2 segmental spinal nerves innervate each facet joint ipsilaterally, and therefore both branches must be ablated per spinal level to denervate each joint. Because of diverse rostral-caudal spine anatomy, ideal cannula location depends on spine region. At the level of the lumbar spine, the radiofrequency probe is best positioned slightly inferior to the junction of the transverse process and the pedicle to approach the medial branches. At the level of the sacral spine, the dorsal ramus of the medial branch of L5 is denervated with the probe in the sacral alar notch. The cannula should be at the S1 contribution to the superior aspect of the ipsilateral S1 neural foramen to capture the dorsal ramus of the L5-S1 joint.[48] At the cervical levels inferior to C3, the active cannula tip must be positioned in the concave aspect of the lateral articular pillar of the transverse process. At C3, the anatomy is similar to the inferior segments, except that it also has a superficial branch that runs immediately posterior to the C2-C3 facet joint as it becomes the third occipital nerve. Partially responsible for the sensory innervation of the posterior skull and scalp, the third occipital nerve can be lesioned in addition to the C2 component of the C2-C3 joint with the lateral articular pillar technique to cover head and neck.[49] The thoracic anatomy can be more involved, but facet-related pain is uncommon in this distribution.[27] The medial branches of the thoracic dorsal rami are lumbar in character at T11 and T12, whereas other thoracic levels assume a different anatomic distribution. Uniquely, at several levels, the medial branch does not exist in the same plane as the transverse process in the thoracic spine and a 2-needle technique is thus advocated for the thoracic spine, where 1 needle is inserted to contact the lateral third of the transverse process and a second needle is positioned at the identical depth but more cephalad via lateral fluoroscopy confirmation to avoid lung puncture.[27,50] To enhance lesion size, decrease technical failure, and decrease pain from the ablation procedure, lidocaine or other local anesthetic is often injected to the site before denervation.[51]

Sacroiliac joint injections and radiofrequency ablations

A typical examination finding for SI joint (see **Fig. 3**)–induced nerve pain reveals buttock pain (only) or buttock pain with referrals to the lower lumbar, groin, and leg areas. Pain originating from the SI joint can account for an estimated 15% to 30% of axial low back pain, especially in individuals with prior lumbar fusion (adjacent segment syndrome), orthopedic irregularities, or spondyloarthropathies.[52] A large, diarthrodial joint with a true synovium, posterior innervation of the SI joint has been shown to arise from lateral branches of S1-S3 and dorsal rami of L3-L5, whereas the anterior aspect may receive contributions from L2-S2.[53] Relief of pain after a diagnostic SI joint block is the gold standard for diagnosing SI joint pain, and radiofrequency ablation of the SI joint after a positive diagnostic examination can be done with multiple probes or single-entry probes with multiple nodes.[54]

Outcomes, risks, and efficacy

Radiofrequency denervation stops neural function by selective coagulation of neuronal contents within the sheath. However, because the neuronal substrate remains, regrowth of the nerve without neuroma formation is expected about 8 to 12 months after the procedure, and a repeat procedure can be performed if pain recurs.[31] Because there is no contraindication to repeating the denervation or increased technical difficulty with subsequent procedures, this minimally invasive route is favored rather than surgical therapy in patients with high medical comorbidity. Done with mild sedation or unsedated, the overall risks are also low for this procedure, with rare case reports of nerve or spinal cord damage, with direct needle trauma from arterial injection causing embolic paralysis, infection, pneumothorax, and tissue burn along the needle path. Postablation neuritis is also possible, although this risk can be mitigated by adding steroids to local injection.[55]

Sympathetic Nerve Blocks

As the fight-or-flight part of the autonomic nervous system, the sympathetic nervous system mediates vasoconstriction, tachycardia, decreased intestinal motility, and piloerection, among other effects. Efferent fibers of the sympathetic nervous system begin in the intermediolateral column of the spinal cord and exit along the ventral roots from T1 to L2. These fibers then leave the ventral root as white rami communicantes and enter the sympathetic chains on the anterolateral aspect of the vertebral bodies, becoming preganglionic fibers that eventually synapse in one of the sympathetic ganglia. Postganglionic fibers leaving the ganglia then travel to their sites of action.[56]

Afferent fibers of the nervous system carry sensory pain back to the spinal cord through 2 routes. Although somatic pain is transmitted alongside the somatic nerves, visceral burning and aching pain from C fibers travel through the sympathetic ganglia but do not synapse there on their way to entering the spinal cord through the dorsal root ganglia. Because of the proximity of sympathetic and visceral sensory pathways near the vertebral bodies, sympathetic blocks anesthetize the visceral sensory nerves as well.[57] Sympathetic nerve blocks do not cause somatic numbness or motor blockade, unlike somatic nerve blocks. Classically, sympathetically maintained pain involves sympathetic symptoms such as vasoconstriction, decreased extremity temperature, and decreased limb perfusion, with the most severe of these manifestations potentially contributing significantly to limb disorders such as complex regional pain syndrome.

Indications and techniques for lumbar sympathetic blocks

Preganglionic fibers from the lower thoracic sympathetic nerves enter the lumbar sympathetic chain. They enter the abdomen between the medial arcuate ligament and the psoas muscle before coursing along the psoas fascia to reach the anterolateral aspect of the vertebral bodies, continuing along the medial border of the psoas muscle. The left and right sympathetic chains lie posterior to the aorta and the vena cava, respectively. The lumbar sympathetic chains synapse within the lumbar sympathetic plexus and then send rami communicantes to the first and second lumbar spinal nerve roots. This separation of the spinal roots and the sympathetic ganglia allows the sympathetic nerves to be blocked with low risk of somatic nerve damage.

There have not been many prospective studies testing the efficacy of lumbar sympathetic blocks for lower extremity pain.[58] Because sympathectomy results in increased body temperature because of vasodilation, many studies attempt to correlate temperature change in the lower extremity to pain relief. Tran and colleagues[59] performed 28 lumbar sympathetic blocks and found that a successful lumbar sympathetic block correlated with ipsilateral toe temperature increase to within 3° C of core temperature, concluding that cutaneous toe temperatures approaching core temperature may predict relief of sympathetically maintained pain. However, another prospective observation study, by van Eijs and colleagues,[60] did not find correlation between temperature change and symptomatic relief.

The lumbar sympathetic chains are commonly approached by the paramedian or lateral approach using fluoroscopic guidance. The needles enter the skin at the level of the transverse process and 5 to 6 cm lateral to the midline in the paramedian approach, whereas the lateral approach begins 9 to 10 cm lateral to the midline. These different approaches are identical in their difficulty and risks.[59] With surprisingly little spillover to the spinal nerve roots with this high-volume block, these injections are performed at a single level, either L1 or L2, with 10 to 20 mL per injection, and rely on the spread of local anesthetic along fascial planes for efficacy.[61] Blocking multiple individual levels with less volume may be more safe if performing neurolysis with phenol or alcohol.

Minimally Invasive Treatment of Lumbar Spinal Stenosis with Interspinous Implants

Lumbar spinal stenosis is a progressive, degenerative process by which pathologic overgrowth of bony, ligamentous, and synovial components of the axial spine narrow the spinal canal and compress neural structures.[62,63] As the nucleus pulposus of the intervertebral discs desiccate and herniate because of aging, repeated mechanical trauma, and supportive muscular atrophy, the disc space collapses and shortens the anterior spinal column.[62] This process results in excessive stress toward the posterior spinal structures, including facet joints and ligaments, generating axial joint overgrowth and spinal canal narrowing from synovial hypertrophy, synovial cysts, osteophyte formation, and posterior ligamentous buckling and thickening.[62] Symptoms range from mild static back pain to severe neurogenic claudication (leg pain; sensation of heavy and weak legs with ambulation), classically improved by lumbar flexion (such as climbing stairs or sitting) and worsened by lumbar extension.[63] Occupational hazards, high body mass index, and genetic predisposition all contribute to development of lumbar spinal stenosis, with up to 30% of adults more than 40 years of age affected with severe stenosis.[62] Although, in 2013, the North American Spine Society guidelines suggested that the use of ESI can provide short-term relief for neurogenic claudication or radiculopathy,[64] a later review suggested that ESI resulted in minimal, if any, symptomatic relief or walking improvement, and that steroid injections seemed to have no benefit compared with lidocaine injections alone.[18] In addition, physical therapy has shown little efficacy as a stand-alone intervention, but it seems to improve outcomes after surgical decompression.[65] Patients often seek surgical intervention when they are functionally debilitated and lack relief from noninvasive treatments such as physical therapy and ESIs. Recently, interspinous implants have been investigated as an additional minimally invasive, percutaneous, nonsurgical option for spinal stenosis. Requiring only a 15-mm skin incision, little to no sedation under fluoroscopy, and minimal blood loss, interspinous implants are inserted between adjacent spinous processes or lamina and expanded to prop open the compressed space.[66] Although still under investigation, industry-sponsored publications suggest that these devices, such as the Superion Vertiflex, had benefit for a small number of patients with less than 50% reduction of central canal diameter.[67] In addition, implantation of a device such as the Superion Vertiflex for pain caused by lumbar spinal stenosis may provide an opportunity to decrease opioid use for this population.[68]

MINIMALLY INVASIVE PROCEDURES FOR NONSPINE NEUROLOGIC DISORDERS
Trigeminal Neuralgia

Indications and diagnosis
The trigeminal nerve (fifth cranial nerve [CN V]) is 1 of 12 cranial nerves that provide sensory and motor function to the face. It has 3 branches: ophthalmic (V1), maxillary (V2), and mandibular (V3). The International Association for the Study of Pain (IASP) defines neuralgia as pain in the distribution of a nerve or nerves. Trigeminal neuralgia (TN) is a neuropathic pain that is characterized by unilateral electric shock–like pain in the distribution of CN V. It is typically sudden in onset/termination and can affect 1 or more divisions of CN V. One of the defining characteristics of classic TN is that the patient is pain free between episodes. If the patient has constant facial pain between these episodes, this is defined as TN type 2. In addition, a patient may also have secondary TN, which is classic TN that is caused by an underlying disease, such as multiple sclerosis or a space-occupying lesion.

Although the overall prevalence of TN in the general population is 0.015%, the incidence of TN is estimated to be 4.3 to 27 per 100,000 annually.[69–71] It is more common in women and age is a primary risk factor for developing TN.[70] TN is most commonly diagnosed in individuals between the ages of 50 and 70 years, but the onset can be earlier.[70] The most common distribution for this pain is in the V2 and V3 divisions of CN V, and the left side is more frequently affected.[71]

It is thought that nerve compression at the cerebellopontine cistern by a blood vessel, vein, or more often an artery is the cause for TN.[69–71] However, such findings are also present in patients with persistent idiopathic facial pain, and often in asymptomatic patients, thus suggesting that this finding may be a normal variant. The compression can be primary or secondary, with primary being defined as visual compression of the nerve without a secondary cause. Secondary causes include space-occupying lesions to include meningiomas, schwannomas, aneurysms, arteriovenous malformations, and cysts. Other medical conditions may increase the likelihood of developing TN, including chronic sinusitis, multiple sclerosis, and diabetes.[69]

TN is primarily a diagnosis based on the patient's history, clinical presentation, along with an appropriate physical examination. The diagnosis of TN can be made based on meeting the criteria from the International Headache Society (International Classification of Headache Disorders, Third Edition [ICHD-3]).[72] The following criteria must be met to diagnose a patient with classic TN: recurrent paroxysms of unilateral facial pain in the distribution of 1 or more divisions of the trigeminal nerve, with no radiation beyond, and the pain has the characteristics of lasting from a fraction of a second to 2 minutes; severe intensity and electric shock–like, shooting, sharp, or stabbing in quality; precipitated by innocuous stimuli within the affected trigeminal distribution; and not better accounted for by another ICHD-3 diagnosis. Secondary TN must meet the following criteria: characteristics of classic TN; an underlying disease has been shown that is known to be able to cause the neuralgia; not better accounted for by another ICHD-3 diagnosis.

Techniques for trigeminal neuralgia procedures

Although numerous treatment options exist, the first-line treatment of TN is pharmacologic, with carbamazepine being the gold standard. However, other medication options include oxcarbazepine, phenytoin, baclofen, lamotrigine, gabapentin, levetiracetam, topiramate, botulinum toxin A, and sodium valproate.[69,70] Note that these medications can have serious side effects, ranging from sleepiness and dizziness to Stevens-Johnson syndrome, as may be seen with carbamazepine.[69]

If the pharmacologic therapies do not provide satisfactory benefit, then other invasive modalities are typically considered. Minimally invasive anesthetic techniques for TN treatment include diagnostic, therapeutic, or neurolytic blocks. The trigeminal or gasserian ganglion, located in the Meckel cave, is the target for the anesthetic techniques and is accessed via the foramen ovale with computed tomography or fluoroscopic guidance.[73] The Meckel cave is bordered by the cavernous sinus medially, inferior surface of the temporal lobe superiorly, and the brain stem posteriorly.[74] The patient is placed supine and the fluoroscope is positioned with a steep cephalad tilt and slight oblique positioning to visualize the foramen ovale, located just medial to the medial edge of the mandible. After appropriate skin and subcutaneous anesthesia, needle entry is typically made approximately 2 to 3 cm lateral to the ipsilateral corner of the mouth. The needle is advanced until the tip is seen adjacent to the foramen, at which point a lateral image is obtained to confirm placement. If the Meckel cave is entered, it is common to encounter cerebrospinal fluid because of dural puncture. At this point, contrast is injected to confirm appropriate placement before injection of local anesthetic, corticosteroid, or phenol depending on the goal of the injection.

Invasive techniques include surgical interventions, neuromodulation, or subdermal therapies.[75] The surgical interventions can include Gamma Knife radiosurgery, percutaneous radiofrequency rhizotomy, balloon decompression, and microvascular decompression.[75] Neuromodulation options include stimulation of the trigeminal branch of the gasserian ganglion. In addition, stimulation of the central structures such as motor cortex or deep brain stimulation may also be considered. Neurosurgeons often do neurolysis or nerve decompression under significant sedation or general anesthesia.

Other Minimally Invasive Anesthetic Techniques

Trigger point injections

Trigger points, associated with myofascial pain syndrome, are defined as hyperirritable tissue points that are tender when compressed.[76] Pain from trigger points may then give rise to referred pain. Although physical therapy, heat therapy, and ultrasonography therapy have been attempted, the most common invasive therapy is trigger point injections. Described as direct wet needling, injection of fluid (often a local anesthetic but also corticosteroids, vitamin B, acetylsalicylate, ketorolac, or botulinum toxin) is directed into the trigger point in an attempt to deactivate it. A systematic review of small, published trials concluded that, although there is no clear evidence for either benefit or ineffectiveness, it was able to relieve symptoms regardless of injectate type used.[77] Although there is a small risk of pneumothorax in the thoracic areas, trigger point injections are widely regarded as a safe technique.

SUMMARY

This article reviews the management of back, lower extremity, and TN pain through anesthetic and percutaneous techniques. The introduction of fluoroscopy and ultrasonography has led to the ability to precisely deliver various medications to the correct target, whether local anesthetic, steroid, cryoanalgesia, thermal energy, or neurolytic agents. Using local anesthetic and having early feedback on whether a patient's pain has improved allow clinicians to narrow large differential diagnosis to a smaller and even single source of pain generation that could serve as an interventional or surgical target. Further, multimodal therapy, including physical therapy, psychosocial counseling, and procedural care, seems to be most efficacious in many studies for successful pain treatment.

Pain procedures are also now routinely conducted not just by anesthesiologists but also by rehabilitation providers, interventional radiologists, and neurologists. This article is by no means comprehensive in describing pain management in neurosurgery, and each practitioner has a subset of expertise ranging from pure medication management to pure procedural assessments.

CLINICS CARE POINTS

- Chronic back pain is defined as pain lasting longer than 12 weeks. It can originate from 3 distinct sources: axial, radicular, or referred.
- Diagnostic injections attempt to localize a pain source to specific nerve roots for therapeutic planning, while therapeutic procedures have the goal of alleviating pain to decrease opioid use and increase quality of life.
- Minimally invasive pain procedures are most effective if combined with multimodal therapy, and may delay but not obviate the potential need for neurosurgery.
- Sympathetic nerve blocks can be efficacious for treating pain from the celiac plexus for advanced abdominal cancer, or for treating complex regional pain syndrome in limbs.

REFERENCES

1. Chou R, Deyo R, Friedly J, et al. Nonpharmacologic therapies for low back pain: a systematic review for an american college of physicians clinical practice guideline. Ann Intern Med 2017;166(7):493–505.
2. Steffens D, Maher CG, Pereira LS, et al. Prevention of low back pain: a systematic review and meta-analysis. JAMA Intern Med 2016;176(2):199–208.
3. Hoy D, Bain C, Williams G, et al. A systematic review of the global prevalence of low back pain. Arthritis Rheum 2012;64(6):2028–37.
4. Urits I, Burshtein A, Sharma M, et al. Low back pain, a comprehensive review: pathophysiology, diagnosis, and treatment. Curr Pain Headache Rep 2019; 23(3):23.
5. Cohen SP, Wallace M, Rauck RL, et al. Unique aspects of clinical trials of invasive therapies for chronic pain. Pain Rep 2019;4(3). https://doi.org/10.1097/pr9. 0000000000000687.
6. Cohen SP, Bicket MC, Jamison D, et al. Epidural steroids. Reg Anesth Pain Med 2013;38(3):175–200.
7. King W, Miller DC, Smith CC. Systemic effects of epidural corticosteroid injection. Pain Med 2018;19(2):404–5.
8. Hrobjartsson A, Thomsen ASS, Emanuelsson F, et al. Observer bias in randomised clinical trials with binary outcomes: systematic review of trials with both blinded and non-blinded outcome assessors. BMJ 2012;344:e1119.
9. Savović J, Jones HE, Altman DG, et al. Influence of reported study design characteristics on intervention effect estimates from randomized, controlled trials. Ann Intern Med 2012;157(6):429–38.
10. Wood L, Egger M, Gluud LL, et al. Empirical evidence of bias in treatment effect estimates in controlled trials with different interventions and outcomes: meta-epidemiological study. BMJ 2008;336(7644):601–5.
11. Turner JA. The importance of placebo effects in pain treatment and research. JAMA 1994;271(20):1609–14.
12. Kaptchuk TJ, Miller FG. Placebo effects in medicine. N Engl J Med 2015; 373(1):8–9.
13. Cohen SP, Hayek S, Semenov Y, et al. Epidural steroid injections, conservative treatment, or combination treatment for cervical radicular pain. Anesthesiology 2014;121(5):1045–55.
14. White AH. Injection techniques for the diagnosis and treatment of low back pain. Orthop Clin North Am 1983;14:533–67.
15. Chen CPC, Tang SFT, Hsu T-C, et al. Ultrasound guidance in caudal epidural needle placement. Anesthesiology 2004;101(1):181–4.
16. Manchikanti L, Pampati V, Falco FJE, et al. Growth of Spinal interventional pain management techniques. Spine 2013;38(2):157–68.
17. Bicket MC, Hurley RW, Moon JY, et al. The development and validation of a quality assessment and rating of technique for injections of the spine (AQUARIUS). Reg Anesth Pain Med 2016;41(1):80–5.
18. Friedly JL. A randomized trial of epidural glucocorticoid injections for spinal stenosis. N Engl J Med 2014;371(4):11–21.
19. Bicket MC, Gupta A, Brown CH, et al. Epidural injections for spinal pain. Anesthesiology 2013;119(4):907–31.
20. Sibell DM, Fleisch JM. Interventions for low back pain: what does the evidence tell us? Curr Pain Headache Rep 2007;11(1):14–9.

21. Arden NK, Price C, Reading I, et al. A multicentre randomized controlled trial of epidural corticosteroid injections for sciatica: the WEST study. Rheumatology 2005;44(11):1399–406.
22. Chou R, Hashimoto R, Friedly J, et al. Epidural corticosteroid injections for radiculopathy and spinal stenosis. Ann Intern Med 2015;163(5):373.
23. Cohen SP, Chen Y, Neufeld NJ. Sacroiliac joint pain: a comprehensive review of epidemiology, diagnosis and treatment. Expert Rev Neurother 2013;13(1): 99–116.
24. Chou R. Pain management injection therapies for low back pain. Technology assessment report ESIB0813. (Prepared by the pacific northwest evidence-based practice center under contract No. HHSA 290-2012-00014-I.). Rockville (MD): Agency for Healthcare Research and Quality; 2015.
25. Glaser SE. Root cause analysis of paraplegia following transforaminal epidural steroid injections: the "unsafe" triangle. Pain Physician 2010;13:237–44.
26. Park JW, Nam HS, Cho SK, et al. Kambins triangle approach of lumbar transforaminal epidural injection with spinal stenosis. Ann Rehabil Med 2011;35(6): 833–43.
27. Manchikanti KN, Sairam A, Vijay S, et al. An update of evaluation of therapeutic thoracic facet joint interventions. Pain Physician 2012;15:E463–81.
28. Davis K, Prater A, Fluker S-A, et al. A difficult case to swallow. Am J Ther 2014; 21(1). https://doi.org/10.1097/mjt.0b013e318220500f.
29. Drazin D, Hanna G, Shweikeh F, et al. Varicella-zoster-mediated radiculitis reactivation following cervical spine surgery: case report and review of the literature. Case Rep Infect Dis 2013;2013:1–5.
30. Eisenberg E, Goldman R, Schlag-Eisenberg D, et al. Adhesive arachnoiditis following lumbar epidural steroid injections: a report of two cases and review of the literature. J Pain Res 2019;12:513–8.
31. Choi EJ, Choi YM, Jang EJ, et al. Neural ablation and regeneration in pain practice. Korean J Pain 2016;29(1):3.
32. Bogduk N, Long DM. The anatomy of the so-called "articular nerves" and their relationship to facet denervation in the treatment of low-back pain. J Neurosurg 1979;51(2):172–7.
33. Galiano K, Obwegeser AA, Bodner G, et al. Ultrasound guidance for facet joint injections in the lumbar spine: a computed tomography-controlled feasibility study. Anesth Analg 2005;101(2):579–83.
34. Sibell D. Facet joint procedures for chronic back pain. In: Schmidt R, Willis W, editors. Encyclopedia of pain. Berlin, Heidelberg (NY): Springer; 2007.
35. Ogden A, Winfree C. Facet joint pain. In: Schmidt R, Willis W, editors. Encyclopedia of pain. Berlin, Heidelberg (NY): Springer; 2007.
36. Cohen SP, Doshi TL, Constantinescu OC, et al. Effectiveness of Lumbar Facet Joint Blocks and Predictive Value before Radiofrequency Denervation: The Facet Treatment Study (FACTS), a Randomized, Controlled Clinical Trial. Anesthesiology 2018;129(3):517–35. Erratum in: Anesthesiology 2018;129(3):618.
37. Gupta S, Gharibo CG, Bakshi S, et al. A best-evidence systematic appraisal of the diagnostic accuracy and utility of facet (zygapophysial) joint injections in chronic spinal pain. Pain Physician 2015;18:E497–533.
38. Cohen SP, Huang JHY, Brummett C. Facet joint pain—advances in patient selection and treatment. Nat Rev Rheumatol 2013;9(2):101–16.
39. King W, Ahmed SU, Baisden J, et al. Diagnosis and treatment of posterior sacroiliac complex pain: a systematic review with comprehensive analysis of the published data. Pain Med 2015;16(2):257–65.

40. Moran R, O'Connell D, Walsh MG. The diagnostic value of facet joint injections. Spine 1988;13(12):1407–10.
41. Wilde VE, Ford JJ, Mcmeeken JM. Indicators of lumbar zygapophyseal joint pain: survey of an expert panel with the delphi technique. Phys Ther 2007;87(10): 1348–61.
42. Kapural L, Mekhail N. Radiofrequency ablation for chronic pain control. Curr Pain Headache Rep 2001;5(6):517–25.
43. Bartleson JD, Maus TP. Diagnostic and therapeutic spinal interventions: facet joint interventions. Neurol Clin Pract 2014;4(4):342–6.
44. Manchikanti L, Vijay S, Frank JEF, et al. Comparative outcomes of a 2-year follow-up of cervical medial branch blocks in management of chronic neck pain: a randomized, double-blind controlled trial. Pain Physician 2010;13:437–50.
45. Parsons SJ, Hawboldt GS. Herpes Zoster: a previously unrecognized complication of epidural steroids in the treatment of complex regional pain syndrome (Editorial). J Pain Symptom Manage 2003;25(3):198–9.
46. McDonald GJ, Lord SM, Bogduk N. Long-term follow-up of patients treated with cervical radiofrequency neurotomy for chronic neck pain. Neurosurgery 1999; 45(1):61–8.
47. Manchukonda R, Manchikanti KN, Cash KA, et al. Facet joint pain in chronic spinal pain: an evaluation of prevalence and false-positive rate of diagnostic blocks. J Spinal Disord Tech 2007;20(7):539–45.
48. Lau P, Mercer S, Govind J, et al. The surgical anatomy of lumbar medial branch neurotomy (facet denervation). Pain Med 2004;5(3):289–98.
49. Nguyen T, Chan K, Chryssidis S, et al. CT guided radiofrequency ablation of the cervical medial branch using a lateral approach in the supine patient. J Spine Surg 2017;3(3):463–7.
50. Bogduk N. Practice guidelines for spinal diagnostic and treatment procedures. 2nd edition. San Francisco (CA): International Spine Intervention Society; 2013.
51. Provenzano DA, Lassila HC, Somers D. The effect of fluid injection on lesion size during radiofrequency treatment. Reg Anesth Pain Med 2010;35(4):338–42.
52. Liliang P-C, Lu K, Liang C-L, et al. Sacroiliac joint pain after lumbar and lumbosacral fusion: findings using dual sacroiliac joint blocks. Pain Med 2011;12(4): 565–70.
53. Cohen SP. Sacroiliac joint pain: a comprehensive review of anatomy, diagnosis, and treatment. Anesth Analg 2005;101(5):1440–53.
54. Schmidt PC, Pino CA, Vorenkamp KE. Sacroiliac joint radiofrequency ablation with a multilesion probe. Anesth Analg 2014;119(2):460–2.
55. Dobrogowski J. Radiofrequency denervation with or without addition of pentoxifylline or methylprednisolone for chronic lumbar zygapophysial joint pain. Pharmacol Rep 2005;57:475–80.
56. Alshak MN, M Das J. Neuroanatomy, sympathetic nervous system. Treasure Island: StatPearls; 2019. Available at: https://www.ncbi.nlm.nih.gov/books/NBK542195/. Accessed June 30, 2020.
57. Strong JA, Zhang JM, Schaible H. The sympathetic nervous system and pain. In: Wood JN, editor. The Oxford handbook of the neurobiology of pain. Oxford (United Kingdom): Oxford University Press; 2018. p. 1–25.
58. Gunduz OH, Coskun OK. Ganglion blocks as a treatment of pain: current perspectives. J Pain Res 2017;10:2815–26.
59. Tran KM, Frank SM, Raja SN, et al. Lumbar sympathetic block for sympathetically maintained pain: changes in cutaneous temperatures and pain perception. Anesth Analg 2000;90(6):1396–401.

60. Van Eijs F, Geurts J, Kleef MV, et al. Predictors of pain relieving response to sympathetic blockade in complex regional pain syndrome type 1. Anesthesiology 2012;116(1):113–21.
61. Middleton WJ, Chan VWS. Lumbar sympathetic block: a review of complications. Tech Reg Anesth Pain Manag 1998;2(3):137–46.
62. Bagley C, MacAllister M, Dosselman L, et al. Current concepts and recent advances in understanding and managing lumbar spine stenosis. F1000Res 2019;8:F1000.
63. Deer T, Sayed D, Michels J, et al. A review of lumbar spinal stenosis with intermittent neurogenic claudication: disease and diagnosis. Pain Med 2019;20(2): S32–44.
64. Kreiner DS, Shaffer WO, Baisden JL, et al. North American spine society. An evidence-based clinical guideline for the diagnosis and treatment of degenerative lumbar spinal stenosis (update). Spine J 2013;13(7):734–43.
65. Ammendolia C, Stuber K, de Bruin LK, et al. Nonoperative treatment of lumbar spinal stenosis with neurogenic claudication: a systematic review. Spine (Phila Pa 1976) 2012;37(10):E609–16.
66. Pintauro M, Duffy A, Vahedi P, et al. Interspinous implants: are the new implants better than the last generation? A review. Curr Rev Musculoskelet Med 2017; 10(2):189–98.
67. Gala RJ, Russo GS, Whang PG. Interspinous implants to treat spinal stenosis. Curr Rev Musculoskelet Med 2017;10(2):182–8.
68. Nunley PD, Deer TR, Benyamin RM, et al. Interspinous process decompression is associated with a reduction in opioid analgesia in patients with lumbar spinal stenosis. J Pain Res 2018;11:2943–8.
69. Jones MR, Urits I, Ehrhardt KP, et al. A comprehensive review of trigeminal neuralgia. Curr Pain Headache Rep 2019;23(10):74.
70. Khan M, Nishi SE, Hassan SN, et al. Trigeminal neuralgia, glossopharyngeal neuralgia, and myofascial pain dysfunction syndrome: an update. Pain Res Manag 2017;2017:7438326.
71. Maarbjerg S, Di Stefano G, Bendtsen L, et al. Trigeminal neuralgia - diagnosis and treatment. Cephalalgia 2017;37(7):648–57.
72. Headache classification committee of the international headache society (IHS) the international classification of headache disorders, 3rd edition. Cephalalgia 2018;38(1):1–211.
73. Peters G, Nurmikko TJ. Peripheral and gasserian ganglion-level procedures for the treatment of trigeminal neuralgia. Clin J Pain 2002;18(Issue 1):28–34.
74. Benzon HT, Rathmell JP, Wu CL, et al. Raj's practical management of pain. In: Benzon HT, Wu CL, Argoff CE, et al, editors. Nerve blocks of the head and neck. Philadelphia (PA): Mosby Elsevier; 2008. p. 858–9.
75. Spina A, Mortini P, Alemanno F, et al. Trigeminal neuralgia: toward a multimodal approach. World Neurosurg 2017;103:220–30.
76. Wong CSM, Wong SHS. A new look at trigger point injections. Anesthesiol Res Pract 2012;492452. https://doi.org/10.1155/2012/492452.
77. Scott NA, Guo B, Barton PM, et al. Trigger point injections for chronic nonmalignant musculoskeletal pain: a systematic review. Pain Med 2009;10(1): 54–69.

Basics of Neuromonitoring and Anesthetic Considerations

Shilpa Rao, MD[a],*, James Kurfess, MD[b],
Miriam M. Treggiari, MD, PhD, MPH[c]

KEYWORDS

- Evoked potentials • Electroencephalography • Burst suppression

KEY POINTS

- Amplitude and latency.
- Intraoperative changes in neuromonitoring signals.
- Effect of anesthesia on neuromonitoring.
- Controversies in neuromonitoring.

INTRODUCTION

Neuromonitoring is a modality involving recording electrical potentials generated by neurons or their axons throughout the nervous system. Commonly used modalities include electroencephalography (EEG), somatosensory evoked potentials (SSEPs), motor evoked potentials (MEPs), and brainstem auditory evoked potentials (BAEPs).

Intraoperative neuromonitoring (IONM) modalities are extensively used in adult and pediatric intracranial surgeries to facilitate near complete and safe surgical resection of brain tumors, resection of arteriovenous malformations, aneurysm clipping, and coiling. They are also widely used in spine surgeries to monitor integrity of the spinal cord during spine fusion/fixation and tumor resections. In addition, neuromonitoring techniques are commonly used during carotid endarterectomy surgery. Sudden changes in any signal aids in rapid diagnosis of acute change in clinical condition and alerts the surgeon and anesthesiologist to intraoperative critical events.

In this article, we discuss basics of neuromonitoring, indications, contraindications, and effect of anesthetic medications on various types of neuromonitoring techniques. We also discuss controversies associated with the use of IONM.

[a] Division of Neuroanesthesia, Department of Anesthesiology, Yale School of Medicine, Yale University, PO Box 208051, 333 Cedar Street, TMP 3, New Haven, CT 06510, USA; [b] Department of Anesthesiology, Yale University, PO Box 208051, 333 Cedar Street, TMP 3, New Haven, CT 06510, USA; [c] Department of Anesthesiology, Yale School of Medicine, Yale University, PO Box 208051, 333 Cedar Street, TMP 3, New Haven, CT 06510, USA
* Corresponding author.
E-mail address: shilpa.rao@yale.edu

Anesthesiology Clin 39 (2021) 195–209
https://doi.org/10.1016/j.anclin.2020.11.009   anesthesiology.theclinics.com
1932-2275/21/© 2020 Elsevier Inc. All rights reserved.

ELECTROENCEPHALOGRAPHY
Indications and Contraindications

The EEG records electrical potentials generated by the neurons in cerebral cortex. Electrodes made of silver disks with conductive gel are placed on the scalp or sterilized and placed directly in the surgical field. The most commonly used description for the location of scalp electrodes is the 10- to 20-lead placement system (**Fig. 1**), where the specific electrodes are placed in relation to specific areas of the cerebral cortex.

However, during a craniotomy requiring EEG monitoring, the complete 10 to 20 system cannot be fully used because of surgical incision and exposure, hence the leads are usually placed as close as possible to the surgical site to facilitate monitoring. Each scalp electrode gives a continuous recording of spontaneous superficial brain activity covering an area of 2 to 3 cm in diameter (**Fig. 2**).[1]

Indications of EEG monitoring include the following procedures:

- Surgery involving eloquent cortex
- Carotid endarterectomy to aid in diagnosis of stroke
- Aortic arch surgery to monitor cerebral perfusion
- Certain seizure surgeries

There are no major contraindications for intraoperative EEG monitoring. Presence of scalp infection may preclude the placement of scalp electrodes. Emergency surgeries often proceed without any type of neuromonitoring because of clinical urgency.

Basic EEG waveforms are described next and shown in **Fig. 3**A.

- Delta (0.5–4 Hz): Delta rhythm is physiologically seen in deep sleep states and is prominent in the frontocentral head regions. Pathologic delta rhythm presents in awake states in case of generalized encephalopathy and focal cerebral dysfunction. Frontal intermittent rhythmic delta activity is normally present in adults.[2] Temporal intermittent rhythmic delta activity is seen in patients with temporal lobe epilepsy.[3]
- Theta (4–7 Hz): This is often seen in the frontocentral regions, and travels posteriorly, replacing the alpha rhythm during early drowsiness. This waveform is enhanced by heightened emotional states.

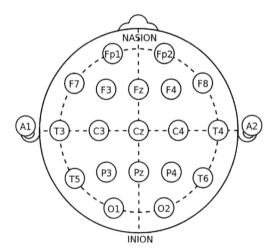

Fig. 1. A 10- to 20-EEG lead placement system.

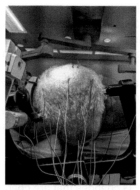

Fig. 2. Photograph showing EEG lead placement in a craniotomy. (*Courtesy of* Courtney Alles, CNIM.)

- Alpha (8–12 Hz): The dominant alpha rhythm is typically present in normal awake EEG recordings in the occipital region. It is best recorded with the eyes closed and during mental relaxation and is attenuated by eye opening.
- Beta (13–30 Hz): This is the most frequently seen rhythm in normal adults and children. Most sedatives increase the amplitude and quantity of beta activity. Beta wave attenuation can occur with cortical injury, and any fluid collection in the brain.

Several factors can affect EEG waveforms including pharmacologic interventions, physiologic factors (mostly sleep and awake status), and disease states.

Pharmacologic interventions

- General anesthesia causes progressive slowing of the raw EEG waveforms and can potentially cause gradual burst suppression in deeper states.
- Inhaled anesthetics (eg, sevoflurane), intravenous anesthetics (eg, propofol), and barbiturates produce slowing of the EEG frequency when used in higher

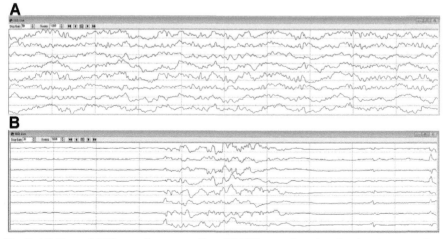

Fig. 3. (*A*) Normal EEG waveform recording. (*B*) EEG recording showing burst suppression. (*Courtesy of* K. Eggan, CNIM, New Haven, CT.)

concentrations. During deep anesthesia with these agents, a "burst suppression" pattern is noticed (**Fig. 3**B), which is characterized by high-frequency "bursts" alternating with flat tracings "suppression."

- Nitrous oxide does not produce burst suppression but produces fast oscillatory activity.
- Ketamine increases theta frequencies and decreases alpha oscillations but does not produce burst suppression.
- Opiates produce loss of beta waves, slow alpha waves, and an increase in delta wave activity. Commonly used opiates do not cause burst suppression in clinical doses.

Pathologic factors

- Hypoglycemia causes EEG changes that are characterized by increased activity in the delta and theta frequencies.
- Any cortical injury that alters the brain homeostasis (eg, trauma, bleeding, or hematoma).
- Diffuse encephalopathy (eg, virus induced, drug induced, or metabolic derangements).
- Hyperventilation-induced hypocapnia ($Paco_2$ <20 mm Hg), which causes generalized slowing of the EEG activity.
- Changes in the cerebral blood flow produce rapid changes in the EEG. With progressive reduction of cerebral blood flow and ischemia, progressive decrease in synaptic activity results in loss of high-frequency activity, loss of power, and ultimately EEG silence (**Table 1**).
- Temperature: Hypothermia with core temperature less than 35°C.
- Seizures: Intraoperative EEG can aid in the diagnosis of focal or generalized seizure, which is seen as polyspike discharges from the affected area.

Clinical Utility

Multichannel EEG is used as a monitor of global or focal cerebral perfusion and to detect epileptiform activity. In the intraoperative period it is indicated for cases with

Table 1			
EEG frequency: beta greater than 12 Hz, theta 4–8 Hz, delta 0–4 Hz			
Cerebral Blood Flow (mL/100 g/min)	EEG Changes	Severity and Neuronal Injury	Time to Cell Death
35–70	Normal	None	
25–35	Loss of fast (beta) frequencies, often not seen during general anesthesia	Mild, reversible	
18–25	EEG slowing into theta range, decrease in amplitude	Mild, reversible	Hours
12–18	Further slowing to delta range, decrease in amplitude	Moderate, reversible	
8–12	Severe amplitude loss at all frequencies	Severe, cell death	Minutes
<8	Loss of activity, isoelectric EEG	Loss of neurons	

Adapted from Jameson LC, Janik DJ, Sloan TB. Electrophysiologic monitoring in neurosurgery. Anesthesiol Clin 2007; 25:605; with permission.

a high potential for cortical ischemia, such as carotid endarterectomy, select supratentorial surgery, and epilepsy surgery for monitoring epileptic activity. EEG analysis can also be used to monitor for isoelectricity under hypothermic arrest. Similarly, it is used to avoid isoelectricity by titrating anesthetics to avoid reaching excessively deep planes of anesthesia.

Processed Electroencephalography

EEG waveform data is "processed" using power spectral analysis. Sine waves extracted at different frequencies are plotted over time and then overlaid using Fourier transformation to produce a single dimensionless value. There are several commercially available processed EEG monitors with slight variations in signal processing and information displayed. In general, all processed EEG uses fewer electrodes (usually one to four) compared with the full EEG. These monitoring modalities have simpler electrode placement in the operating room setting and are more straightforward to analyze and interpret. Each of the commercially available monitors use propriety algorithms to process EEG waveforms (**Table 2**).

The goal of processed EEGs is to monitor the relative density of different waveforms corresponding to the following states: awake, sedated, surgical anesthesia, and burst suppression. Data are then used to titrate anesthetic agents to avoid periods of possible awareness under anesthesia and unnecessary burst suppression. Bispectral index is the most widely used with a typical target goal of 40 to 60 for general anesthesia.

Caveats of Electroencephalography Monitoring

EEG monitoring modalities are expensive, and do not completely guarantee the presence of unconsciousness, lack of awareness, or the absence of cerebral ischemia, especially if there is preexisting neural damage. Furthermore, use of intraoperative EEG is prone to multiple artifacts, from the use of cautery, skin contact and impedance, patient movement, and location of lead placement.

SOMATOSENSORY EVOKED POTENTIALS

Intraoperatively, SSEPs are used in a variety of surgeries to monitor the integrity of the posterior (dorsal) columns of the spinal cord. An electrical stimulus is applied to a peripheral nerve, typically the median or ulnar nerve at the wrist for upper extremity SSEPs and the posterior tibial nerve at the ankle for lower extremity SSEPs, using needle or surface electrodes near the nerve.[4] Impulses ascend primarily in the dorsal column fibers of the spinal cord, which then synapse in the lower medulla. These then decussate at the level of the medulla and travel up the brainstem as the medial lemniscus to synapse in the contralateral thalamus. From there, relay neuron nerve fibers form the thalamocortical radiations, which travel through the internal capsule and synapse in the primary sensory cortex of the parietal lobe. SSEPs are useful in assessing the integrity of the sensory system from the peripheral nerves through to the cerebral cortex (**Figs. 4** and **5**).

Common indications for use of SSEPs include:

- A wide variety of spine surgeries, including scoliosis repair and posterior spinal instrumentations/fixations
- Carotid endarterectomies
- Some intracranial tumors
- Cardiovascular surgeries

Table 2
Commercially available processed EEG monitors

	Index	Company	Index Range	Works with Agents	Not Work with Agents/Disadvantages
1	Bispectrum Index (BSI)	Aspect Medical Systems (now Covidien), United States, 1992	0–100	Propofol, midazolam, and isoflurane Outperformed all	Nitrous oxide and ketamine Problems with EMG
2	Narcotrend Index NCT	MonitorTechnik, Germany, 2000	0–100	Children, sevoflurane propofol/remifentanil EMG susceptibility Good artifact removal	Neuromuscular blocking agents Complex algorithm Slowest response to a change in sedation
3	Entropy Index	Datex-Ohmeda Company, United States, 2003	0–100 1–91	Desflurane, sevoflurane propofol, thiopental	Ketamine
4	Patient State Index (PSI) or (PSA)	Physiomatrix (now SED Line Systems), United States, 2001	0–100	Propofol, alfentanil, nitrous oxide EMG susceptibility	—
5	AEP-Monitor (AAI)	Danmeter, Denmark, 2001	0–100 or 1–60	Propofol, midazolam, and isoflurane	No effects of nitrous oxide and ketamine
6	Snap Index	Everest Biomedical Instruments, United States, 2002		Sevoflurane and sevoflurane/nitrous oxide	Sensitive to unintentional awareness
7	Cerebral State Index (CSI)	Danmeter A/S, Denmark, 2004	0–100	Propofol	Nitrous oxide

Abbreviation: EMG, electromyographic.
Data from Al-Kadi MI, Reaz MB, Ali MA. Evolution of electroencephalogram signal analysis techniques during anesthesia. Sensors 2013;13(5): 6605-35.

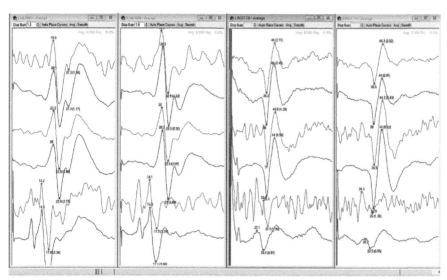

Fig. 4. Normal SSEP waveform during a spine surgery. (*Courtesy of* K. Eggan, CNIM, New Haven, CT.)

Factors Affecting the Amplitude and Latency of Somatosensory Evoked Potentials Waveforms

Similar to the EEG waveform, several factors including pharmacologic and physiologic and disease states influence SSEP signals.

Pharmacologic agents

- Halogenated inhalational agents cause dose-dependent reduction in amplitude and increase in latency, with a greater effect on cortex compared with spinal, peripheral, and subcortical tracings.[5]
- Nitrous oxide works synergistically with inhalational and most intravenous agents to decrease amplitude and increase latency of SSEPs.
- Intravenous agents with the notable exceptions of ketamine and etomidate decrease amplitude and increase latency of SSEP recordings.
- Barbiturates cause dose-dependent decreases in amplitude and increases in latency. Barbiturate doses that induce coma are still compatible with SSEP monitoring[6] even when they are dosed to produce burst suppression in the EEG.
- Propofol causes amplitude decrease and increased latency, although less pronounced than inhalational agents including nitrous oxide, or midazolam administered in doses to achieve comparable planes of anesthesia. Propofol is used for SSEP monitoring especially with opioids.[7]
- Etomidate causes increased amplitude with increased latency on SSEP cortical recordings.
- Ketamine causes increased amplitude with no change in latency or cortical potentials.[8]
- Opioids mildly decrease cortical SSEP amplitude and mildly increase latency with minimal effect on subcortical and peripheral potentials. Bolus dosing of opioids has a greater impact on SSEP changes than continuous infusion.[9]
- Benzodiazepines alone have little effect on SSEPs but may increase latency with the concomitant administration of nitrous oxide.

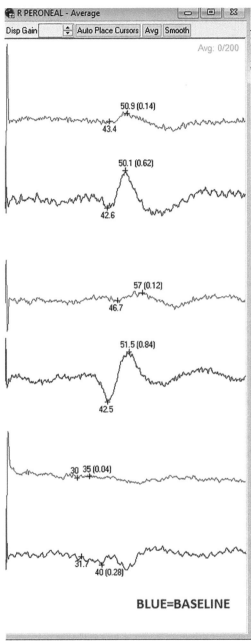

Fig. 5. Loss of greater than 50% amplitude in SSEP waveform during the placement of a spine fixator device, which was immediately removed. (*Courtesy of* K. Eggan, CNIM, New Haven, CT.)

Physiologic factors

- Temperature: Mild hypothermia increases SSEP latency but not amplitude. Although profound hypothermia silences SSEPs completely, mild hyperthermia decreases latency without affecting amplitude.[10]
- Tissue perfusion: Similar to EEG changes, cerebral blood flow less than 18 mL/min/100 g of tissue affects SSEPs. Amplitude is initially reduced and cortical SSEPs is lost with worsening hypotension. Regional ischemia caused by vascular injury, surgical traction, clipping, embolic effects, or positioning are common causes of altered SSEP monitoring during surgery. If mild, anemia can actually cause a mild increase in SSEP amplitude and reduced latency caused by improved viscosity effects, but worsening anemia causes decreases in amplitude and increased latency.[11]
- Although early responses to ischemia or hypoxia can manifest as a transient increase in SSEP amplitude, severe, progressive hypoxemia is associated with a decrease in SSEP amplitude and an increase in latency, eventually resulting in complete loss of cortical SSEP waves. Ventilation and $Paco_2$ levels have little effect on SSEP monitoring.[6]
- Intracranial hypertension causes decreased SSEP monitoring and eventual loss of responses in conjunction with uncal herniation.

MOTOR EVOKED POTENTIALS

MEPs are measured by exciting the motor cortex and subsequently measuring the electrical activity in the muscles of the hands or feet. MEP monitoring is a method of assessing the integrity of the corticospinal tract and the anterior segments of the spinal cord during spinal surgery. It has a high sensitivity and specificity to detect intraoperative neurologic deficits.[12]

Muscle responses to stimulation of the motor cortex are especially impacted by increasing concentrations of inhaled anesthetics and use of neuromuscular blockade, because MEPs are extremely sensitive to these medications. Special stimulation techniques and certain anesthetic regimens are used to optimize MEPs. Monitoring techniques are divided according to the site of stimulation (motor cortex or spinal cord), method of stimulation (electrical potential or magnetic field), and the site of recording (spinal cord or peripheral mixed nerve and muscle).

MEP monitoring is new compared with SSEPs monitoring and has gained popularity after isolated motor injury without sensory changes was described following idiopathic scoliosis procedures. MEP monitoring is now the standard of care in spinal deformity surgeries. Importantly, MEP changes were noted in 6% of spine deformity surgeries and 72% of these changes were reversible.[13] The ability to maintain neural integrity and prevent devastating injury has led to MEP monitoring in a growing number of surgical cases. When intraoperative use of MEPs is planned, soft bite blocks should be placed between the upper and lower molars to prevent the patient from biting either the tongue or the endotracheal tube during stimulation.

CRANIAL NERVE ELECTROMYOGRAM MONITORING

Often, individual cranial nerves may be monitored depending on the location of surgical resection. Examples include cranial nerve V and VII during the resection of cerebellopontine angle tumors and/or acoustic neuroma resection. Lower cranial nerves (VII, IX, X, XII) are monitored in certain thyroid resections and brainstem tumor resections. The hypoglossal nerve is monitored during open carotid endarterectomy.

A single nerve electromyography aids in successfully isolating the "at risk" nerve during establishment of surgical access and while performing the resection, allowing preservation of its vital function. The anesthetic considerations focus solely on the avoidance of neuromuscular blockade during the monitoring period. A specialized neural integrity monitor electromyographic (EMG) endotracheal tube may be required in instances that require monitoring cranial nerve X and its laryngeal nerves.

BRAINSTEM AUDITORY EVOKED POTENTIALS

BAEPs are recorded using a loud acoustic stimulus in the ear canal with an ear insert device. The sound is transduced by ear structures, with information conducted to the brainstem via the eighth cranial nerve. Recording electrodes are placed at the head near the mastoid process or ear lobe. Five main short-latency peaks (I to V) are usually seen within the first 10 milliseconds after stimulation (**Fig. 6**).[14]

BAEPs are commonly used in conjunction with other neuromonitoring modalities during posterior fossa surgeries to assess brainstem function. BAEPs are typically resistant to anesthesia as compared with other evoked potentials.

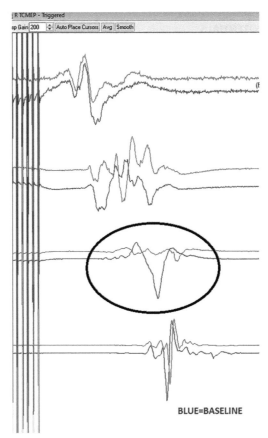

Fig. 6. The circled area captures the intraoperative change in waveform with greater than 50% decrease in MEP amplitude, during spine surgery. (*Courtesy of* K. Eggan, CNIM, New Haven, CT.)

RECOMMENDATIONS FOR CHOICE OF ANESTHETICS DURING THE USE OF VARIOUS NEUROMONITORING MODALITIES

The effects of medications used for induction of anesthesia typically do not persist long enough to influence IONM. Conversely, it is important to use an appropriate intraoperative maintenance regime to facilitate monitoring techniques. The authors recommend considering the following approaches:

- Use of SSEP monitoring: Propofol infusion at anesthetic doses (titrated to patient age and comorbidities; eg, 80–120 μg/kg/min) along with an opioid infusion (eg, remifentanil at 0.1–0.2 μg/kg/min, fentanyl infusion at 2–3 μg/kg/h, or sufentanil infusion at 0.15–0.4 μg/kg/h). An alternative to this is the use of a volatile anesthetic, such as sevoflurane at approximately 0.5 minimum alveolar concentration (MAC) along with propofol infusion and opioid. Neuromuscular blocking agents are used as necessary if SSEP monitoring is the only monitor that is being used intraoperatively.
- Use of SSEPs and MEPs monitoring: Propofol infusion at anesthetic doses (titrated to patient age and comorbidities; eg, 80–120 μg/kg/min) along with an opioid infusion (eg, remifentanil at 0.1–0.2 μg/kg/min, fentanyl infusion at 2–3 μg/kg/h, or sufentanil infusion at 0.15–0.4 μg/kg/h). Volatile anesthetics are typically avoided because of the exquisite sensitivity of MEPs to them. Neuromuscular blocking agents are avoided during the period of monitoring. A short-acting neuromuscular blocking agent may be used to facilitate intubation.
- Use of SSEPs and cranial nerve EMG: The approach to the anesthetic to what has already been described for MEP monitoring.
- Use of isolated cranial nerve EMG: No neuromuscular blocking agent during the period of monitoring. Up to 1.5 MAC volatile anesthetic and no restriction in opioid administration.
- Use of EEG, SSEPs, and MEPs: Volatile anesthetics are administered at approximately 0.5 MAC, and/or a propofol infusion is used in combination with an opioid infusion (eg, remifentanil at 0.1–0.2 μg/kg/min, fentanyl infusion at 2–4 μg/kg/h, or sufentanil infusion at 0.15–0.4 μg/kg/h). Alternatively, fentanyl boluses may be used to maintain analgesia. Dexmedetomidine is a valuable adjunct when this combination is being used and aids in reducing the dose of propofol required. Neuromuscular blocking agents are avoided during the period of monitoring. A short- or intermediate-acting neuromuscular blocking agent may be used to facilitate intubation.

CONTROVERSIES IN NEUROMONITORING

With the increasing use of neuromonitoring modalities in various types of surgeries, several studies have analyzed the benefits and cost effectiveness of their routine use.

According to the guidelines for the use of electrophysiologic monitoring for human spinal cord surgery,[15] the use of multimodal IONM including SSEPs and MEPs during spinal cord/spinal column surgery is a level I recommendation because of its reliability and validity in assessing spinal cord integrity. MEP recordings are superior to SSEP recordings during spinal cord/spinal column surgery as diagnostic adjuncts for assessment of spinal cord integrity and are recommended if used for this purpose. Use of multimodal IONM, including SSEPs and MEP recording, during spinal cord/spinal column surgery does not improve gross total tumor resection or improve neurologic outcome, when used during intramedullary tumor resection procedures (Level II evidence).[15]

Daniel and colleagues[16] performed a literature review and meta-analysis of six studies comparing neurologic events with and without IONM. Based on the evidence provided in the studies reviewed, they concluded that IONM did not result in fewer neurologic events compared with no monitoring (Level 2 evidence). For surgeries involving intramedullary lesions, there was a trend to fewer neurologic events in patients who underwent surgery with IONM.[16]

A literature search of Medline database was performed and relevant studies from all levels were included in a narrative review by Charalampidis and colleagues.[17] Nearly all of these studies investigated the use of IONM in the setting of spine surgery. Overall, these reports support the use of multimodal IONM in spinal tumor resections. The combined use of SSEPs and MEPs seems to provide increased accuracy for detecting injury to sensory and motor pathways, reaching a high sensitivity, specificity, positive predictive value, and negative predictive value.[17]

In 2010, Ayoub and colleagues[18] performed a cost-effectiveness analysis on a cohort of 210 patients who underwent cervical spine surgery with SSEP monitoring. The total cost of the surgery, hospital stay, neuromonitoring, and medical expenditures associated with postoperative neurologic injury was accounted for in the cost analysis. Given an incidence of 0.1% for spinal cord injury, the authors assumed that without SSEP monitoring 1 out of 201 patients would have had a permanent spinal cord injury. In their estimation, the total annual cost savings for a single injured patient would range from $64,074 to $102,192 for their institution, whereas the yearly expenditure on SSEP amounted to only $31,546.[18]

Recently, Ney and colleagues[19] constructed a simulated cost-effectiveness model to estimate the value of IONM to avert postoperative neurologic deficits. The model assumptions included parameters, such as the surgical risk, frequency of cases averted, and cost per case estimates. The authors concluded that use of IONM in spinal procedures was associated with a 49% reduction in relative risk for neurologic complications. They further estimated that the cost of monitoring to prevent a single neurologic injury was $63,387.[19]

Conversely, Traynelis and colleagues,[20] in a single-center study, reported a case series of 720 consecutive patients who underwent routine cervical spine procedures without the use of IONM. The authors reported a 0.4% rate of postoperative neurologic deficits. Furthermore, at 1-year follow-up, all patients had significantly improved, and their neurologic deficits had complete resolution. The authors, therefore, questioned the utility of IONM during routine cervical spine surgery. Additionally, further analysis was performed to explore the economic impact of IONM during cervical spine procedures. This cost analysis was based on the Current Procedural Terminology reimbursement codes. They concluded that significant savings could be achieved by not using IONM in simple cervical spine procedures.[20]

In a large retrospective propensity score matched analysis, using a national database, Cole and colleagues[21] investigated single-level spinal procedures, with and without the use of IONM, with the goal of comparing the occurrence of neurologic complications. Trauma, spinal tumors, and revisions were excluded from the analysis. A total of 85,640 patients were included in the analysis with a minority (13%) receiving IONM during the surgery. The authors found no differences in neurologic complications between those who did and did not receive IONM. They concluded that the use of IONM was associated with higher costs ranging from $2859 to $3841.[21]

In summary, currently there is conflicting evidence regarding the cost effectiveness of use of IONM in routine spine surgeries. Additional expenditures in terms of training neuromonitoring personnel, use of specialized equipment for monitoring, and choice of anesthetic techniques would further complicate the evaluation of these monitoring modalities.

Multimodal IONM is also commonly used in carotid endarterectomies. Hong and colleagues[22] analyzed 668 carotid endarterectomy cases at six surgical centers, and found that a decrease in amplitude of 50% or more in any EEG or SSEP channel should be used as the criteria to indicate the need for shunting or to initiate a neuro-protective protocol. A reduction of 50% or greater in the beta band of the EEG or amplitude of the SSEP was observed in 150 cases, most of which occurred during cross-clamping. No patient showed signs of a cerebral infarct after surgery. Selective shunting based on EEG and SSEP monitoring can reduce carotid endarterectomy intraoperative stroke rate to a near zero level if trained personnel practice with standardized protocols.

In conclusion, the role of multimodal monitoring for the intraoperative detection of physiologic changes allows the care team to decrease the likelihood of potential cell or nerve injury. However, with the possible exception of certain spinal procedures and carotid endarterectomies, the benefits in terms of prevention of permanent neurologic complications or cost effectiveness are not well documented and data are generally inconclusive because of the absence of rigorously controlled trials.

DISCLOSURE

No conflicts of interest.

CLINICS CARE POINTS

- With the increasing use of neuromonitoring modalities during intracranial, carotid and spine procedures, it is important to understand the effects of physiological changes and pharmacologic interventions on these monitoring modalities.
- There is currently a level I recommendation for the use of multimodal intraoperative neuromonitoring (including SSEPs and MEPs) during procedures involving the spine. This recommendation is based on the reliability and validity of these monitoring modalities in assessing spinal cord integrity.
- MEPs are superior to SSEP recordings as diagnostic adjuncts for the assessment of spinal cord integrity.
- There is insufficient evidence for routine use of neuromonitoring for routine cervical spine procedures in neurologically intact patients.
- Controversies continue to exist regarding the cost effectiveness of use of intraoperative multimodal neuromonitoring for procedures other than spine surgery.

REFERENCES

1. Jameson LC, Janik DJ, Sloan TB. Electrophysiologic monitoring in neurosurgery. Anesthesiol Clin 2007;25(3):605–30.
2. Cordeau JP. Monorhythmic frontal delta activity in the human electroencephalogram: a study of 100 cases. Electroencephalogr Clin Neurophysiol 1959;11:733–46.
3. Reiher J, Beaudry M, Leduc CP. Temporal intermittent rhythmic delta activity (TIRDA) in the diagnosis of complex partial epilepsy: sensitivity, specificity and predictive value. Can J Neurol Sci 1989;16(4):398–401.
4. Toleikis JR, American Society of Neurophysiological Monitoring. Intraoperative monitoring using somatosensory evoked potentials. A position statement by the

American Society of Neurophysiological Monitoring. J Clin Monit Comput 2005; 19(3):241–58.

5. Sloan TB, Heyer EJ. Anesthesia for intraoperative neurophysiologic monitoring of the spinal cord. J Clin Neurophysiol 2002;19(5):430–43.

6. Banoub M, Tetzlaff JE, Schubert A. Pharmacologic and physiologic influences affecting sensory evoked potentials: implications for perioperative monitoring. Anesthesiology 2003;99(3):716–37.

7. Borrissov B, Langeron O, Lille F, et al. Combination of propofol-sufentanil on somatosensory evoked potentials in surgery of the spine. Ann Fr Anesth Reanim 1995;14:326–30.

8. Schubert A, Licina MG, Lineberry PJ. The effect of ketamine on human somatosensory evoked potentials and its modification by nitrous oxide [published correction appears in Anesthesiology 1990;72(6):1104]. Anesthesiology 1990; 72(1):33–9.

9. Becker A, Amlong C, Rusy DA. Somatosensory-evoked potentials. In: Koht A, Sloan TB, Toleikis JR, editors. Monitoring the nervous system for anesthesiologists and other health care professionals. Springer; 2017. p. 3–18.

10. Stecker MM, Cheung AT, Pochettino A, et al. Deep hypothermic circulatory arrest: II. Changes in electroencephalogram and evoked potentials during rewarming. Ann Thorac Surg 2001;71(1):22–8.

11. Zanatta P, Bosco E, Comin A, et al. Effect of mild hypothermic cardiopulmonary bypass on the amplitude of somatosensory-evoked potentials. J Neurosurg Anesthesiol 2014;26(2):161–6.

12. Nagao S, Roccaforte P, Moody RA. The effects of isovolemic hemodilution and reinfusion of packed erythrocytes on somatosensory and visual evoked potentials. J Surg Res 1978;25(6):530–7.

13. Ushirozao H, Yoshida G, Hasegawa T, et al Characteristics of false-positive alerts on transcranial motor evoked potential monitoring during pediatric scoliosis and adult spinal deformity surgery: an "anesthetic fade" phenomenon, J Neurosurg Spine 32(3); 423-431.

14. Holdefer RN, Skinner SA. Motor evoked potential recovery with surgeon interventions and neurological outcomes: a meta-analysis and structural causal model for spine deformity surgeries. Clin Neurophysiol 2020;131(7):1556–66.

15. Hadley MN, Shank CD, Rozzelle CJ, et al. Guidelines for the use of electrophysiological monitoring for surgery of the human spinal column and spinal cord. Neurosurgery 2017;81(Issue 5):713–32.

16. Daniel JW, Ricardo Vieira B, Jerônimo Buzetti M, et al. Intraoperative neurophysiological monitoring in spine surgery. A systematic review and meta-analysis. Spine 2018;43(Issue 16):1154–60.

17. Charalampidis A, Jiang F, Jamie R, et al. The use of intraoperative neurophysiological monitoring in spine surgery. Global Spine J 2020;10(1 Suppl):104S–14S.

18. Ayoub C, Zreik T, Sawaya R, et al. Significance and cost-effectiveness of somatosensory evoked potential monitoring in cervical spine surgery. Neurol India 2010; 58:424–8.

19. Ney JP, van der Goes DN, Watanabe JH. Cost-effectiveness of intraoperative neurophysiological monitoring for spinal surgeries: beginning steps. Clin Neurophysiol 2012;123:1705–7.

20. Traynelis VC, Abode-lyamah KO, Leick KM, et al. Cervical decompression and reconstruction without intraoperative neurophysiological monitoring. J Neurosurg Spine 2012;16:107–13.
21. Cole T, Veeravagu A, Zhang M, et al. Intraoperative neuromonitoring in single-level spinal procedures: a retrospective propensity score-matched analysis in a national longitudinal database. Spine (Phila Pa 1976) 2014;39:1950–9.
22. Hong L, Di Giorgio AM, Williams ES, et al. Protocol for electrophysiological monitoring of carotid endarterectomies. J Biomed Res 2010;24(6):460–6.

Intraoperative MRI for Adult and Pediatric Neurosurgery

Dean Laochamroonvorapongse, MD, MPH[a],*, Marie A. Theard, MD[a],
Alexander T. Yahanda, MS[b], Michael R. Chicoine, MD[b]

KEYWORDS

- Neurosurgery • Intraoperative magnetic resonance imaging
- Pediatric anesthesiology • MRI safety

KEY POINTS

- Intraoperative MRI (iMRI) has advanced significantly over the past 25 years, allowing neurosurgeons to account for brain shift and maximize the extent of surgical resection in near-real time.
- Combining the operating room environment with a mobile magnetic field presents multiple challenges for the perioperative team, requiring increased safety protocols and training.
- By understanding the anesthetic considerations for iMRI procedures and the limitations of monitors and equipment in this environment, anesthesiologists play a crucial role in ensuring patient safety.

INTRODUCTION

Intraoperative MRI (iMRI) technology has advanced significantly since its invention in 1994, allowing neurosurgeons to obtain diagnostic-quality imaging in near real-time to account for brain shift, evaluate the extent of surgical resection, and detect complications. Although initially used primarily for brain tumor resections, iMRI is now used for a variety of neurosurgical procedures in both adults and children, including epilepsy surgery, laser interstitial thermal therapy (LITT), awake craniotomies, cyst aspirations, deep brain stimulators, and spinal cord tumor resections. Combining the risks of an MRI suite with an operating room (OR) environment creates a challenging workspace for the anesthesiologist to safely care for patients. This article provides an overview of the evidence supporting the use of iMRI in neurosurgery and reviews the major equipment and safety considerations anesthesiologists must recognize to plan and deliver optimal perioperative care.

[a] Department of Anesthesiology and Perioperative Medicine, Oregon Health and Science University, 3181 Southwest Sam Jackson Park Road, Mail Code-UH2, Portland, OR 97239, USA;
[b] Department of Neurosurgery, Washington University School of Medicine, 660 South Euclid Avenue, St Louis, MO 63110, USA
* Corresponding author.
E-mail address: laochamr@ohsu.edu

Anesthesiology Clin 39 (2021) 211–225
https://doi.org/10.1016/j.anclin.2020.11.010   **anesthesiology.theclinics.com**
1932-2275/21/© 2020 Elsevier Inc. All rights reserved.

HISTORY OF INTRAOPERATIVE MRI

Before the invention of iMRI, neurosurgeons relied on stereotactic navigation systems to precisely map the location of brain lesions. These stereotactic navigation systems were initially bulky, frame-based systems that impeded access to the patient's airway. Over time, frame-based navigation was replaced by modern frameless stereotactic systems that use an infrared stereoscopic camera or electromagnetic field to determine the 3-dimensional position of structures. Frameless navigation systems require a "registration" process that involves either placing fiducials or using a face-tracing system in order to layer a series of fixed points of the patient's head in surgical position over preoperative imaging to increase operative precision.[1]

Despite these advances, stereotactic navigation systems registered to preoperative imaging alone cannot account for brain shift, which is the movement of intracranial structures after opening the cranium and dura. The brain can shift more than 1 cm intraoperatively, depending on the patient's position, degree of hyperventilation, cerebrospinal fluid drained, surgical bleeding, and volume of tissue resected. Brain shift worsens as surgery progresses, decreasing the accuracy of stereotactic navigation, especially for deep-seated brain lesions or those near eloquent regions. IMRI works synergistically with stereotactic navigation, because imaging obtained in the OR can be used to account for brain shift and increase the volume of tumor that can be safely resected.

The first iMRI system was the SIGNA SP, a midstrength 0.5-T MRI that was built in 1994 at the Brigham and Women's Hospital in collaboration with General Electric Medical Systems (Milwaukee, WI, USA). With this system, the patient remained inside the bore of the MRI during the entire operation, requiring surgeons to operate through a small space between 2 donut-shaped magnets. Although this enabled surgeons to perform certain operations with the patient in the MRI scanner, other surgical approaches were impossible given the limited access to the patient. The main advantage of this system was its ability to generate frequent, real-time MRIs within minutes without moving the patient or altering the surgical field. This real-time imaging enabled the prompt detection and definitive treatment of unexpected surgical complications, such as intracranial hemorrhage.[2,3] However, surgeons using the SIGNA SP operated *within* the 5-G line, necessitating the use of only MR safe equipment for anesthesia and surgery, including titanium surgical instruments that were reportedly brittle and difficult to sterilize. For these reasons, this iMRI system is no longer commercially available. Current iMRI systems have evolved so that most surgery occurs *behind* the 5-G line, which allows for the routine use of MR unsafe items ubiquitous to modern neurosurgical practice, such as regular (stainless steel) surgical instruments, an operating microscope, and neurophysiologic monitoring.

INTRAOPERATIVE MRI FIELD STRENGTHS

Modern iMRI systems that allow surgeons to operate behind the 5-G line can be broadly divided into low field (0.15–0.3 T) and high field (1.5 or 3T) based on their magnetic field strengths.

Low-Field Intraoperative MRI

With low-field iMRI systems like the Medtronic PoleStar N-20 (Medtronic, Louisville, CO, USA), the field strength of the magnet is greatly reduced, allowing it to remain near the patient during surgery at the expense of image quality and resolution. The PoleStar has 2 vertical magnetic discs on a U-shaped arm that is kept under the OR table near the patient's head during surgery. These discs generate minimal magnetic field, permitting the use of regular surgical instruments.[2] During intraoperative imaging, the discs are raised up to the level of the patient's head, and an accordion-shaped radiofrequency (RF) shield (StarShield; Medtronic) slides over the entire patient, minimizing the effects of external electrical noise on image quality. As a result, the anesthesiologist is unable to directly visualize the patient during intraoperative imaging, which can take up to 20 minutes.[4] Low-field iMRI systems are portable and much less expensive than high-field iMRI systems. However, patients with brain tumor having surgery with low-field iMRI typically require a postoperative MRI in a diagnostic-quality scanner because of the limited resolution of these low-field magnets. Obtaining this postoperative MRI for infants and young children may require an additional anesthetic and its concomitant risks.

High-Field Intraoperative MRI

High-field iMRI systems use a diagnostic-quality magnet (1.5 or 3 T) supercooled with liquid helium or nitrogen that is kept further away from the patient during surgery, allowing neurosurgeons to operate *behind* the 5-G line using regular surgical instruments, microscope, and neuromonitoring in a way resembling a conventional OR. High-field iMRI provides diagnostic-quality imaging that can be used to update the stereotactic navigation system to account for brain shift. High-field iMRI devices have gained prominence because of their ability to perform advanced imaging techniques, such as perfusion imaging, diffusion tensor imaging (DTI), and MR spectroscopy. These techniques can be helpful in identifying residual tumor, outlining critical white matter tracts, or locating areas of ischemia.

When intraoperative imaging is needed, the magnet can either move into the OR via overhead ceiling-mounted rails and over the patient's head (ie, stationary-patient, mobile-magnet iMRI suite), or the patient can be moved on an MR-safe trolley into a nearby magnet (ie, stationary-magnet, mobile-patient iMRI suite). Regardless of configuration, the main disadvantage of high-field iMRI is that safely moving a surgical patient into the magnet to obtain imaging takes time and preparation. To maintain sterility of the surgical field, the patient must be sheathed in an additional sterile plastic drape before scanning. All ferromagnetic surgical instruments and MR unsafe equipment must also be accounted for and moved behind the 5-G line or out of the OR before the magnet enters the room. After intraoperative imaging is obtained, the process must be reversed before the operation can resume. As a result of the time delay, imaging is obtained in near real-time, limiting the amount of iMRI scans that can practically be performed during a single operation. Studies have found that iMRI adds a significant amount of time to the typical neurosurgical case.[5] Fortunately, this added operative time has not been associated with an increase in surgical or anesthetic complications.[6]

Another disadvantage is the initial cost of $5 to 10 million required to build an RF-shielded iMRI suite, which may prove prohibitive for many institutions.[5] As a result, these suites are often built with versatility in mind and can be used for conventional surgical procedures when iMRI is not needed. With proper design and planning, high-field iMRI scanners can also be used for diagnostic imaging to help recoup initial costs and improve patient throughput. For example, Pamir and colleagues[7] successfully performed 19,000 outpatient MRIs over 3 years using a 3-T iMRI. For stationary-patient, mobile-magnet iMRI devices, the IMRIS Hybrid Operating Suite (IMRIS Deerfield Imaging Inc, Minnetonka, MN, USA) is currently used at more than 75 institutions worldwide. This suite has a ceiling-mounted mobile magnet that is housed in a separate garage between 2 ORs. The magnet may move between each OR, allowing for better efficiency and resource utilization.[8]

EVIDENCE SUPPORTING INTRAOPERATIVE MRI USE IN NEUROSURGERY

A comprehensive review of the neurosurgical literature supporting iMRI use is beyond the scope of this article; however, a short overview of the benefits of iMRI is presented to provide background for the anesthesiologist caring for iMRI patients.

In 2011, Senft and colleagues[9] published the first prospective randomized controlled iMRI trial, which used the PoleStar N-20 low-field iMRI to assess the impact of iMRI on extent of resection (EOR) for adult glioma patients. Out of 49 patients, 24 had surgical resection with iMRI and 25 controls had surgical resection without iMRI. Of iMRI patients, 33% had further resection after intraoperative imaging, and 96% of patients in this group had gross total tumor resection (GTR) on postoperative MRI compared with 68% of the control group ($P = .023$). There were no statistically significant differences in postoperative neurologic deficits between the 2 groups. They also found that increasing EOR was a significant predictor of improved progression-free survival.

Many retrospective and prospective studies, including some large, multicenter studies, have assessed the impact of iMRI on EOR and survival in tumor patients.[10–14] These studies have found that iMRI is a useful tool for identifying residual tumor, increasing the EOR, and increasing rates of GTR for many kinds of brain tumors. Increased EOR, especially GTR, was a common prognostic factor for overall and progression-free survival, indicating that iMRI may be useful for enabling safe maximal resection of tumor and for prolonging survival.

For ethical reasons, no randomized controlled trials using iMRI have been conducted in pediatric patients, so most of the available evidence consists of case series or comparisons of prospectively acquired iMRI patients with retrospective controls that underwent conventional surgery. Kremer and colleagues[15] published a case series in which a 0.2-T low-strength iMRI was used on 41 patients having 45 neurosurgical procedures; in this group, 31 patients underwent a total of 35 craniotomies for tumor resection. iMRI led to further resection in 60% of craniotomies, increasing the rate of gross total resection to 83% of brain tumor patients. Similarly, in a retrospective, multicenter series of 280 pediatric glioma patients, 46.8% of patients had additional tumor resection after their first iMRI scan.[16] In a single-center study of 65 low-grade glioma patients, 71% of iMRI patients had total resection compared with 41% of retrospective controls having conventional surgery, leading the investigators to suggest the routine use of iMRI for any pediatric LGG resection.[17] Shah and colleagues[5] found that use of iMRI significantly decreased the proportion of pediatric patients requiring early reoperation for additional tumor resection (0% for iMRI, 7.8% for conventional surgery).

In addition to minimizing anxiety and stress associated with reoperation, iMRI may be cost-effective, saving an estimated $23,778 per patient where repeat surgery is prevented.[5] Despite a large body of evidence to date supporting the use of iMRI and other advanced surgical techniques, a recent Cochrane review concluded that higher-level evidence is still needed to prove the benefits of iMRI.[18] Additional prospective trials are required to fully elucidate the relationship between iMRI use and overall and progression-free survival.

ANESTHETIC CONSIDERATIONS FOR INTRAOPERATIVE MRI

An iMRI suite combines the risks of an MR environment with those of a surgical OR, which makes it challenging for the anesthesiologist to deliver safe anesthetic care. In 2015, the American Society of Anesthesiologists published an updated practice advisory for anesthetic care in MRI, but these do not specifically address the iMRI, which requires increased vigilance and the creation of safety protocols unique to this environment.[19] The American College of Radiology (ACR) recently published an updated guidance document on MR safe practices that addresses intraoperative and nonstandard MR environments.[20] The authors recommend that all anesthesiologists working in the iMRI suite review these guidelines.

There are many considerations specific to the iMRI environment that the anesthesiologist must be aware of in order to deliver optimal care. These considerations can be broadly categorized as the physical forces of MRI, equipment and monitoring issues, patient positioning, and contraindications to iMRI.

THE PHYSICAL FORCES OF MRI

The anesthesiologist must be familiar with the 3 major physical forces generated in MRI that may pose a safety risk for patients and staff: the static magnetic field, the dynamic magnetic field, and the RF electromagnetic field. The static magnetic field is always "on" and can lead to ferromagnetic items becoming projectiles. Its strength is measured in Gauss or Tesla, with 20,000 G equaling 1 T. The magnetic field generated by a 3-T iMRI scanner is 60,000 times stronger than that of the earth.[21] Ferromagnetic items are unaffected by static magnetic fields of 5 G and under, which is also a safe level of exposure for humans. Thus, it is essential that the 5- G line surrounding the scanner is clearly outlined in the iMRI suite and that the anesthesiologist is always aware of his or her position and the position of anesthesia equipment in relation to the 5-G line. Clear demarcation of Gauss lines is particularly important for stationary-patient, mobile-magnet iMRI suites, where the 5-G line is a moving entity and may extend into the OR when the magnet is docked in the garage (**Fig. 1**).

The dynamic magnetic field is a smaller magnetic field applied over the static magnetic field during image acquisition, which can induce current in tissues or implants, such as pacemakers.[22] It generates the loud noise commonly heard in the MR environment, which may exceed 100 dB, so earplugs are required for both the patient and the staff during intraoperative scanning. The RF electromagnetic field is one thousand times stronger than the dynamic magnetic field and induces proton excitation, which generates heat and can cause burns, interfere with electrical equipment, and induce current in looped wires. As a result, the axilla and skin creases must be padded with gauze to avoid skin-to-skin contact, and loops must be avoided in electrical wires or intravenous (IV) tubing. This risk can be mitigated by limiting the energy generated by the RF field, which is known as the specific absorption rate.

EQUIPMENT AND MONITORING ISSUES

It is recommended that the specific terms "MR safe," "MR conditional," and "MR unsafe" established in 2005 by the Food and Drug Administration and American Society Testing of Materials be used to describe the relative safety of items in the MR environment.[23] MR safe items pose no known hazards in all MRI environments. MR conditional items have been demonstrated to pose no known hazards in a specified MR environment with specified conditions of use. For instance, the commonly used MR conditional Aestiva/5 MRI anesthesia machine (Datex-Ohmeda, Madison, WI, USA) can be safely used in fields up to 300 G in a 1.5- or 3-T magnet. MR unsafe items are those known to be unsafe in all MR environments and include ferromagnetic items.

Patients undergoing neurosurgical procedures in the iMRI suite are often subject to numerous iatrogenic hemodynamic and physiologic disturbances over the course of the operation (eg, surgical hemorrhage, controlled hyperventilation, diuresis) and require more extensive monitoring compared with patients in diagnostic MRI.

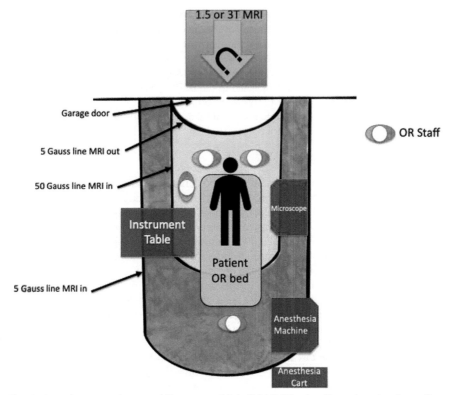

Fig. 1. A stationary-patient, mobile-magnet high-field iMRI suite. Note that the Gauss lines change with the position of the magnet.

Because of this, it is necessary to use MR safe or conditional anesthesia machines, physiologic monitors, infusion pumps, and IV poles that can remain in the OR within the 5-G line during intraoperative scanning. Similarly, the neurosurgeon must also use MR safe pins for head fixation.

Many commonly used pieces of modern anesthesia equipment are MR unsafe, including portable ultrasound machines, train-of-four monitors, video laryngoscopes, fiberoptic bronchoscopes, convective warming devices, and IV fluid warmers. These items can be routinely used in most iMRI suites, but safety protocols must be created to ensure they are moved behind the 5-G line or out of the OR before the magnet enters the room.

LIMITATIONS OF MONITORING IN THE INTRAOPERATIVE MRI ENVIRONMENT

Obtaining reliable electrocardiogram (ECG) monitoring in the iMRI suite may be challenging because of electrical interference. MR conditional monitors come with preset filters that minimize interference but cannot overcome all artifacts. The battery-powered MR conditional ECG modules used in the iMRI suite consist of 4 short electrical wire leads that are connected to ECG electrodes and transmit data wirelessly to the monitor using a fiberoptic converter box. The wires are short to minimize the potential for burns, so the ECG leads are placed on the left side of the chest during iMRI cases. This suboptimal lead placement combined with electrical interference makes

ST segment analysis impossible during scanning, so iMRI-guided surgery is relatively contraindicated in patients at significant risk of myocardial ischemia. Despite this, a recent study of 31 anesthesiologists found that they could correctly detect and identify arrhythmias on ECG rhythm strips with simulated electrical interference.[24] Similarly, the fiberoptic MR conditional pulse oximeters used in the iMRI suite are more sensitive to motion artifact compared with conventional pulse oximeters.

In general, neurophysiologic monitoring can be used for iMRI cases but needs to be completed before scanning, because the leads used during somatosensory and motor-evoked potential monitoring can generate burns or become dislodged during scanning. Most institutions use a checklist to ensure that all neuromonitoring leads are removed, counted, and moved behind the 5-G line. Despite this, pilot studies have reported successfully leaving platinum/iridium neuromonitoring leads in situ during intraoperative scanning in order to maintain neuromonitoring during the final stages of tumor resection, with the only reported complication being first-degree burns on the shoulders of 2 patients in 1 report.[25,26]

At the authors' institutions, a nondisposable MR conditional core temperature probe is placed in the patient's axilla for each iMRI case. Temperature probe urinary catheters are MR unsafe and cannot be used for iMRI cases. Overall, the cooler ambient OR temperature needed to maintain an optimal magnetic field, intermittent application of convective warming, and longer anesthetic duration do not lead to an increased incidence of intraoperative hypothermia during iMRI cases. A study of 76 adults having high-strength iMRI craniotomy found that patients had a mean temperature of 36.7°C in post-anesthesia care unit[27]; similarly, a retrospective review of 105 pediatric iMRI procedures noted a mean temperature of 37°C.[28] It is equally important to avoid hyperthermia during iMRI craniotomy, which has been shown to worsen neurologic outcome in stroke and brain injury patients.[29]

PATIENT POSITIONING AND ACCESS CONSIDERATIONS DURING INTRAOPERATIVE MRI CASES

Overall, patient access is quite limited in the iMRI suite compared with a standard OR. For most stationary-patient, mobile-magnet iMRI suites, the OR table is in a fixed position and the patient is rotated 180° away from the anesthesiologist. As a result, the patient's head is more than 10 feet away from the anesthesia machine, which requires the use of 2 breathing circuits joined together with a straight connector and extra extension tubing on IV, arterial, and gas sampling lines in order to safely reach the patient. This increased dead space may delay inhaled or IV drug administration, requiring higher fresh gas flows or a saline flush if rapid changes in anesthetic depth or hemodynamic parameters are needed. All lines, including temperature probe, urinary catheter, and cerebrospinal fluid drain, should be labeled and easily accessible near the anesthesiologist's workspace. The location of the ECG and pulse oximetry modules under the surgical drapes should also be noted by the anesthesiologist in case their batteries need to be replaced intraoperatively.

Access to the patient's airway is limited with the head being 180° away, often prone in fixation pins or further obscured by the placement of the MRI coil, so the endotracheal tube must be well secured to prevent inadvertent extubation. For this reason, some anesthesiologists prefer nasal intubation, particularly for pediatric patients, because it may be more stable when moving the patient's head. The pilot balloon in standard cuffed PVC endotracheal tubes contains a small metallic spring, so it should be taped near the circuit away from the patient's head to minimize any image artifact during scanning. Armored endotracheal tubes are MR unsafe and cannot be used.

There are certain patients at the extremes of size that may not be able to receive iMRI-guided surgery. Severely obese patients that have successfully received diagnostic MRI may not be able to fit into the bore of the iMRI magnet because of surgical positioning and the added bulk of surgical drapes. These patients require meticulous padding to prevent pressure sores and burns from skin-to-skin contact. A ring-shaped alignment tool (VISIUSeye; IMRIS Deerfield Imaging Inc) that has the exact inner diameter of the magnet bore can be used to ensure that the fully draped patient will fit into the bore of the magnet before scanning. Infants less than 5 kg are typically excluded from having surgery in the iMRI suite, because of the difficulty of obtaining accurate monitoring and adequate ventilation in this population given the limitations of the MR conditional equipment and increased dead space.

CONTRAINDICATIONS TO INTRAOPERATIVE MRI

Before surgery, patients should complete an MR screening form that is reviewed by the MR technologist to ensure that there are no ferromagnetic implants or devices that could become dislodged, malfunction, or cause burns when exposed to the magnetic field. If no one is available to provide a reliable patient history, then patients should undergo radiography to rule out the presence of ferromagnetic implants or devices. Absolute contraindications to iMRI-guided surgery include most cardiac implantable electronic devices (CIED), cochlear implants, vagal nerve stimulators, ferrous intracranial aneurysm clips, and metal joints.[30] Although patients with MR conditional CIED have safely received diagnostic MRIs, each MR conditional device is unique and may require certain limitations or alteration of sequences that may preclude iMRI-guided surgery in a high-field magnet.[31] The device manufacturer's recommendations should always be followed, and the potential risks and benefits of iMRI in these patients should be considered and discussed with the patient.

CREATING A CULTURE OF SAFETY IN THE INTRAOPERATIVE MRI SUITE

The physical forces of MRI can harm patients and staff, leading to serious morbidity and mortality from burns, projectiles, and equipment failure. In 2001, a 6-year-old boy died of intracranial hemorrhage after being struck by a ferromagnetic oxygen tank that was inadvertently brought into the scanner during his sedated MRI.[32] This sentinel event gained national attention, leading to the development of MRI screening protocols and the creation of 4 MRI zones to limit access to the MRI (**Fig. 2**). The entire

MRI Safety Zone	Description
I	Public access area outside of MR environment
II	Interface between Zone I and restricted Zone III; MR screening occurs here
III	Control room; access restricted to those that pass screening (no exceptions)
IV	MRI magnet room; this Zone moves with mobile magnet iMRI systems

Fig. 2. The ACR MRI safety zones. The entire iMRI suite is zone III or IV.

iMRI suite is zone III or IV, so all patients and staff must be screened by the designated MR safety officer before entering.

The increased complexity of the iMRI environment necessitates additional training and safety protocols for the perioperative team beyond those required in diagnostic MRI. It is recommended that key stakeholders in anesthesiology, neurosurgery, radiology, and perioperative nursing work together to create institution-specific protocols that account for type of iMRI used.[33] Evidence from the World Health Organization's Safe Surgery Saves Lives program supports a strong association between a checklist-based, collaborative approach to creating a culture of safety in the OR and improved patient outcomes.[34] As an example, the authors briefly describe the iMRI workflow at Oregon Health and Science University (OHSU).

At OHSU, all members of the iMRI team complete annual MR screening forms and online modules reviewing both the fundamentals of MRI safety and the considerations specific to the stationary-patient, mobile-magnet iMRI suite. To prevent staff injury and accidents, door access to the iMRI suite is limited to only those that have completed this training. Before each iMRI case, an additional perioperative nurse is designated the MR safety officer and is responsible for completing the Room Zero checklist (**Fig. 3**), ensuring that there are no extra ferromagnetic items in the OR. Any MR unsafe items brought into the OR are added to the checklist and removed from the OR at the end of the case. If it is unclear whether an item is ferromagnetic, it should be tested with a handheld magnet before entering the room.

A substerile room adjacent to the OR serves as a safe space beyond the 5-G line to store routinely used equipment and ferromagnetic personal items, like pagers, phones, watches, and stethoscopes (**Fig. 4**).

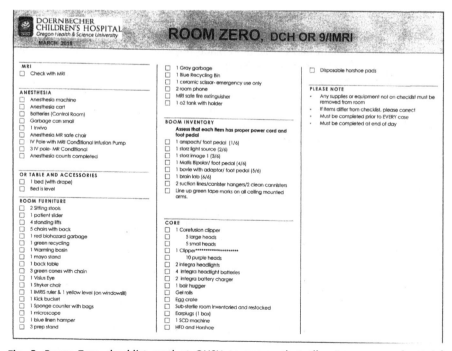

Fig. 3. Room Zero checklist used at OHSU to ensure that all extraneous equipment is removed from the OR before an iMRI case.

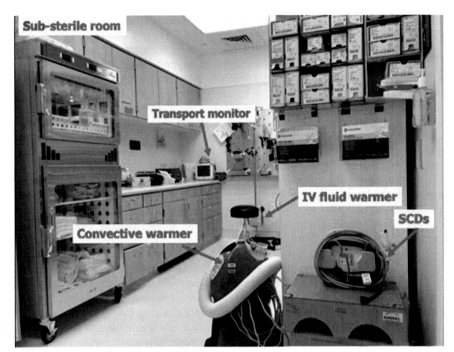

Fig. 4. Substerile room immediately behind the iMRI suite, where commonly used MR unsafe equipment is stored before scanning. SCDs, sequential compression devices.

Before draping the anesthetized patient, the MR safety officer completes a pre-drape checklist to ensure that MR safe items are used, all pressure points are padded, and the patient has earplugs in place (**Fig. 5**). Before the magnet enters the OR for intraoperative imaging, all surgical instruments are counted, and the instrument table is moved against the wall outside the 5-G line. All MR-unsafe equipment, including sharps used for line placement, are counted, witnessed, and then removed to outside the 5-G line. All discrepancies must be resolved before the magnet is allowed to enter the OR. The anesthesiologist who will remain with the patient during the iMRI should wear earplugs and perform a self-check to ensure that no ferromagnetic items remain on his or her person. A prescan checklist is helpful in facilitating this process (**Fig. 6**A, B).

If the patient requires emergency resuscitation during intraoperative scanning, the anesthesiologist may sound an alarm audible in the control room, which alerts the MR technologist to begin docking the magnet, which can take up to 90 seconds. Once the magnet is out of the OR and the garage doors close, the code cart and defibrillator may be brought into the OR for cardiopulmonary resuscitation.[22] Members of the responding code team must be quickly screened before the entering the OR. To reinforce this specialized emergency response, simulated codes in the iMRI suite are routinely performed at some institutions. A process for reporting adverse events and debriefing staff is critical to the success any iMRI program.

FUTURE DIRECTIONS FOR INTRAOPERATIVE MRI IN NEUROSURGERY

Intraoperative imaging has made great strides since the implementation of the early iMRI systems, and further innovations, such as intraoperative DTI, resting-state and

Pre-Drape Checklist, DCH OR 9/iMRI

Visual Patient Check- must occur before patient draped for surgery
Patient gown removed
Visual skin check for any pads, adhesive, medication patches, jewelry, etc.
ET tube padded and taped
Wires, leads and tubing padded as necessary, with no loops
Foley placed, draining evident and no skin contact
Arterial line is MRI compatible, padded with no loops
Skin padded with no skin to skin contact (chin, armpits, breast, groin, thighs, fingers, etc)
Earplugs with string inserted and secured with tape. Pt. Is not laying on string.
Fiducial placed to mark L/R
Arm boards are removed from table- if used
Bovie pad site is accessible for removal prior to scanning
Bair Hugger is placed to allow patient heating/cooling
Visius eye check, if in doubt
MRI compatible pins for HFD
Anesthesia counts completed

Fig. 5. Predrape checklist used at OHSU before surgical incision.

functional MRI, continue to increase its utility. DTI is a specialized MRI sequence that allows for noninvasive mapping of important white matter tracts in the brain. In neurosurgery, this is used most often preoperatively to identify critical areas that may be abutted or surrounded by tumor, for instance, corticospinal tracts, optic radiations, or arcuate fasciculus. Resting-state and functional MRI seeks to identify important connections and networks throughout the brain that may be associated with particular tasks (as in functional MRI) or that are associated during task-negative states when no

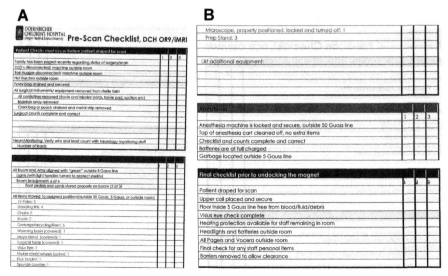

Fig. 6. (*A*, *B*) Prescan checklist used at OHSU to ensure safety before undocking the magnet.

explicit action is being performed (resting-state MRI).[35] These sequences are used primarily before surgery to identify the proximity of certain areas of the brain to tumors. However, using iMRI, intraoperative DTI is being used increasingly more often as a way to provide a clearer picture of the surgical margins surrounding white matter tracts. Intraoperative corticospinal tract mapping is being used to reassess motor pathways during surgery. Moving forward, intraoperative imaging of optic tracts and the arcuate fasciculus may be routinely used for tumors that may encroach on vision or speech areas, respectively. Similarly, intraoperative resting-state and functional MRI will be used to enable more precise resection of tumors while minimizing postoperative neurologic deficits.

LITT is another emerging area that is intimately related to iMRI. LITT offers a less-invasive option for treating tumors, epileptogenic foci, cavernous malformations, and areas of radiation necrosis.[36,37] Using a small burr hole, an optical fiber probe is placed near the lesion of interest, and laser energy is focused through that probe to a precise area. This energy heats the surrounding tissue to a sufficient degree and duration to cause cell death.[38] These less-invasive LITT procedures often facilitate treatment of deep, inaccessible lesions, and patients often can be discharged from the hospital within 24 hours of the procedure.

The use of iMRI has been integral to the success of this technology. After insertion of the laser probe, the patient is placed in the iMRI scanner. From this point, firing of the probe can be monitored in real-time using both T1-weighted images and MR thermography, which enables surgeons to measure the temperatures of surrounding tissues in order to determine whether these areas are being heated to an adequate temperature. To fully treat a tumor or lesion, the laser probe must be manipulated many times to provide sufficient thermal energy to the entire region of interest, which would be nearly impossible without the iMRI guidance.

SUMMARY

In the more than 25 years since the early development of iMRI, great advances have been made in the treatment of brain tumors, epilepsy, movement disorders, cavernous malformations, and other conditions. Advanced imaging techniques have improved the ability to identify and preserve critical areas of brain function. The introduction of laser interstitial thermotherapy has further increased the therapeutic utility of the iMRI surgical suites. Because of the complexity of the iMRI suite, in order to optimize patient outcomes, the anesthesiologist must recognize and account for the major equipment, monitoring, and safety considerations before administering an anesthetic in this environment.

DISCLOSURE

The authors have no commercial or financial conflicts of interest to disclose.

CLINICS CARE POINTS

- The anesthesiologist should be familiar with the specific iMRI system being used, the location of the 5 Gauss line, and the limitations of MR conditional anesthesia equipment before working in this environment.
- Anesthesiologists should work collaboratively with key stakeholders in neurosurgery, radiology, and nursing to create site-specific iMRI workflows and checklists to ensure patient safety while facilitating care.

- Despite the added complexity of the iMRI suite, the overall anesthetic management and complication rate is similar to patients having conventional neurosurgical procedures.

REFERENCES

1. Mezger U, Jendrewski C, Bartels M. Navigation in surgery. Langenbecks Arch Surg 2013;398(4):501–14.
2. Mutchnick I, Moriarty TM. Intraoperative MRI in pediatric neurosurgery-an update. Transl Pediatr 2014;3(3):236–46.
3. McClain CD, Soriano SG, Goumnerova LC, et al. Detection of unanticipated intracranial hemorrhage during intraoperative magnetic resonance image-guided neurosurgery: report of two cases. J Neurosurg Pediatr 2007;106(5):398–400.
4. Barua E, Johnston J, Fujii J, et al. Anesthesia for brain tumor resection using intraoperative magnetic resonance imaging (iMRI) with the Polestar N-20 system: experience and challenges. J Clin Anesth 2009;21(5):371–6.
5. Shah MN, Leonard JR, Inder G, et al. Intraoperative magnetic resonance imaging to reduce the rate of early reoperation for lesion resection in pediatric neurosurgery: clinical article. J Neurosurg Pediatr 2012;9(3):259–64.
6. Schroeck H, Welch TL, Rovner MS, et al. Anesthetic challenges and outcomes for procedures in the intraoperative magnetic resonance imaging suite: a systematic review. J Clin Anesth 2019;54:89–101.
7. Pamir MN, Özduman K, Dinçer A, et al. First intraoperative, shared-resource, ultrahigh-field 3-Tesla magnetic resonance imaging system and its application in low-grade glioma resection. J Neurosurg 2010;112(1):57–69.
8. Chicoine MR, Lim CCH, Evans JA, et al. Implementation and preliminary clinical experience with the use of ceiling mounted mobile high field intraoperative magnetic resonance imaging between two operating rooms. In: Pamir M, Seifert V, Kiris T, editors. Intraoperative Imaging. Acta Neurochirurgica Supplementum, vol. 109. Vienna: Springer; 2011. p. 97–102. https://doi.org/10.1007/978-3-211-99651-5_15.
9. Senft C, Bink A, Franz K, et al. Intraoperative MRI guidance and extent of resection in glioma surgery: a randomised, controlled trial. Lancet Oncol 2011;12(11):997–1003.
10. Senft C, Franz K, Blasel S, et al. Influence of iMRI-guidance on the extent of resection and survival of patients with glioblastoma multiforme. Technol Cancer Res Treat 2010;9(4):339–46.
11. Napolitano M, Vaz G, Lawson TM, et al. Glioblastoma surgery with and without intraoperative MRI at 3.0T. Neurochirurgie 2014;60(4):143–50.
12. Sylvester PT, Evans JA, Zipfel GJ, et al. Combined high-field intraoperative magnetic resonance imaging and endoscopy increase extent of resection and progression-free survival for pituitary adenomas. Pituitary 2015;18(1):72–85.
13. Yahanda AT, Patel B, Shah AS, et al. Impact of intraoperative magnetic resonance imaging and other factors on surgical outcomes for newly diagnosed grade II astrocytomas and oligodendrogliomas: a multicenter study. Neurosurgery 2020. https://doi.org/10.1093/neuros/nyaa320.
14. Yahanda AT, Patel B, Sutherland G, et al. A multi-institutional analysis of factors influencing surgical outcomes for patients with newly diagnosed grade I gliomas. World Neurosurg 2020;135:e754–64.

15. Kremer P, Tronnier V, Steiner HH, et al. Intraoperative MRI for interventional neurosurgical procedures and tumor resection control in children. Childs Nerv Syst 2006;22(7):674–8.

16. Karsy M, Akbari SH, Limbrick D, et al. Evaluation of pediatric glioma outcomes using intraoperative MRI: a multicenter cohort study. J Neurooncol 2019;143(2): 271–80.

17. Roder C, Breitkopf M, et al. Beneficial impact of high-field intraoperative magnetic resonance imaging on the efficacy of pediatric low-grade glioma surgery. Neurosurg Focus 2016;40(3):E13.

18. Jenkinson MD, Barone DG, Bryant A, et al. Intraoperative imaging technology to maximise extent of resection for glioma. Cochrane Gynaecological, Neuro-oncology and Orphan Cancer Group, ed. Cochrane Database Syst Rev 2018. https://doi.org/10.1002/14651858.CD012788.pub2.

19. Practice advisory on anesthetic care for magnetic resonance imaging: an updated report by the American Society of Anesthesiologists Task Force on anesthetic care for magnetic resonance imaging. Anesthesiology 2015;122:495–520.

20. Greenberg TD, Hoff MN, Gilk TB, et al. ACR guidance document on MR safe practices: updates and critical information 2019. J Magn Reson Imaging 2020; 51(2):331–8.

21. Panych LP, Madore B. The physics of MRI safety. J Magn Reson Imaging 2018; 47(1):28–43.

22. Johnston T, Moser R, Moeller K, et al. Intraoperative MRI: safety. Neurosurg Clin N Am 2009;20(2):147–53.

23. Shellock FG, Woods TO, Crues JV. MR labeling information for implants and devices: explanation of terminology. Radiology 2009;253(1):26–30.

24. Bailey M, Kirchen G, Bonaventura B, et al. Intraoperative MRI electrical noise and monitor ECG filters affect arrhythmia detection and identification. J Clin Monit Comput 2012;26(3):157–61.

25. Dias S, Sarnthein J, Jehli E, et al. Safeness and utility of concomitant intraoperative monitoring with intraoperative magnetic resonance imaging in children: a pilot study. World Neurosurg 2018;115:e637–44.

26. Darcey TM, Kobylarz EJ, Pearl MA, et al. Safe use of subdermal needles for intraoperative monitoring with MRI. Neurosurg Focus 2016;40(3):E19.

27. Archer DP, Cowan RAM, Falkenstein RJ, et al. Intraoperative mobile magnetic resonance imaging for craniotomy lengthens the procedure but does not increase morbidity. Can J Anesth 2002;49(4):420–6.

28. Cox RG, Levy R, Hamilton MG, et al. Anesthesia can be safely provided for children in a high-field intraoperative magnetic resonance imaging environment: anesthesia for intraoperative MRI in children. Pediatr Anesth 2011;21(4):454–8.

29. Malpas G, Taylor JA, Cumin D, et al. The incidence of hyperthermia during craniotomy. Anaesth Intensive Care 2018;46(4):368–73.

30. Henrichs B, Walsh RP. Intraoperative MRI for neurosurgical and general surgical interventions. Curr Opin Anaesthesiol 2014;27(4):448–52.

31. Munawar DA, Chan JEZ, Emami M, et al. Magnetic resonance imaging in non-conditional pacemakers and implantable cardioverter-defibrillators: a systematic review and meta-analysis. Europace 2020;22(2):288–98.

32. Hu W. Hospital fined by health dept. in death of boy during M.R.I. The New York Times. Available at: https://www.nytimes.com/2001/09/29/nyregion/hospital-fined-by-health-dept-in-death-of-boy-during-mri.html. Accessed October 1, 2020.

33. Rahmathulla G, Recinos PF, Traul DE, et al. Surgical briefings, checklists, and the creation of an environment of safety in the neurosurgical intraoperative magnetic resonance imaging suite. Neurosurg Focus 2012;33(5):E12.
34. Haynes AB, Weiser TG, Berry WR, et al. A surgical safety checklist to reduce morbidity and mortality in a global population. N Engl J Med 2009;360(5):491–9.
35. Roder C, Charyasz-Leks E, Breitkopf M, et al. Resting-state functional MRI in an intraoperative MRI setting: proof of feasibility and correlation to clinical outcome of patients. J Neurosurg 2016;125(2):401–9.
36. Holste KG, Orringer DA. Laser interstitial thermal therapy. Neurooncol Adv 2020; 2(1):vdz035.
37. Shimamoto S, Wu C, Sperling MR. Laser interstitial thermal therapy in drug-resistant epilepsy. Curr Opin Neurol 2019;32(2):237–45.
38. Lee I, Kalkanis S, Hadjipanayis CG. Stereotactic laser interstitial thermal therapy for recurrent high-grade gliomas. Neurosurgery 2016;79(Suppl 1):S24–34.

Anesthetic Considerations for Functional Neurosurgery

Lane Crawford, MD[a,1,*], Dorothee Mueller, MD[b,1], Letha Mathews, MBBS[a]

KEYWORDS

- Functional neurosurgery • Anesthesia • Deep brain stimulation • Parkinson disease
- Epilepsy

KEY POINTS

- Stereotactic frames or intraoperative imaging may impede access to the airway during many neurofunctional procedures.
- When deep brain stimulator implantation is performed under minimum alveolar concentration, anesthetics should be chosen to minimize tremor suppression while maintaining patient comfort and respiratory drive.
- Intraoperative electrocorticography requires careful anesthetic management to facilitate successful monitoring and to prevent and manage intraoperative seizure.

INTRODUCTION

Stereotactic and functional neurosurgery is a rapidly growing branch of neurosurgery. It uses structural and functional neuroimaging to identify and target discrete areas of the brain and to perform specific interventions (eg, ablation, neurostimulation, neuromodulation, neurotransplantation, and others), aiming to relieve symptoms of neurologic and other disorders and to improve function of both structurally normal and abnormal nervous systems.[1] Functional neurosurgery initially was undertaken primarily for the treatment of medically refractory Parkinson disease (PD), but, with advances in the science of neuromodulation and neuroimaging, its applications have extended to other movement disorders, epilepsy, chronic pain, and psychiatric conditions.[2] Functional neurosurgical procedures and the patients who require them can present special challenges for the anesthesiologist. This article reviews the perioperative management of patients undergoing functional neurosurgery for movement disorders and epilepsy.

The authors have no conflicts of interest to disclose.
[a] Department of Anesthesiology, Vanderbilt University Medical Center, 1301 Medical Center Drive, 4648 TVC, Nashville, TN 37232, USA; [b] Department of Anesthesiology, Vanderbilt University Medical Center, 1211 21st Ave S, 422 MAB, Nashville, TN 37212, USA
[1] Both of them are first authors.
* Corresponding author.
E-mail address: Lane.c.crawford@vumc.org

Anesthesiology Clin 39 (2021) 227–243
https://doi.org/10.1016/j.anclin.2020.11.013
1932-2275/21/© 2020 Elsevier Inc. All rights reserved.

FUNCTIONAL NEUROSURGERY FOR MOVEMENT DISORDERS

The field of movement disorders encompasses a variety of disease processes, with the most common being PD, essential tremor (ET), and dystonia. Successful surgical treatment of patients with a movement disorder is dependent on careful patient selection and preparation. A multidisciplinary team approach that includes neurologists, neurosurgeons, anesthesiologists, psychiatrists, and neurophysiologists is critical for good surgical outcomes. Patients should be evaluated by an anesthesiologist preoperatively, because the procedures and a patient's disease can pose unique challenges in the perioperative period.

Parkinson Disease

PD is a multisystem degenerative process caused by dopamine deficiency in the substantia nigra. Diminished inhibition of the extrapyramidal motor system causes characteristic features of the disease, such as resting tremor, bradykinesia, and cogwheel rigidity, as well as shuffling gait, facial immobility, and a monotonous voice. Due to widespread neurodegeneration, many patients also suffer from nonmotor features, which can include seborrhea, orthostatic hypotension, bladder dysfunction, dementia, and depression.[3]

Medical management is geared toward increasing the activity of dopamine relative to acetylcholine in the brain while minimizing negative side effects of dopamine in the periphery. The most effective drug is levodopa, often combined with carbidopa, a peripheral decarboxylase inhibitor, to avoid side effects, such as nausea, vomiting, and hypotension. Other medical management options are dopamine receptor agonists, such as bromocriptine and pramipexole, and selegiline, a type B monoamine oxidase inhibitor (MAOI).[4]

When patients experience wearing-off phenomena or dyskinesias unresponsive to medical management, surgical interventions, such as deep brain stimulation (DBS) and focused ultrasound (FUS) thalamotomy, represent highly effective alternatives.[3]

Anesthetic considerations in PD are numerous and relate both to the underlying disease and treatment regimen (**Table 1**). Preoperative evaluation should include detailed questioning about disease severity and symptoms, especially bulbar dysfunction and autonomic insufficiency. PD medications should be reviewed, including the timing of last doses and when next doses are due.

Essential Tremor

ET is the most common tremor disorder. It usually appears in adulthood but can have an early onset in childhood and may coexist with other movement disorders. In the vast majority of patients, it affects the upper limbs with a low-amplitude, bilateral action and postural tremor. ET less commonly affects the head, legs, or voice. It often starts by affecting fine motor coordination, such as threading a needle, but later progresses to involve gross motor function. Cognitive dysfunction and gait abnormalities also may be features of ET, but the impairment does not correlate to tremor severity. Although the brains of ET patients do not appear to have any structural abnormalities, several features point to an underlying cerebellar or brainstem pathology.[5,6]

Some patients develop exacerbations of ET only with stressful triggers, such as public performances, and thus require only intermittent treatment. For others, ET causes persistent disability and requires continuous treatment. First-line treatment is medical management with propranolol, a β-blocker, or primidone, an anticonvulsant. Other medical management options include other β-blockers or anticonvulsants

Table 1
Anesthetic considerations in patients with movement disorders

Movement Disorder	Anesthetic Considerations
Parkinson disease	Airway concerns
	• Airway obstruction and laryngospasm
	• Restrictive lung disease due to chest wall rigidity
	• Increased risk of aspiration due to dysphagia and dysmotility (consider antacids or promotility agents)
	• Avoid metoclopramide (dopamine receptor antagonist)
	Autonomic insufficiency
	• Orthostatic hypotension and genitourinary dysfunction can be warning sign
	• Hemodynamic instability
	• Altered response to vasopressors
	Neurologic decline
	• Dementia
	• Impaired cooperation during monitored anesthesia care
	Medication interactions
	• Antidopaminergic drugs can worsen PD symptoms (metoclopramide, promethazine, prochlorperazine, haloperidol, and droperidol)
	• Serotonergic drugs may increase risk of serotonin syndrome in patients taking an MAOI
	• Acetylcholinesterase inhibitors (rivastigmine, donepezil, and galantamine) may cause prolonged effect of succinylcholine and resistance to nondepolarizing neuromuscular blocking agents.
	PD medication in perioperative period
	• Minimize interruptions to avoid symptom exacerbation
	• Should hold medications if patient presents for DBS or ablative procedure
Essential tremor	Bradycardia due to use of β-blockers as treatment
Dystonia	Difficult positioning due to deformities or constant movements
	• Might require creative positioning
	• Additional padding, such as foam or pillows, required
	Cervical dystonia
	• Difficult airway, consider awake fiberoptic intubation

Data from Sapir S, Ramig L, Fox C. Speech and swallowing disorders in Parkinson disease. Curr Opin Otolaryngol Head Neck Surg. 2008;16(3):205-210; and Katus L, Shtilbans A. Perioperative management of patients with Parkinson's disease. Am J Med. 2014;127(4):275-280.

(eg, gabapentin, topiramate, phenobarbital, and levetiracetam), benzodiazepines, or injection with botulinum toxin.[7]

If medical management is unsuccessful, DBS and FUS unilateral thalamotomy are good alternatives.[7]

Severe ET may make it difficult for patients to hold still during procedures under light sedation. Other anesthetic considerations are related to medication side effects (see **Table 1**).

Dystonia

Dystonia is a movement disorder characterized by sustained or intermittent muscle contractions that result in abnormal postures or movements; it can be classified based on clinical manifestations or etiology.[8] Usually, dystonia is worsened by voluntary movements, whereas rest or sleep can abolish the symptoms. Common locations include the neck (cervical dystonia or torticollis), eyelids (blepharospasm), and vocal cords (spasmodic dysphonia).[9]

There is no cure for dystonia, and the treatment options mainly are symptomatic. The most promising medications include levodopa in the dopa-responsive group of patients, anticholinergic medications (often limited by side effects), and, to a lesser extent, baclofen, benzodiazepines, muscle relaxants, and anticonvulsant therapy. Although injections with botulinum toxin are considered first-line treatment of cervical dystonia, it also has been used with success for blepharospasm and spasmodic dysphonia.[9]

For patients failing medical management, surgical treatments are a valid alternative. The main treatment option currently is DBS, but in certain patient populations ablative procedures also might be reasonable.[9]

Anesthetic challenges for patients with dystonia may include difficulty with positioning or airway management (see **Table 1**).

SPECIFIC PROCEDURES AND ANESTHETIC CONSIDERATIONS

By far, the most common surgical treatment of movement disorders is DBS (discussed later). For patients who are not candidates for DBS, ablative techniques, such as laser interstitial thermal therapy (LITT) and FUS, may be used. These techniques are discussed in detail alter.

Deep Brain Stimulation

High-frequency DBS therapy originally was developed in the 1980s as an alternative to thalamic lesioning for patients with advanced movement disorders, because it mimicked the effects of ablation in a reversible and titratable manner.[10] Its indications since have expanded greatly. DBS has revolutionized the management of movement disorders, such as medically refractory PD, and improved the quality of life of patients suffering from debilitating neurologic disorders and some neuropsychiatric conditions. As of 2019, it is estimated that more than 160,000 patients worldwide have received DBS implants.[11] The target nuclei selected for stimulation is determined by the underlying disease conditions. The subthalamic nucleus and globus pallidus internus (GPi) are targeted for management of PD, ventral intermediate nucleus for ET, GPi for dystonia, and the anterior limb of internal capsule for obsessive compulsive disorder. The most common DBS target for epilepsy is the anterior nucleus of the thalamus (**Fig. 1**).

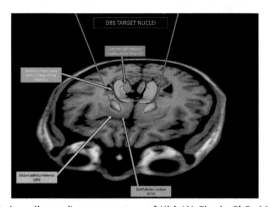

Fig. 1. DBS targets in epilepsy. (Image courtesy of Kirk W. Finnis, PhD, Medtronic ©2020.)

The exact mechanism of action of DBS still is not fully understood, but it causes neuro-modulation[12] of pathologically altered or dysfunctional neuronal circuits.[2] It is hypothesized that electrical stimulation of these altered neurons may revert them to a more physiologic state.[13]

DBS surgery typically is undertaken in multiple stages. During the first stage, bone markers or a stereotactic frame is placed on the skull, followed by imaging (computed tomography [CT)] and magnetic resonance imaging [MRI] for brain mapping and target planning. This is done with local anesthesia (LA) and sedation or general anesthesia (GA) based on institutional practice and the patient's ability to lie still for MRI and CT. This is followed by electrode implantation into the target nuclei in the brain. In the final stage, the leads are internalized and the implantable pulse generator (IPG) implanted (**Fig. 2**). The success of the procedure is highly dependent on appropriate patient selection, accurate localization of the targets, implantation of electrodes with precision, and good perioperative management. Intraoperative localization of target is achieved by frame-based navigation; microelectrode recording (MER), which displays specific firing patterns for each nucleus; and macrostimulation to observe clinical benefits and detect side effects. Stereotactic frames, such as Cosman, Roberts, and Wells (CRW) (Integra Radionics, Burlington, Massachusetts) and Leksell (Elekta AB, Stockholm, Sweden) frames commonly are used to locate intracranial structures. Some centers use a frameless stereotaxy system known as the microTargeting Platform[14] (MTP) (FHC Inc, Bowdoin, Maine), which is customized for each patient and offers the advantage of easier airway management from the anesthesiologist's perspective (**Fig. 3**). The details of the surgical

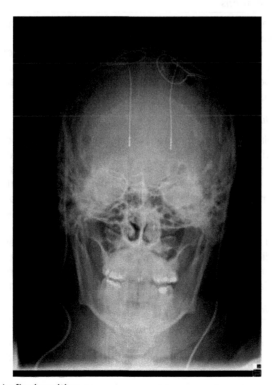

Fig. 2. DBS leads in final position.

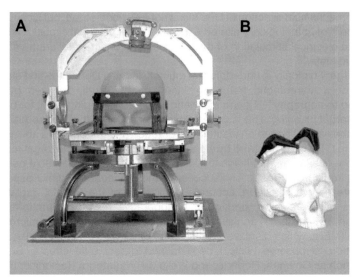

Fig. 3. (A) CRW stereotactic frame versus (B) MTP system.

procedure are beyond the scope of this article and can be found in the published literature.[10,15]

Anesthetic Considerations

The goal of anesthetic management is to provide patient comfort while facilitating safe surgical conditions for mapping and implantation of DBS systems. Historically, DBS procedures have been done in awake patients with LA or with conscious sedation to facilitate MER and patient cooperation during macrostimulation. Now, with advances in intraoperative CT and intraoperative MRI yielding increased accuracy of target localization, many centers routinely use GA for DBS placement.[16-18]

Preoperative Evaluation

Patients undergoing DBS surgery often are medically complex and present unusual challenges related to anesthesia (see **Table 1**). In addition to the disease-specific concerns (discussed previously), clinicians also must evaluate for comorbidities like hypertension that could affect the risk of intracranial hemorrhage (ICH). The anesthesiologist must consider the impact of a stereotactic frame on airway management, a concern that can be complicated further by obstructive sleep apnea or obesity.

Patients should be given clear instructions on medication management. Anti Parkinson Disease medications generally are withheld for 24 hours if lead insertion is performed under minimum alveolar concentration (MAC) so that the patient is in a drug-off state to facilitate intraoperative mapping and physiologic testing.

Anesthetic Techniques

Awake with local anesthesia or monitored anesthesia care

Thorough LA infiltration or scalp blocks are crucial for patient comfort during awake lead implantation.[19,20] LA often is supplemented with intravenous sedation. Patients usually are placed in a semisitting position, with standard monitors applied and oxygen delivered via nasal cannula. Invasive blood pressure monitoring may be indicated

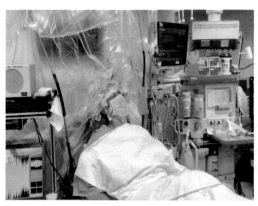

Fig. 4. DBS lead implantation under MAC.

in select patients due to their comorbidities or for tighter hemodynamic control (**Figs. 4** and **5**).

After brief sedation for the creation of burr holes, the patient is awakened for neurologic testing. There is no ideal sedation agent, but the effects of commonly used drugs on MER and respiratory drive should be considered. Because airway management of patients in stereotactic frames can be extremely challenging, drugs that cause respiratory depression should be used with extreme caution and plans should be in place for rescuing the airway. When dosing cautiously, however, it also is important to control anxiety and pain. Patients with PD who present for surgery are in an drug-off state due to discontinuation of drugs, making their symptoms worse, which, combined with anxiety, can cause hypertension. Patients with ET may be taken off their β-blockers, which also can lead to hypertension. Uncontrolled hypertension can increase the risk of ICH.[21]

Drugs that commonly are used for sedation are propofol, fentanyl, remifentanil, and dexmedetomidine. Benzodiazepines, such as midazolam, generally are avoided because they can affect MER and abolish tremors in movement disorder patients.[22,23] Although all the drugs discussed also can have an impact on MER, their effect varies based on the dose and timing of administration, and there is inadequate evidence to

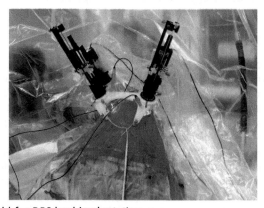

Fig. 5. Surgical field for DBS lead implantation.

recommend any particular drug. A detailed review of the literature on the effect of commonly used drugs on MER has been published by Bos and colleagues.[24]

General anesthesia

Lead implantation under GA has become more common and usually is done with intraoperative CT or intraoperative MRI. GA provides the advantage that patients can continue their routine medications and have less discomfort and anxiety during surgery. Anesthesiologists are not limited in the choice of drugs that can be administered and standard general endotracheal anesthesia can be utilized. When the surgical procedure occurs in the radiology suite, however, the challenges associated with out–of–operating room (OR) anesthesia require additional preparation in the event of complications. Guidelines for management of patients in MRI have been published previously.[25,26]

Randomized controlled trials comparing asleep versus awake DBS procedures are lacking due to low enrollment[27] and to the limited number of institutions that can do both with equipoise.[28] The data on the clinical and surgical outcomes for asleep DBS for PD are comparable to those for awake DBS.[29]

IPG implantation, during which the tunneled DBS leads are connected to the IPG (typically placed in the pectoral region of chest wall), usually is done done under GA. IPGs have seen significant improvement over the years with rechargeable batteries and MRI compatibility.

Perioperative Complications of Deep Brain Stimulation Procedures

Anesthesiologists should be aware of the potential risks associated with DBS procedures. It is vital to be familiar with a patient's coexisting medical conditions and to be prepared to treat any complications promptly. The incidence of reported complications varies significantly, from 1% to 25%.[30] The commonly reported intraoperative complications are reviewed by Khatib and colleagues.[31] These include airway obstruction, apnea, aspiration, confusion, agitation, uncontrolled hypertension, cardiac ischemia, venous air embolism, and neurologic complications, such as ICH, seizures, and stroke.

Future Directions

DBS treatment has contributed significantly to the management of several medically refractory diseases. The indications for DBS continue to expand. Advances in understanding of neurophysiological mechanisms and neuroanatomic structures through better imaging and technology and improved cooperation between neuroscientists and clinicians are furthering the development of DBS for targeted treatments.

FUNCTIONAL NEUROSURGERY FOR EPILEPSY

Epilepsy is a clinical condition characterized by a lasting predisposition to recurrent, unprovoked seizures. It is one of the most common serious neurologic disorders, with a prevalence of approximately 6 per 1000 people worldwide.[32] The etiology of epilepsy is diverse and includes genetic mutations, developmental abnormalities, head trauma, infectious disease, cerebrovascular disease, and structural abnormalities, such as mesial temporal sclerosis, focal cortical dysplasia, vascular malformation, and tumor. Up to one-third of patients with epilepsy have drug-resistant disease, defined as persistent seizures despite trial of 2 antiepileptic drug (AED) regimens.[33] Many of these individuals ultimately are candidates for surgical therapy.

The armamentarium of surgical treatment options for epilepsy has expanded significantly in recent years.[34] Resection via craniotomy remains the preferred treatment when seizures originate from a focal epileptogenic zone (EZ). Ablative techniques, however, offer a minimally invasive alternative to craniotomy. Neuromodulatory techniques may be used when complete resection or ablation is not possible (eg, in cases of EZ proximity to eloquent cortex or generalized/multifocal epilepsy). Finally, disconnective surgery, such as corpus callosotomy, remains a palliative option for some patients.

Choosing and executing the best treatment modality for a given patient require a multidisciplinary team approach.[35] Presurgical evaluation includes a thorough history and physical examination and both interictal and long-term video electroencephalogram (EEG). MRI may allow for radiographic identification of the EZ, sometimes in conjunction with other imaging modalities. If noninvasive techniques fail to adequately localize the EZ, intracranial EEG, also called electrocorticography (ECoG), becomes necessary. Traditionally, subdural electrode (SDE) grid or strip placement via craniotomy has been the most common technique for ECoG in the United States, but in recent years stereotactic EEG (SEEG) depth electrodes have been used more widely.[36] When the EZ is in close proximity to brain areas responsible for language, movement, vision, or memory, additional studies are required to map the region precisely. The mapping may be achieved with imaging, such as functional MRI, or may require invasive techniques, such as the Wada test or electrical stimulation mapping (ESM) of the functional cortex.

Anesthetic Considerations in Epilepsy

Anesthesiologists who care for patients undergoing diagnostic or therapeutic surgery for epilepsy should familiarize themselves with this growing array of procedures. First, however, they must be aware of the considerations for providing anesthesia to patients with epilepsy. Confusingly, most anesthetic drugs have been shown to exhibit both proconvulsant and anticonvulsant properties at different doses, with varying degrees of clinical relevance.[37,38] Propofol, thiopental, and benzodiazepines suppress seizure activity, especially at higher doses. Etomidate, methohexital, and ketamine can potentiate seizure activity and should be used with caution in patients with epilepsy. Synthetic opioids, such as fentanyl and its congeners, are proconvulsant at high doses. Sevoflurane has been shown to cause epileptiform activity in some settings, whereas isoflurane and desflurane appear to be primarily anticonvulsants, making them the preferred volatile anesthetics for patients with epilepsy. Nitrous oxide has minimal proconvulsant or anticonvulsant effects.[39]

Patients should continue their AED regimen through the morning of surgery unless intraoperative monitoring of seizure activity is planned. Many AEDs, especially older agents, are prone to numerous drug interactions based on induction or inhibition of hepatic enzymes. Relevant to the anesthesiologist is the decreased duration of action of nondepolarizing neuromuscular blocking agents that results from enzyme induction by phenytoin, carbamazepine, and phenobarbital.[40] Although resistance to fentanyl has been observed in patients taking AEDs,[41] patients who experience sedation as a side effect of their AED regimen can be expected to have decreased anesthetic requirements.

Specific Procedures and Anesthetic Considerations

Subdural electrode or depth electrode placement
ECoG with SDE grid or strip is most useful for localizing a superficial EZ or for functional cortical mapping.[36] Placement is accomplished via craniotomy under GA. Assuming no intraoperative ECoG or mapping is planned, anesthetic considerations are similar to those for any craniotomy in a patient with epilepsy. The grid or strip is

removed via repeat craniotomy, often at the time of resective surgery. SEEG depth electrodes are preferable to SDE when monitoring of deeper or multifocal structures is required.[36] Depth electrodes are placed via burr holes with stereotactic guidance under GA. During the procedure, a stereotactic frame is affixed to the patient's head, allowing precise 3-dimensional placement of electrodes based on previously obtained brain imaging (**Fig. 6**). Extra care should be taken when securing the endotracheal tube due to limited access to the airway once the frame is in place. Patient immobility is critical for accurate stereotactic guidance, and intraoperative monitoring of neuromuscular blockade is recommended. Invasive monitoring typically is not required unless indicated by patient comorbidities; however, perioperative hypertension should be avoided because ICH is a risk of this procedure.[42] Venous air embolism is a rare but possible complication.

Intraoperative electrocorticography and electrical stimulation mapping

ECoG often is performed extraoperatively with SDE or depth electrode implantation followed by long-term monitoring in an epilepsy monitoring unit. ECoG also may be performed intraoperatively, however, to localize the EZ immediately before resection and to determine adequacy of resection. Because it is unlikely for a spontaneous seizure to occur during the relatively short monitoring period, intraoperative ECoG

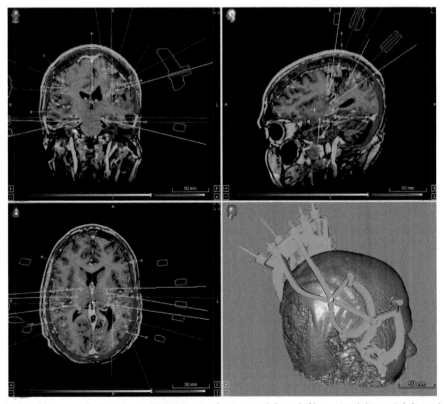

Fig. 6. Shown are planning trajectories in the coronal (*top left*), sagittal (*top right*), and axial (*bottom left*) planes, and a 3D reconstruction showing the final frame plan (*bottom right*).

relies primarily on the pattern of interictal epileptiform discharges (IEDs) to identify the EZ. Direct cortical stimulation via the ECoG electrodes or a handheld wand also may be used. A similar technique is used when performing ESM of functional cortex in order to define the limits of resection.

Because most sedative-hypnotic agents interfere with ECoG signals, intraoperative ECoG ideally is performed via awake craniotomy. When this is not possible due to patient factors, light GA with volatile or intravenous maintenance may be acceptable, but the anesthetic must be weaned prior to monitoring and patients should be warned about the risk of awareness. ESM of eloquent cortex often requires patient participation (eg, when mapping cortex responsible for language) and thus necessitates awake craniotomy. The anesthetic considerations for awake craniotomy are extensive and reviewed elsewhere. Whether sedation or GA is employed, anesthetic agents must be selected and titrated carefully to minimize interference with ECoG or ESM **(Table 2)**. Commonly used agents include propofol, dexmedetomidine, and opioid infusions. Benzodiazepines suppress IEDs and should be avoided. Volatile agents should be limited to less than 1 MAC. High doses of synthetic opioids have a proconvulsant effect, and alfentanil bolus may be used during ECoG to increase cortical excitability and stimulate IEDs.[43]

Intraoperative seizure is an important complication of intraoperative ECoG and ESM. Cortical stimulation can trigger electrographic or clinical seizure activity, which can interfere with the planned procedure and cause serious patient harm. The first-line treatment of intraoperative seizure is the application of ice-cold saline to the cortex by the surgeon. If this fails to terminate the seizure, small doses of propofol or benzodiazepine should be administered, but these medications may interfere with further monitoring. Prolonged seizure during awake craniotomy necessitates prompt securement of the airway.

Ablative techniques
Ablative techniques offer a less invasive alternative to craniotomy when permanent destruction of brain tissue is desired. Their primary application in epilepsy is treatment of focal epileptogenic lesions, such as mesial temporal sclerosis, vascular

Table 2
Effects of anesthetic agents on intraoperative electrocorticography and electrical stimulation mapping

Anesthetic Agent	Effect on Electrocorticography
Benzodiazepines	Suppress IEDs. Avoid use.
Propofol	Suppresses IEDs at high doses. Limit to lower doses and pause 15 min prior to monitoring.
Dexmedetomidine	Minimal effect on IEDs
Volatile anesthetics	In general, suppress IEDs. Limit to concentrations <1 MAC and pause 15 min prior to monitoring.
Nitrous oxide	Mixed data but used in many centers
Synthetic opioids (fentanyl, remifentanil, sufentanil, and alfentanil)	Minimal effect on IEDs at conventional doses. Proconvulsant at high doses. Alfentanil bolus may be used for pharmacologic cortical stimulation.
Etomidate Methohexital	Proconvulsant at high doses. May be used for pharmacologic cortical activation.

Data from Chui J, Manninen P, Valiante T, Venkatraghavan L. The anesthetic considerations of intraoperative electrocorticography during epilepsy surgery. Anesth Analg. 2013;117(2):479-486.

malformations, and hamartomas. Although neuromodulatory techniques like DBS largely have supplanted ablative techniques for treatment of movement disorders, ablation may be preferable for patients who are not candidates for DBS or who wish to avoid implanted devices. Other applications include brain tumors, psychiatric disease, and chronic pain.

Radiofrequency thermoablation Radiofrequency thermoablation (RFTA) first was reported in the 1950s. RFTA for unilateral pallidotomy was one of the most efficacious procedural therapies for PD but has fallen out of favor with the advent of DBS.[44,45]

RFTA is one of the most straightforward of the lesioning techniques. Patients usually are awake and able to participate. A stereotactic frame is placed, and targets are chosen based on previously acquired CT scans. A wire then is passed to the desired target and position is confirmed using either MER or macrostimulation with clinical evaluation. After confirmation, heat is applied to the tip of the electrode to induce thermoablation.

Because patients usually are awake, special consideration should be given to positioning to ensure patients' comfort and ability to remain motionless for a prolonged period of time. The stereotactic frame can compromise airway access.

Stereotactic radiosurgery For stereotactic radiosurgery (SRS), multiple beams of low-dose ionizing radiation are converged on 1 target to induce radionecrosis. For this procedure, the patient's head is secured in a frame and the coordinates of the radiation exposure fields are set using CT and MRI technology. The advantage of SRS is that it is noninvasive, because the patient does not require an incision or burr holes. It is not possible, however, to confirm improvement of symptoms during the procedure because both the desired effect and adverse effects do not fully develop for several days to weeks, with some complications presenting months to years after the initial treatment. The extent of adverse effects can vary widely, and in some cases may be mitigated by the slow pace of necrosis, which allows for neuroplastic compensatory changes.[46]

SRS usually is performed under general endotracheal anesthesia. Special consideration should be given to the challenges of out-of-OR anesthesia in the radiation suite, such as the potential lack of immediate help in an emergency.

Laser interstitial thermal therapy LITT is a minimally invasive procedure used mainly to treat epilepsy, gliomas, and brain metastases. The procedure involves a small burr hole for insertion of a cooled catheter through which laser energy is delivered. The key advantages involve the minimally invasive nature of the procedure, which does not require a large incision or bone flap, and shorter hospital stay with faster return to usual activities compared with other approaches. MRI thermography allows for a real-time visualization of the ablation volume. Due to the steep temperature drop off at the outer edge of the ablation zone, a larger zone can be ablated with a single pass, eliminating the need for the multiple passes needed with RFTA.[47]

This procedure can be performed awake or under GA, depending on the preference and comorbidities of the patient. Because the lesion is confirmed by MRI thermography, participation of the patient is not necessarily required.

Magnetic resonance imaging–guided focused ultrasound thermal ablation MRI-guided FUS (MRgFUS) ablation is a noninvasive treatment that recently has gained approval for thalamotomy in ET and tremor-dominant PD. Emerging applications include other movement disorders, epilepsy, brain tumors, and psychiatric disease. In this technique, CT and MRI thermography images are overlaid to localize a precise treatment target while monitoring ablation temperatures in real time. This allows for a slow increase in temperature while monitoring the patient's tremor and/or any adverse effects in a time frame at which they are still presumed reversible. MRgFUS usually is performed only unilaterally, because, in some cases gait, speech, or sensory disturbances can persist chronically. The major advantage of MRgFUS is that it is noninvasive, reducing the risk of infection, bleeding, or need for follow-up because no permanent hardware is installed.[48,49]

This procedure usually is performed awake. Special consideration should be given to positioning the patient in the MRI scanner as well as the challenges of out-of-OR anesthesia, when relevant.

Neuromodulatory techniques

Implanted neuromodulatory systems can reduce seizure burden in patients who are not candidates for resective or ablative techniques or who continue to have inadequate control after surgery.

Vagal nerve stimulation The longest-standing neuromodulatory treatment of epilepsy is vagal nerve stimulation (VNS), which, after 2 years of therapy, decreases seizure burden by at least 50% in 50% of patients.[50] Its mechanism of efficacy is thought to involve modulation of cerebral neuronal excitability via stimulation of action potentials in the cervical vagus nerve. VNS consists of a generator implanted in the chest wall and a lead, which is tunneled through the subcutaneous tissue of the neck to electrodes coiled around the vagus nerve. Stimulation usually occurs according to a preprogrammed schedule, although recently developed closed-loop VNS systems allow for stimulation in response to sensed seizure activity.[51] VNS implantation typically is performed under general endotracheal anesthesia. Procedural considerations include the rare risk of hemorrhage or airway-compromising neck hematoma resulting from vascular injury. Damage to the recurrent laryngeal nerve can lead to postoperative hoarseness or dyspnea. Rare instances of severe bradycardia and asystole with initial stimulation have been reported. Preoperative cardiology consultation may be indicated in patients with a preexisting conduction abnormality, and anesthesia providers should be prepared to treat intraoperative arrhythmia. Finally, VNS can worsen

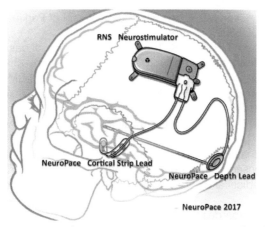

RNS Neurostimulator

NeuroPace Cortical Strip Lead

NeuroPace Depth Lead

NeuroPace 2017

Fig. 7. Implanted RNS® System. (© 2017 NeuroPace, Inc. Image used with permission from NeuroPace, Inc.)

symptoms of obstructive sleep apnea, warranting extra vigilance for respiratory complications in the immediate postoperative period.[52]

Deep brain stimulation DBS of the anterior nucleus of the thalamus has been shown to decrease seizure burden by 40% with increasing efficacy over time and is Food and Drug Administration approved for the treatment of medically refractory partial-onset epilepsy.[53] Other anatomic targets are under investigation, including the centromedian thalamus and the hippocampus.[54] DBS implantation for epilepsy is performed under general endotracheal anesthesia. Anesthetic considerations for DBS implantation are discussed previously.

Responsive neurostimulation Responsive neurostimulation (RNS) uses a closed-loop system consisting of an intracranial stimulator connected to SDE strips or depth electrodes located in the EZ or other anatomic targets (**Fig. 7**). The electrodes allow for both continuous ECoG monitoring as well as targeted stimulation to abort any sensed seizure activity. RNS has been shown to decrease seizure burden in partial epilepsy by 38% with increasing efficacy over time.[55] RNS implantation is performed via craniotomy under general endotracheal anesthesia. Anesthetic considerations are similar to those for any craniotomy in a patient with poorly controlled epilepsy.

SUMMARY

Functional neurosurgery has entered a new era with advances in neuroscience, neuroimaging, surgical techniques, and devices. MRI-guided targeting for DBS, FUS, and LITT procedures have reduced the need for patients to be awake during surgery without compromising quality and accuracy. Anesthesiologists should familiarize themselves with the various surgical therapies for movement disorders and epilepsy and be actively involved in developing guidelines for perioperative management of these patients.

REFERENCES

1. World Society for Stereotactic and Functional Neurosurgery. Available at: https://www.wssfn.org/about-us. Accessed August 5, 2020.
2. Lozano AM, Lipsman N. Probing and regulating dysfunctional circuits using deep brain stimulation. Neuron 2013;77(3):406–24.
3. Armstrong MJ, Okun MS. Diagnosis and Treatment of Parkinson Disease: A Review. JAMA 2020;323(6):548–60.
4. Olanow CW, Stern MB, Sethi K. The scientific and clinical basis for the treatment of Parkinson disease. Neurology 2009;72(21 Suppl 4):S1–136.
5. Shanker V. Essential tremor: diagnosis and management. BMJ 2019;366:l4485.
6. Ondo WG. Current and emerging treatments of essential tremor. Neurol Clin 2020;38(2):309–23.
7. Haubenberger D, Hallett M. Essential tremor. N Engl J Med 2018;378(19):1802–10.
8. Albanese A, Bhatia K, Bressman SB, et al. Phenomenology and classification of dystonia: a consensus update. Mov Disord 2013;28(7):863–73.
9. Jinnah HA. Medical and surgical treatments for dystonia. Neurol Clin 2020;38(2):325–48.
10. Benabid AL, Chabardes S, Mitrofanis J, et al. Deep brain stimulation of the subthalamic nucleus for the treatment of Parkinson's disease. Lancet Neurol 2009;8(1):67–81.

11. Lozano AM, Lipsman N, Bergman H, et al. Deep brain stimulation: current challenges and future directions. Nat Rev Neurol 2019;15(3):148–60.

12. Jakobs M, Fomenko A, Lozano AM, et al. Cellular, molecular, and clinical mechanisms of action of deep brain stimulation-a systematic review on established indications and outlook on future developments. EMBO Mol Med 2019;11(4). https://doi.org/10.15252/emmm.201809575.

13. McIntyre CC, Anderson RW. Deep brain stimulation mechanisms: the control of network activity via neurochemistry modulation. J Neurochem 2016;139(Suppl): 338–45.

14. Konrad PE, Neimat JS, Yu H, et al. Customized, miniature rapid-prototype stereotactic frames for use in deep brain stimulator surgery: initial clinical methodology and experience from 263 patients from 2002 to 2008. Stereotact Funct Neurosurg 2011;89(1):34–41.

15. Venkatraghavan L, Luciano M, Manninen P. Review article: anesthetic management of patients undergoing deep brain stimulator insertion. Anesth Analg 2010;110(4):1138–45.

16. Cui Z, Pan L, Song H, et al. Intraoperative MRI for optimizing electrode placement for deep brain stimulation of the subthalamic nucleus in Parkinson disease. J Neurosurg 2016;124(1):62–9.

17. Aziz TZ, Hariz M. To sleep or not to sleep during deep brain stimulation surgery for Parkinson disease? Neurology 2017;89(19):1938–9.

18. Aviles-Olmos I, Kefalopoulou Z, Tripoliti E, et al. Long-term outcome of subthalamic nucleus deep brain stimulation for Parkinson's disease using an MRI-guided and MRI-verified approach. J Neurol Neurosurg Psychiatry 2014;85(12):1419–25.

19. Girvin JP. Resection of intracranial lesions under local anesthesia. Int Anesthesiol Clin 1986;24(3):133–55.

20. Osborn I, Sebeo J. "Scalp block" during craniotomy: a classic technique revisited. J Neurosurg Anesthesiol 2010;22(3):187–94.

21. Xiaowu H, Xiufeng J, Xiaoping Z, et al. Risks of intracranial hemorrhage in patients with Parkinson's disease receiving deep brain stimulation and ablation. Parkinsonism Relat Disord 2010;16(2):96–100.

22. Lin S-H, Chen T-Y, Lin S-Z, et al. Subthalamic deep brain stimulation after anesthetic inhalation in Parkinson disease: a preliminary study. J Neurosurg 2008; 109(2):238–44.

23. Komur M, Arslankoylu AE, Okuyaz C. Midazolam-induced acute dystonia reversed by diazepam. J Anaesthesiol Clin Pharmacol 2012;28(3):368–70.

24. Bos MJ, Buhre W, Temel Y, et al. Effect of anesthesia on microelectrode recordings during deep brain stimulation surgery: a narrative review. J Neurosurg Anesthesiol 2020. https://doi.org/10.1097/ANA.0000000000000673.

25. Rahmathulla G, Recinos PF, Traul DE, et al. Surgical briefings, checklists, and the creation of an environment of safety in the neurosurgical intraoperative magnetic resonance imaging suite. Neurosurg Focus 2012;33(5):E12.

26. The American Society of Anesthesiologysits Task Force on Anesthetic Care for Magetic Resonacce imaging. Practice advisory on anesthetic care for magnetic resonance imaging: a report by the Society of Anesthesiologists Task Force on Anesthetic Care for Magnetic Resonance Imaging. Anesthesiology 2009; 110(3):459–79.

27. Chen T, Mirzadeh Z, Ponce FA. "Asleep" deep brain stimulation surgery: a critical review of the literature. World Neurosurg 2017;105:191–8.

28. Kochanski RB, Sani S. Awake versus asleep deep brain stimulation surgery: technical considerations and critical review of the literature. Brain Sci 2018;8(1). https://doi.org/10.3390/brainsci8010017.
29. Wang J, Ponce FA, Tao J, et al. Comparison of awake and asleep deep brain stimulation for parkinson's disease: a detailed analysis through literature review. Neuromodulation 2020;23(4):444–50.
30. Fenoy AJ, Simpson RK. Risks of common complications in deep brain stimulation surgery: management and avoidance. J Neurosurg 2014;120(1):132–9.
31. Khatib R, Ebrahim Z, Rezai A, et al. Perioperative events during deep brain stimulation: the experience at cleveland clinic. J Neurosurg Anesthesiol 2008;20(1): 36–40.
32. Fiest KM, Sauro KM, Wiebe S, et al. Prevalence and incidence of epilepsy: A systematic review and meta-analysis of international studies. Neurology 2017;88(3): 296–303.
33. Kwan P, Arzimanoglou A, Berg AT, et al. Definition of drug resistant epilepsy: consensus proposal by the ad hoc Task Force of the ILAE Commission on Therapeutic Strategies. Epilepsia 2010;51(6):1069–77.
34. Englot DJ. A modern epilepsy surgery treatment algorithm: Incorporating traditional and emerging technologies. Epilepsy Behav 2018;80:68–74.
35. Tripathi M, Ray S, Chandra PS. Presurgical evaluation for drug refractory epilepsy. Int J Surg 2016;36(Pt B):405–10.
36. Chauvel P, Gonzalez-Martinez J, Bulacio J. Presurgical intracranial investigations in epilepsy surgery. Handb Clin Neurol 2019;161:45–71.
37. Modica PA, Tempelhoff R, White PF. Pro- and anticonvulsant effects of anesthetics (Part I). Anesth Analg 1990;70(3):303–15.
38. Modica PA, Tempelhoff R, White PF. Pro- and anticonvulsant effects of anesthetics (Part II). Anesth Analg 1990;70(4):433–44.
39. Shetty A, Pardeshi S, Shah VM, et al. Anesthesia considerations in epilepsy surgery. Int J Surg 2016;36(Pt B):454–9.
40. Kofke WA. Anesthetic management of the patient with epilepsy or prior seizures. Curr Opin Anaesthesiol 2010;23(3):391–9.
41. Tempelhoff R, Modica PA, Spitznagel EL. Anticonvulsant therapy increases fentanyl requirements during anaesthesia for craniotomy. Can J Anaesth 1990;37(3): 327–32.
42. Rajkalyan C, Tewari A, Rao S, et al. Anesthetic considerations for stereotactic electroencephalography implantation. J Anaesthesiol Clin Pharmacol 2019; 35(4):434–40.
43. Chui J, Manninen P, Valiante T, et al. The anesthetic considerations of intraoperative electrocorticography during epilepsy surgery. Anesth Analg 2013;117(2): 479–86.
44. Crowell JL, Shah BB. Surgery for Dystonia and Tremor. Curr Neurol Neurosci Rep 2016;16(3):22.
45. Walters H, Shah BB. Focused ultrasound and other lesioning therapies in movement disorders. Curr Neurol Neurosci Rep 2019;19(9):66.
46. Martínez-Moreno NE, Sahgal A, De Salles A, et al. Stereotactic radiosurgery for tremor: systematic review. J Neurosurg 2018;130(2):1–12.
47. Missios S, Bekelis K, Barnett GH. Renaissance of laser interstitial thermal ablation. Neurosurg Focus 2015;38(3):E13.
48. Elias WJ, Lipsman N, Ondo WG, et al. A randomized trial of focused ultrasound thalamotomy for essential tremor. N Engl J Med 2016;375(8):730–9.

49. Chang JW, Park CK, Lipsman N, et al. A prospective trial of magnetic resonance-guided focused ultrasound thalamotomy for essential tremor: Results at the 2-year follow-up. Ann Neurol 2018;83(1):107–14.

50. Englot DJ, Rolston JD, Wright CW, et al. Rates and Predictors of Seizure Freedom With Vagus Nerve Stimulation for Intractable Epilepsy. Neurosurgery 2016;79(3): 345–53.

51. Hamilton P, Soryal I, Dhahri P, et al. Clinical outcomes of VNS therapy with AspireSR® (including cardiac-based seizure detection) at a large complex epilepsy and surgery centre. Seizure 2018;58:120–6.

52. Hatton KW, McLarney JT, Pittman T, et al. Vagal nerve stimulation: overview and implications for anesthesiologists. Anesth Analg 2006;103(5):1241–9.

53. Fisher R, Salanova V, Witt T, et al. Electrical stimulation of the anterior nucleus of thalamus for treatment of refractory epilepsy. Epilepsia 2010;51(5):899–908.

54. Salanova V. Deep brain stimulation for epilepsy. Epilepsy Behav 2018;88S-(Supplement):21–4.

55. Skarpaas TL, Jarosiewicz B, Morrell MJ. Brain-responsive neurostimulation for epilepsy (RNS® System). Epilepsy Res 2019;153:68–70.

Moving?

Make sure your subscription moves with you!

To notify us of your new address, find your **Clinics Account Number** (located on your mailing label above your name), and contact customer service at:

Email: journalscustomerservice-usa@elsevier.com

800-654-2452 (subscribers in the U.S. & Canada)
314-447-8871 (subscribers outside of the U.S. & Canada)

Fax number: 314-447-8029

**Elsevier Health Sciences Division
Subscription Customer Service
3251 Riverport Lane
Maryland Heights, MO 63043**

*To ensure uninterrupted delivery of your subscription, please notify us at least 4 weeks in advance of move.

9780323796248